AF844707

Developing Anti-Racist Practices in the Helping Professions: Inclusive Theory, Pedagogy, and Application

Kaprea F. Johnson
Narketta M. Sparkman-Key
Alan Meca • Shuntay Z. Tarver
Editors

Developing Anti-Racist Practices in the Helping Professions: Inclusive Theory, Pedagogy, and Application

palgrave
macmillan

Editors
Kaprea F. Johnson
Department of Educational Studies,
Counselor Education Program
The Ohio State University
Columbus, OH, USA

Alan Meca
Department of Psychology
The University of Texas at San Antonio
San Antonio, TX, USA

Narketta M. Sparkman-Key
Department of Counseling and Human Services
Old Dominion University
Norfolk, VA, USA

Shuntay Z. Tarver
Department of Counseling and Human Services
Old Dominion University
Norfolk, VA, USA

ISBN 978-3-030-95450-5 ISBN 978-3-030-95451-2 (eBook)
https://doi.org/10.1007/978-3-030-95451-2

© The Editor(s) (if applicable) and The Author(s), under exclusive licence to Springer Nature Switzerland AG 2022
This work is subject to copyright. All rights are solely and exclusively licensed by the Publisher, whether the whole or part of the material is concerned, specifically the rights of translation, reprinting, reuse of illustrations, recitation, broadcasting, reproduction on microfilms or in any other physical way, and transmission or information storage and retrieval, electronic adaptation, computer software, or by similar or dissimilar methodology now known or hereafter developed.
The use of general descriptive names, registered names, trademarks, service marks, etc. in this publication does not imply, even in the absence of a specific statement, that such names are exempt from the relevant protective laws and regulations and therefore free for general use.
The publisher, the authors and the editors are safe to assume that the advice and information in this book are believed to be true and accurate at the date of publication. Neither the publisher nor the authors or the editors give a warranty, expressed or implied, with respect to the material contained herein or for any errors or omissions that may have been made. The publisher remains neutral with regard to jurisdictional claims in published maps and institutional affiliations.

This Palgrave Macmillan imprint is published by the registered company Springer Nature Switzerland AG.
The registered company address is: Gewerbestrasse 11, 6330 Cham, Switzerland

Contents

Notes on Contributors

Bridget L. Anderson is Associate Professor of Applied Linguistics & English at Old Dominion University. She specializes in sociolinguistics, acoustic phonetics, and forensic linguistics. Her research and teaching focus on "everyday" varieties of American English, with attention to ethnicity, gender, regional orientation, stance, and ideology. Her second book, *Mountain Talk: the Language of Appalachia* is forthcoming from University of Tennessee Press. She also directs PECAR (People Educating Citizens Against Racism) which studies the language of white nationalists with the goal of confronting and disrupting a growing neo-fascist threat.

T'Airra Belcher is an Assistant Professor at Loyola University New Orleans. She is a licensed professional counselor in the states of Louisiana and Virginia. Dr. Belcher has established her career working with children and families in community mental health settings with a focus on interprofessional collaboration to identify best practices and techniques for serving these populations.

Ne'Shaun Borden is a Licensed Mental Health Counselor in the state of Florida, a Nationally Certified Counselor, and a faculty member in the Department of Clinical Mental Health Counseling on the JU Palm Coast instructional site. Prior to joining the JU faculty, she worked as an elementary school teacher, a school based mental health counselor, and as a counselor with justice involved youth. Dr. Borden's research interests include school based mental health counseling, counseling children and adolescents and increasing access to resources for underserved populations. In her free time, she enjoys spending time with family and friends, being an aunt, traveling, and reading.

Rawn Boulden is an assistant professor in the Department of Counseling and Learning Sciences at West Virginia University in Morgantown, WV. Additionally, he provides outpatient counseling services to children in the Greater Morgantown region. His scholarship focuses primarily on school counseling and counseling youth and adolescents. His research interests include school counseling, students with diverse learning needs, counselor education, rural school communities, school climate, resilience, cultural competence, and psychometric research. He has published numerous articles related to counseling and school settings, and has procured $500,000 in federal funding to support his research.

Dana L. Brookover, PhD: Dana Brookover, PhD, NCC, is an assistant professor in the Counseling and Human Services Department at the University of Scranton. A licensed school counselor and national certified counselor, Dr. Brookover worked as a professional school counselor in Virginia. She was an instructor at DePaul University, Villanova University, and Virginia Commonwealth University prior to beginning at the University of Scranton. She has published over a dozen articles in refereed academic journals on topics that include the social health needs of college students and factors that influence the preparedness of first-generation college students.

Melissa E. Buckley, PhD has extensive social work experience in the areas of trauma, child welfare and grief. She is currently an Assistant Professor at Coppin State University in the Social Work Department. She is a steering committee member of Healing City Baltimore, a movement that is responsible for passing the Elijah Cummings Healing City Act, a legislation that addresses the trauma and systemic racism that impacts racially and economically disenfranchised communities in Baltimore city.

Sarah Earlene Burford is both an educator and student. As a graduate student in the Old Dominion University Applied Linguistics program (sociolinguistics), her areas of research include white nationalist extremist language, African American English, and the trajectory of student language choices as they move through K-12 education. Sarah also teaches in a predominantly Black and low-socioeconomic demographic setting, seeking to transform the classroom experience through her integration of sociolinguistic principles.

Catherine Y. Chang (Catharina) is a Professor at Georgia State University and the director of International Programs for the College of Education and Human

Development. Dr. Chang's primary areas of interest include social justice and advocacy, multicultural counseling competence, counselor training and supervision, and counseling implications related to Asian American and Korean American clients.

Stephanie Z. Chen is a Chinese American cisgender woman, immigrant and licensed clinical psychologist who has worked in community mental health, hospitals, schools, and has a private practice. Chen also works as an associate professor of counseling psychology Chen's clinical work and teaching interests include integration and interplay of the intrapsychic, and sociocultural and political systems.

Marvin T. Chiles, PhD, is the Assistant Professor of African American History at Old Dominion University. His research deals broadly with race relations, and the disconnect between harmony and equity within urban, Southern, educational, and political life. His current projects involve racial reconciliatory efforts in the twentieth century U.S. South.

Krystal L. Clemons is an assistant professor in the Counselor Education and Family Studies department at Liberty University. Previously, Dr. Clemons served as a professional school counselor for 6 years. Her research interests include the Black church, Black student achievement in K-12 schools, anti-racism in school counseling and counselor education, and self-care among school counselors and school counseling students. Dr. Clemons has given over 25 presentations on the state, national, and international levels.

Raven K. Cokley (she/her) is currently a tenure-track Assistant Professor at Clark Atlanta University. She earned her PhD in Counseling and Student Personnel Services from the University of Georgia. She is a National Certified Counselor (NCC), with clinical expertise in school-based clinical mental health counseling, Sista Circle group counseling practices with Black girls and women, and individual counseling practices with minoritized clients. Her research agenda includes: 1) exploring the socioemotional and sociocultural experiences of Black girls and women; 2) eradicating anti-Blackness in counselor preparation programs; and 3) utilizing critical theories and methodologies in qualitative study.

Danna Demezier, PhD is an Assistant Professor in Counseling and Co-Coordinator of Clinical Mental Health Counseling at Barry University, Miami, FL, USA. She is a Licensed Mental Health Counselor in Florida and a National Certified Counselor. Her teaching and research interests center on culturally responsive practices and culturally competent supervision in counselors and counselors-in-training. Dr. Demezier presents and publishes on topics related to social justice, culturally responsive, and antiracist practices in counseling.

Adriana Díaz is a Program Specialist with SEAL. She is an impassioned educator with over 25 years advocating for underserved students and their families. She has served as a community coordinator, Spanish bilingual teacher from elementary through high school, academic counselor, and professor of communications for over 7 years. She received her master's degree in Mass Communications from San Jose State University.

Guadalupe Díaz is a Research Associate at Sobrato Early Academic Language (SEAL), Oakland, CA, USA, with extensive experience researching early educational programs for Dual Language Learners. She worked as Postdoctoral Fellow at the University of California, Irvine, where she focused on early education outcomes and parenting for bilingual families. She received her PhD in Human Development and Family Sciences from Oregon State University. Her research is primarily focused on the individual and ecological factors that influence children and their families' educational experiences.

Malcolm Drewery is an Assistant Professor of Sociology at Coppin State University in Baltimore, Maryland. He is considered a specialist in survey methodology and quantitative data analysis. Dr. Drewery has worked at some of the top Think Tanks and Government agencies in the United States conducting social science research. His areas of interest include gentrification, health disparities among minority populations, and race, class, and gender issues in sports.

Erin Durrah is a PhD candidate in the Counselor Education and Supervision program at the University of Arkansas in Fayetteville. Erin is also a licensed Marriage and Family Therapist whose research interests include reducing barriers to mental healthcare access particularly within Black and marginalized communities, and the evaluation of counseling intervention efficacy for diverse populations.

Dashawn Ealey is pursuing an MA in Psychology from the New School for Social Research. He received an M.S.ED in Higher Education from the University of Pennsylvania and a BA in African, African American Diaspora Studies from Wheaton College, MA. He has converging interests in culture, race, and identity and task-sharing approaches to increase access to mental health services. He is interested in using the minority stress model and the intersectionality framework to understand experiences of stigma and marginalization encountered by sexual minority populations of color and the negative health outcomes of intrapersonal, interpersonal, and structural levels of stigma and discrimination to develop dynamic and effective individual and scaleable task-sharing community interventions.

Leslie Ekpe is a third year PhD student at Texas Christian University in Higher Educational Leadership. Ekpe is an alumna of Alabama A&M University where she earned her B.S. in Management and the University of Alabama at Birmingham where she obtained her M.A. in Communication Management. She also holds an M.B.A. from Sam Houston State University. Her research seeks to promote access for marginalized students in education, with a specific focus on college access policies and racial politics in education.

Lucine Francis, PHD, RN Dr. Lucine Francis is an Assistant Professor at Johns Hopkins School of Nursing, a public health nurse, and a solutions-oriented researcher with expertise in health promotion and innovation in child care and schools. Dr. Francis is focused on identifying ways children from low-resourced communities are provided with the best environment to support their health and well-being. Her work has been funded by the National Institutes of Health and the Johns Hopkins Center for Health Disparities Solutions.

Jessica A. Fripp is an Associate Professor in the Department of Psychological Science & Counseling and the Associate Dean for the College of Behavioral and Health Sciences at Austin Peay State University. Her research interests include strategies for engaging African Americans in counseling services. Prior to working in higher education, Dr. Fripp spent the past 11 years working with low-income, ethnically diverse individuals and families in communities where engagement to mental health treatment is low.

Daniel José Gaztambide, PsyD, is assistant director of clinical training in the department of clinical psychology at the New School for Social Research, where he is director of the Frantz Fanon Center for Intersectional Psychology. He is a practicing psychologist and analytic candidate at the NYU Postdoctoral Program. He was featured in the documentary *Psychoanalysis in el Barrio*, and is the author of the book *A People's History of Psychoanalysis: From Freud to Liberation Psychology*.

Eva M. Gibson is currently an Assistant Professor at Austin Peay State University. Prior to becoming a counselor educator, she served 11 years in the public school system as a licensed school counselor. Dr. Gibson previously served as the President of the Tennessee Counseling Association as well as the Tennessee School Counseling Association. Her research areas include school counseling, social justice, and advocacy.

Cassidy Griffith, MSN, RN is a pediatric nurse at Johns Hopkins Children's Center and recent graduate of the Johns Hopkins Masters Entry into Nursing Practice Program. During her time in school at Hopkins, she contributed to several public health and research committees, one being the Teaching and Learning as a Pathway to Diversity, Equity, and Inclusion. She is passionate about health equity, anti-racism, and recently submitted a poster to the annual ACHNE conference about uncovering racism in nursing education.

Andrea Hampton Hall is a PhD student in the Counselor Education and Supervision program at the University of Arkansas in Fayetteville. Andrea is a certified Rehabilitation Counselor whose research interests include women of color and mental health care access, the use of CBD and medical marijuana to treat chronic pain, and social justice advocacy.

Janice Hawkins, PhD, RN is a Clinical Associate Professor at Old Dominion University where she is the Director of Community and Global Initiatives for the School of Nursing. She serves as a United Nations Liaison for Sigma Theta Tau International and as a State Leader for the United Nations Foundation Shot@Life Campaign. In these roles, she works directly with international organizations to address health challenges of marginalized communities worldwide.

Leslie Hoglund, PhD, MEd, is a Clinical Assistant Professor at Old Dominion University in the School of Community and Environmental Health. She desires to deconstruct inequitable systems that protect and perpetuate racism and poor health outcomes such as food apartheid, maternal and child health inequities, and population health assessment and evaluation. She was selected for the 2020 Culture of Health Leaders Program, sponsored by the Robert Wood Johnson Foundation.

Anya Hurwitz is the Executive Director of SEAL. Dr. Hurwitz has worked as a teacher, school leader, district administrator, and within the educational non-profit sector. She spent the early part of her career in New York City and in 2010 moved to Northern California. She holds an MA from Teachers College Columbia University, and a doctorate from UC Berkeley's Leadership for Educational Equity Program.

Taylor J. Irvine, M.Ed., Ed.S., LMHC is a licensed mental health counselor and doctoral candidate in the Counselor Education and Supervision program at

Florida Atlantic University. She has clinical experience working with diverse client populations and presenting issues in community mental health and residential treatment settings. Taylor's research interests include couples and infidelity, eating disorders and body image concerns, and decolonizing multicultural education and pedagogical practices across counselor education programs. Taylor has presented and published on these topics, centering on culturally responsive and equity-based practices across counseling research, training, and practice domains.

Keilah A. Jacques (she/her) is the CEO of Kei-Impact, Group LLC., and an adjunct instructor at the University of North Texas, Dallas in Human Services Management and Leadership. Additionally, she serves as faculty development consultant and adjunct instructor at Johns Hopkins, Bloomberg School of Public Health—where she teaches on Social Justice in Policy, Practice, and Research. Keilah works across multiple disciplines and sectors to examine the intersection of racism and health and specializes in social justice, anti-oppression, curriculum, and pedagogy. She draws from numerous schools of thought to inform her justice orientation including critical pedagogies', anti-oppressive frameworks, transformative education, liberation theology, structural competence, social innovation, moral resilience, collective impact, participatory appraisal, and human-centered design. She received her undergraduate degree in social work from The University of North Texas and is a graduate of The University of Connecticut and Oxford, Brooks University for her graduate and post graduate work. She is an accomplished and award-winning health education researcher and practitioner. As an indicator of her impact, Keilah was recognized with the Delta Omega in Innovation Public Health Curricular Award, at the 2019 American Public Health Association National Conference.

Camille R. Jensen, DNP, RN-CENP has over 15 years of nursing experience in acute care, public health and ambulatory care. She is an informatics nurse specialist interested in data systems and their use in addressing social determinants of health. She is currently an Assistant Professor at Michigan State University in the College of Nursing as well as the Director of Informatics for MSU Health Care. She served as an organizing committee member for Baltimore Neighbors Network, a community-based organization utilizing telehealth to provide social support and outreach to older adults in Baltimore City during the COVID-19 pandemic.

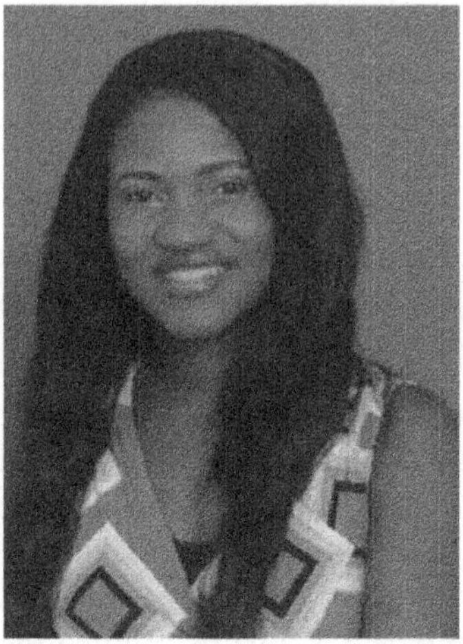

Kaprea F. Johnson, PhD, is a tenured Full Professor of Counselor Education at The Ohio State University in the Department of Educational Studies. Dr. Johnson is a counselor educator, who specializes in both school and mental health counseling, having taught masters level school counseling, mental health, and doctoral level courses during her tenure in academia. Dr. Johnson is currently the Director of the *Equity Research Lab*, in which she has students at the undergraduate and graduate level collaborating on projects that focus on equity issues in screening children and transitional aged youth for social inequities (i.e., discrimination, food and housing insecurity, income inequality), school and mental health practitioner training needs to address social inequities, and interrogation of systems that perpetuate inequities (i.e., education and healthcare systems). These innovative lines of research have assisted Dr. Johnson and her team of collaborators in garnering approximately 5 million in grant funding. In addition, Dr. Johnson has over 100 international, national, regional, community, and invited presentations. She is the co-author of two books, both on implementing diverse, equitable, and inclusive school counseling programs. These books have been chosen (2012 and 2020 edition) to be a part of *the American School Counselor Association* Cultural Competency Specialist training, in which thousands of people across the United States have been trained. Dr. Johnson also engages practitioners through her encyclopedia entries, non-refereed practitioner focus publications, white papers, podcast appearances, and information sharing via social media. In addition to her practitioner focused pieces, she has 54 peer reviewed publications in national and international journals in counseling, education, and allied health. As an active contributor to her profession, Dr. Johnson has served in several service and leadership positions at the national and regional levels. Dr. Johnson is nationally recognized in her field of counselor education and because of interdisciplinary focus she is nationally recognized across many helping professions and subspecialties. As a leader in her field she was sought after to become an editor of a national, long standing journal in counseling in the subspecialty of adult development and aging. In July of 2021, Dr. Johnson became the Editor of *the Adultspan Journal*, a national journal with thousands of readers. In addition to her editorial role she is also the Associate Editor of the Journal of

Humanistic Counseling, which is also a national journal in the Counseling field. As an expert on antiracism and social justice she was recently sought after to serve as an invited Special Guest Editor of the Journal of Mental Health Counseling (Special Topic: Social Justice, Equity, and Action, Spring 2021) another nationally recognized journal. Dr. Johnson, also serves in national elected positions, such as Secretary of the Southern Association of Counselor Education & Supervision, Association of Multicultural Counseling & Development Writers Consortium Chair, and the American Counseling Association Research and Knowledge committee. Dr. Johnson is a nationally recognized scholar, public facing academic, who is energized by the ability to discover and change inequitable systems to support and serve communities across the lifespan. If interested you can keep up with Dr. Johnson via twitter @ DrKaprea.

Gary Jones, PhD, LMSW Assistant Professor of Social Work, practice and research experiences are in the areas of child welfare, family formation, and racial equity and the role of social determinants on well-being. He is currently the Director of Field Education at Coppin State University, College of Behavioral and Social Sciences.

Janelle L. Jones, NCC is a fourth-year doctoral student in the Counselor Education and Supervision program at the University of Alabama. Janelle is a National Board of Certified Counselors Doctoral Fellow and serves as Member at Large for the Association for Adult Development and Aging. Her research interests include social determinants of health and equity, gerontological counseling, racial trauma, trauma informed counseling, and mentorship in counselor education.

Adriana C. Labarta, M.Ed., Ed.S., LMHC is a licensed mental health counselor and doctoral candidate at Florida Atlantic University's Counselor Education program. She has experience treating diverse clients with various mental health concerns in residential, partial hospitalization, intensive outpatient, and university counseling center settings. Adriana's research interests include eating disorders, body image concerns, and multicultural/social justice in counseling and counselor education. Adriana is particularly passionate about addressing barriers and disparities that impact marginalized groups, and promoting equity in research and higher education.

Sarah E. LaFave is a registered nurse and a doctoral candidate in the Johns Hopkins University School of Nursing. As a Robert Wood Johnson Foundation

Future of Nursing Scholar, Sarah's dissertation research focuses on the impact of structural racial discrimination on older African Americans' health. Through her teaching, Sarah engages students in equity-promoting community and public health practice, including through the service-learning organization she co-founded, Lori's Hands.

Aliza H. Lambert, M.Ed., CRC, is a doctoral candidate in the Counselor Education and Supervision program at Virginia Commonwealth University in Richmond, VA. In her clinical work, she provides supported employment for individuals with intellectual and developmental disabilities in the ACE-IT in College program at Virginia Commonwealth University. Her research is primarily focused on inclusive postsecondary education, pre-employment transition services, and community integrated employment for individuals with intellectual and developmental disabilities. She currently serves as the editorial assistant for the Counseling and Values Journal. Aliza's dissertation is on the lived experience of Jewish youth intellectual and developmental disabilities as they experience rituals and practices in the home.

Lea A. Marineau, MSN, ANP-BC, CNE Lea Marineau (she/her) is a PhD candidate at Johns Hopkins University School of Nursing. Her research is focused on further understanding risk factors, including structural racism, associated with recurrent violent injury. She is board certified as an Adult Nurse Practitioner and has been working in a level I trauma center in Baltimore City. Prior to starting the PhD program, she received her MSN from Johns Hopkins University School of Nursing and her BSN from the University of Florida.

Jamela M. Martin, PhD, RN is an Assistant Professor of Nursing at Old Dominion University with extensive experience in community health, global health, and health inequities. Dr. Martin oversees a Centers for Disease Control funded Population Health Learning Hub which enhances partnerships with health departments, non-health sector entities, and community agencies to address social determinants of health for low-income, uninsured, individuals locally. Her recently published manuscripts include examinations of healthcare implicit bias and social determinants of health education models.

Martha I. Martinez is the Director of Research and Evaluation at SEAL. She has over 15 years of experience researching programs and policies designed to improve educational outcomes for underserved populations, and over 10 years of experience examining English Learner issues specifically. Her research interests include linguistically diverse students in PK-12 schools, bilingual education, race/ethnicity, and education systems change.

C. Peeper McDonald, PhD, LPC, ACS, NCC, Assistant Professor at Mercer University, Macon, GA, USA, works as a counselor educator teaching and supervising counselors-in-training and future counselor educators. Her work has propelled her to specifically focus her teaching on issues of: Professional identity, social justice and advocacy, and multiculturalism in counseling. She has presented and published on these topics, with specific focus on the racial mislabeling, color-blindness and discrimination, and identity development of Multiracial individuals.

Joanna Meadvin is a Program Coordinator with SEAL. She has taught in Nicaragua, New York City, Mississippi and California from second grade through university. She holds a master's degree in Bilingual/Bicultural education from Teachers College, Columbia University and a PhD in Literature from the University of California at Santa Cruz.

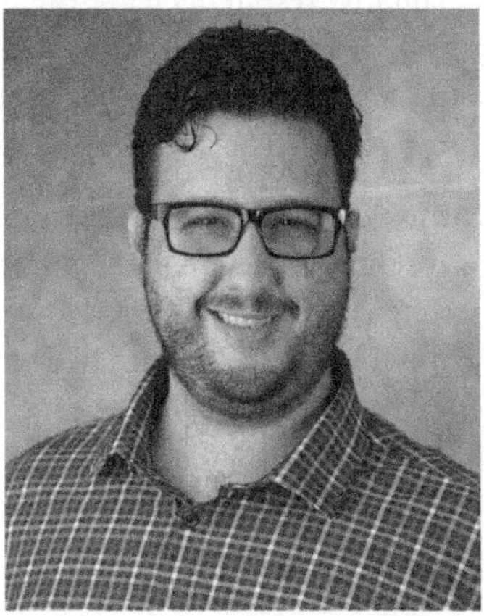

Alan Meca, PhD, is an Assistant Professor in the Department of Psychology at the University of Texas at San Antonio. Dr. Meca received his PhD in Applied Developmental Science from Florida International University in 2014 and completed a postdoctoral fellowship on a NIAAA-funded minority supplement (R01AA021888- 02S2) in the Department of Public Health Sciences at the University of Miami, Miller School of Medicine. Dr. Meca's research is largely focused on identity development and on the links between identity and psychosocial functioning. Although Dr. Meca's research has focused on identity development broadly, the bulk of his work has sought to establish an understanding of the links between identity development, acculturation, and socio-cultural/nativist stressors among ethnic/racial minority youth, particularly within Hispanic/Latinx populations. In pursuing this research agenda, Dr. Meca has published over 70 peer-reviewed manuscripts in national and international journals in developmental, counseling/clinical, cross-cultural, multicultural, and social/personality psychology. As a whole, Dr. Meca's teaching, mentorship, and scholarship has been rooted in a dedication towards anti-racism and anti-oppression seeking to address diversity, inclusion, equity, and justice.

Bora Meraj is a psychology graduate student researcher at the New School for Social Research. She's a member of the Trauma and Global Mental Health Lab and has spent time in Malaysia, developing a global mental health research project on the impact of traumatic events, dehumanization and religious freedom on Rohingya refugees in Selayang and Georgetown.

Francisca Rivas is a doctoral candidate in Counselor Education and Supervision at Old Dominion University, Norfolk, VA, USA. She works full time as a professional counselor with the Department of Veteran's Affairs and part-time as an Adjunct Professor. Ms. Rivas's clinical work is in substance use, serious mental health, trauma, and crisis interventions. Along with Ms. Rivas's professional work, her research interests are in multicultural care and pedagogy, historically minority population issues, as well as topics related to diversity and equity.

Lauren B. Robins, PhD: Dr. Lauren B. Robins is an Assistant Professor and researcher at Old Dominion University. Lauren has been a research associate for several research labs, conducting quantitative and qualitative research. Her research focuses on interprofessional collaboration, underserved populations, equity, social justice, and social determinants of health. She realizes and emphasizes the importance of equity that is centered upon an anti-racist approach and framework.

Waleed Y. Sami is a third-year doctoral student at Virginia Commonwealth University's Counselor Education program. His past clinical experiences involve acute care settings, locked residential facilities, group homes, and correctional settings for adolescents and their families. He is interested in looking at how inequality and the political economy impact mental health. He also is developing novel interventions through Rough and Tumble Play theory to help manage aggression in adolescents and children. Lastly, he is interested in improving mental health professionals' ability to work with Muslim-American clients within counseling. His dissertation examines the impact and decline of labor unions on mental health outcomes.

Corina Sapien is a Program Coordinator and District Relations Administrator at SEAL. She was a public-school educator for over 28 years and began her career as a middle school teacher. Corina obtained her BA in English, three teaching credentials, administrative credential and MA in Educational Administration from Santa Clara University.

Mona Shattell, PhD, RN, FAAN is Chair of the Department of Nursing Systems, Hugh F. and Jeannette G. McKean Endowed Chair, and Professor at the University of Central Florida, Orlando, FL, USA. She is the Editor of the

Journal of Psychosocial Nursing and Mental Health Services, and the author of more than 150 journal articles and book chapters. Her published work focuses on patient-provider relationships, various environments of care, and underserved populations such as long-haul truckers. Dr. Shattell is a Fellow of the Institute of Medicine Chicago, and the American Academy of Nursing.

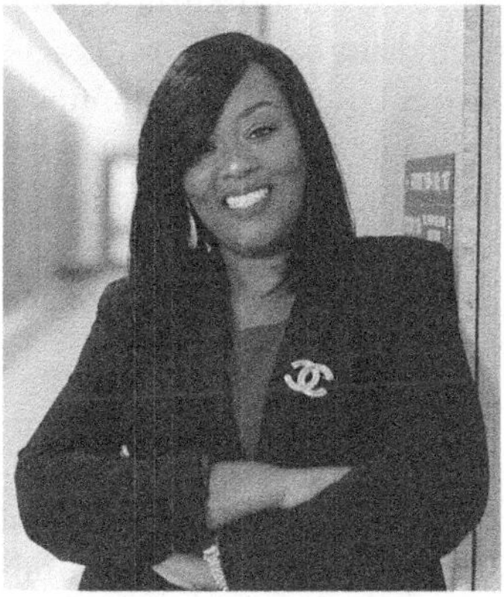

Narketta M. Sparkman-Key, PhD, is a tenured Associate Professor of Human Services at Old Dominion University. She also holds the inaugural position of Academic Affairs Director of Faculty Diversity and Retention. Dr. Sparkman-Key is a human services scholar and practitioner with over 20 years of practitioner experience in the field of human services with a background that spans from foster care case management to program evaluation. She addresses barriers to inclusion through her research efforts and development of programming focused on creating more inclusive environments. Her work is rooted in anti-racist policies and practices. Her research focuses on further defining the professional identity of human services practitioners & delineating practice with vulnerable populations. She has collaboratively published over 25 peer reviewed studies and numerous other op-eds, monographs, briefs and encyclopedia publications. She has collaboratively been awarded approximately 2.5 Million in grant funding. She has taught and mentored undergraduate, graduate and doctoral students over her 9 years in academia, serving on numerous doctoral dissertation committees. She specializes in teaching program evaluation, human service methods, internship, practicum and diversity. She is an affiliated faculty of both Virginia Commonwealth University and the University of West Indies. For the past 8 years she has led students to Montego Bay, Jamaica on a service learning focused study abroad to develop self-esteem among pregnant teens. Dr. Sparkman-Key is currently a self- study reviewer for the Council for Standards in Human Service Education, member of the marketing committee for the National Association of Diversity Officers in Higher Ed and member of the editorial team for the Journal of Trauma Studies in education. Her commitment to the field and to educating her students has earned recognition by the National Organization of Human Services (2013, 2014, 2015 and 2016) and by former students, who nominated her as their "Most Inspiring Faculty" (2015). On a college level she was awarded the Darden College of Education International

Outreach Award (2020) and Community Service Award (2018). At the university level she was awarded the Kate Broderick Educational Accessibility Award (2018), President Broderick Award for Diversity and Inclusion (2016) and the Provost Award for Undergraduate Mentorship (2016). She has been recognized for her work in the community Inside Business News, as a Woman in Business (2020) and "Top 40 under 40 Hampton Roads" (2016). In 2019, Dr. Sparkman-Key was recognized for her community engaged work with students by the Urban League of Hampton Roads, who presented her with the Martin Luther King Community Leader award. In addition, the YWCA of South Hampton Roads presented her with the 2021 Mary Helen Thomas Racial Justice Award and 2019 Woman of Distinction recognition in Research and the Sciences. Dr. Sparkman-Key has a passion for helping others and a strong interest in the advocacy, education, and empowerment of vulnerable populations.

Brittany G. Suggs, M.A., MPH, LPC (VA), is a licensed professional counselor and a doctoral candidate in the Counselor Education and Supervision program at Regent University. Brittany's research centers on collaborative mental health care, multicultural competence, sociocultural advocacy, social determinants of health, race-based traumatic stressors, and emerging adulthood. Broadly, global mental health, spiritual integration, and technology extend into her professional paradigms, coupled with a passionate commitment to diversity and equity promotion.

Sarah L. Szanton, PhD, ANP, FAAN is Health Equity and Social Justice Endowed Professor at the Johns Hopkins School of Nursing. Szanton's work focuses on decreasing barriers to "aging in place" including financial stain and racial discrimination. She co-developed the CAPABLE program, now scaled to 32 sites in 17 States. She received the 2019 Heinz Award for the Human Condition and is a PBS "Next Avenue Influencer in Aging."

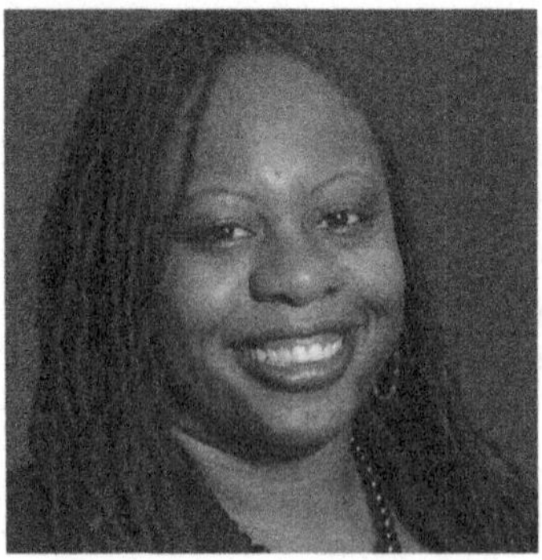

Shuntay Z. Tarver PhD, MSW, earned her PhD in Human Development and Family Studies from the University of North Carolina at Greensboro. She earned her bachelor's degree in social work from the University of Wisconsin-Milwaukee, and her master's degree in social work from the University of Wisconsin-Madison. She is a community-engaged scholar committed to deconstructing and dismantling systemic inequity through

practice and research. Dr. Tarver is an assistant professor at Old Dominion University in the department of Counseling and Human Services. She is also a co-founder and training consultant of The Human Development Group, LLC., where she assists various agencies and organizations with creating equitable and inclusive practices and policies. She serves the City of Hampton (Virginia) as a commissioner on the Citizens Unity Commission to collaboratively promote, sponsor, and facilitate community-wide education and activities to enhance cross-cultural interactions. Dr. Tarver is committed to conducting culturally competent, anti-racist, interdisciplinary research. Her scholarship has three primary objectives: (1) to advance social justice and equity; (2) to unveil the experiences of African Americans within various ecological systems (i.e. schools and families); and (3) to explore the unique intragroup experiences of marginalized populations within society. Dr. Tarver has published in various outlets including the Journal of Human Services, Journal of Diversity in Higher Education, and Journal of Ethnic & Cultural Diversity in Social Work. In addition, Dr. Tarver has conducted over 50 presentations at local, state, national, and international conferences. Dr. Tarver has been recognized as a Diversity Scholar by the University of Michigan's National Center for Institutional Diversity. She was awarded the 2017 Alumni Pacesetter by the University of North Carolina-Greensboro College of Health and Human Services. She also received the 2018 Old Dominion University's President's Diversity Award. Dr. Tarver is dedicated to affirming the inherent worth and dignity of marginalized populations through dismantling systemic inequities and empowering oppressed populations.

Sarah Toutant is a research associate at the University of Southern California's (USC'S) Race and Equity center and a PhD student in the Urban Education Policy program at USC Rossier. Her research examines Black collegiate women's racialized and gendered experiences in their external environments, particularly their encounters with urban nightlife culture. Sarah holds a B.A. in sociology and critical diversity studies from the University of San Francisco and M.Ed. from USC Rossier.

Kimberly Adams Tufts, ND, WHNP-BC, FAAN has an extensive history of working to address health care inequities. Dr. Adams Tufts spearheaded efforts to bring primary care services to underserved residents of inner-urban settings. She designed and implemented a federally sponsored curriculum for community health workers. In addition, she spent several years advocating for the George W. Bush Administration's passage of the initial President's Emergency Plan for AIDS Relief (i.e. PEPFAR) which expanded access to HIV drugs to underserved communities.

Ruth-Alma Turkson-Ocran is a clinical investigator with research interests in health disparities, social determinants of health, and cardiometabolic health. She is a family nurse practitioner by training. Her research portfolio includes examining data from large nationally representative sources, wearable devices including actigraphy and ambulatory blood pressure monitoring (ABPM). She also has experience in immigrant health and has examined nativity differences in biopsychosocial health determinants including stress, discrimination, depression, social support, and resilience. Dr. Turkson-Ocran's current research is centered around hypertension, its associated comorbidities, complications, and prevention. She is also involved in projects examining racial differences in blood pressure patterns from office, ambulatory, and home blood pressure measurements and their associated health outcomes.

Anthony J. Vajda, PhD, NCC Dr. Vajda is an assistant professor in the professional counseling program at the University of Oklahoma. His research focus includes psychosocial determinants of health and wellbeing for people living with HIV and AIDS, racial and ethnic disparities in mental health care and sexual and gender minority mental health especially the impact of violence against transgender and non-binary individuals.

Brittany M. Wake is a LCMHCA and PhD student in the Counseling and Counselor Education Program at NC State. As an anti-oppression activist, counselor, and educator-in-training, Brittany integrates her professional roles through an identity founded upon liberation frameworks such as Relational Cultural Theory and Black Feminist Theory. Brittany's research interests revolve around the historical and current trauma of marginalization as well as educating and supervising minoritized counselors-in-training.

Cory Weschler is a Program Specialist with SEAL. She has spent the past 25 years examining nonviolence, community building, youth development, restorative justice and, most recently, ELs and language development. At the heart of all this work is Cory's desire to support young people accessing their voice. She received her master's in Education from San Francisco State University.

List of Figures

List of Tables

1

Introduction

Alan Meca, Narketta M. Sparkman-Key, Kaprea F. Johnson, and Shuntay Z. Tarver

Racial conflicts and engagement in oppressive practices have existed within the United States from its very conception and resulted in a long, complicated, and continued history with institutional racism (Myrdal, 2001; Sandifer et al., 2021). Despite substantive changes as a result of the civil rights movement in the 1960s, racism, which is systemic and

---

A. Meca (✉)
Department of Psychology, The University of Texas at San Antonio, San Antonio, TX, USA
e-mail: alan.meca@utsa.edu

N. M. Sparkman-Key • S. Tarver
Department of Counseling and Human Services, Old Dominion University, Norfolk, VA, USA
e-mail: nsparkma@odu.edu; smccoy@odu.edu

K. F. Johnson
Department of Educational Studies, Counselor Education Program, The Ohio State University, Columbus, OH, USA
e-mail: Johnson.9545@osu.edu

© The Author(s), under exclusive license to Springer Nature Switzerland AG 2022
K. Johnson et al. (eds.), *Developing Anti-Racist Practices in the Helping Professions: Inclusive Theory, Pedagogy, and Application*,
https://doi.org/10.1007/978-3-030-95451-2_1

institutionalized, plays a prevalent role within the United States today. Indeed, in 2017 we saw a public display of racism in Charlottesville as White supremacists took the street shouted a variety of denigrating racial epithets (Posner, 2017). Additionally, we have publicly witnessed the impact of over policing and police brutality on Black people as a result of the murders of George Floyd, Breonna Taylor, Ahmaud Arbery, and countless others.

It is also critical to acknowledge pervasive health, educational, and economic disparities within the United States. Indeed, ethnic and racial minorities are more likely to experience a number of poor health outcomes (e.g., diabetes, maternal mortality, child suicide) as a result of a variety of disadvantages rooted in systemic racism (Alegria et al., 2010; Kaholokula, 2016; Liese et al., 2019; Spanakis & Golden, 2013). The COVID-19 pandemic has further amplified these inequities within the healthcare system as Black and Brown communities disproportionately experienced the brunt of the detrimental impact of COVID-19 early within the pandemic (Abedi et al., 2021; Khazanchi et al., 2020). Education within the United States has also had a long history rooted in institutionalized racism ranging from the Native American Boarding Schools that were created to forcibly strip indigenous youths' cultural identities to anti-literacy laws and segregation laws (Kohli et al., 2017). These, and the other ways systemic racism has historically shaped our education system, has resulted in institutionalized inequities that have long-term impacts on students of color and account for pervasive educational disparities. Additionally, a variety of meta-analysis have documented the detrimental impact of racism and discrimination on educational attainment, mental health (including depression, anxiety, and stress), and physical health, including cardiovascular diseases, and other potential risk factors for disease such as obesity and substance use (e.g., Benner et al., 2018; Carter et al., 2019; Paradies et al., 2015; Pascoe & Smart Richman, 2009).

Collectively, these recent events, which have clearly illustrated systemic inequalities and racial discrimination (e.g., murders at the hands of police) have resulted in the nation-wide reflection on the role of systemic racism within health professions and topics directly related to diversity, equity, inclusion and social justice. Building on this critical self-reflection and out of the recognition that it is insufficient to have "good intentions" and not be racist (Kendi, 2019), there has been an emphasis on moving towards an intentional anti-racist paradigm that seeks to disrupt oppressive systems and practices that perpetrate systems of inequity and racism. However, limited resources exist for guiding helping professionals toward becoming anti-racist. Addressing this critical gap, the purpose of this edited book is to provide examples of theories, practices, strategies, interventions, and actions that dismantle racism through an anti-racist approach and paradigm in disciplines including counseling, social work, education, psychology and health care under the umbrella of helping professionals. Given that helping professionals often serve individuals who have been historically marginalized, it is imperative that helping professionals implore anti-racist mandates and practices that meet the needs of marginalized populations.

Understanding Racism Within Helping Professions

Several helping professions, from social work to nursing, have unique credentials and/or ethical guidelines that often mandate inclusivity and cultural competence in practice, educational standards, and call to actions centered on establishing anti-racist paradigms within their professional practices. However, in light of recent events highlighting systemic inequalities and racial discrimination, several professional, including the American Public Health Association (2020), American Medical Association (2020), American Psychological Association (2020), the American School Counselor Association (2021), and others, have identified racism as a critical health determinant. However, racism has greatly impacted the healthcare field and health professionals, or occupations that provide health and education services to individuals and groups. Indeed, studies have indicated that healthcare professionals exhibit comparable levels of racism to that of the general population (Hall et al., 2015; Paradies et al., 2015). In part, this is due to fact education and training of helping professions is rooted in White supremacy that has focused on dismissing the values and identities of others, pathologize Black and Brown communities, and reproducing the racist status quo (Arroyo & Gasman, 2014; Chung & Bemak, 2012). In sum, the history of many helping professions is steeped in White supremacy, which upholds White normativity through racist policies, ideologies, pedagogies, and practices. Out of the recognition that it is insufficient to have "good intentions" and not be racist (Kendi, 2019), there has been a recent push across a variety of fields focused on moving towards an intentional anti-racist paradigm that seeks to disrupt oppressive systems and practices that perpetrate systems of inequity and racism.

The Need for Interdisciplinary Integration

Since the recent release of Ibram Kendi's (2019) *How to be Antiracist* book, helping professionals have begun to respond to the call to action by examining how racist practices have been embedded within discipline specific theories, pedagogy, and practice. Racial inequities related to state sanctioned violence, access to resources, existing health disparities, and challenges to mental health have intensified the urgency of helping professionals such as counselors, social workers, educators, and health care providers to reexamine both historical foundations of their professions, and current practices that create systemic inequity through the integration of research, policy and practice (Blitz et al., 2014; Knowles & Hawkman, 2020). However, limited resources exist for guiding helping professionals toward becoming anti-racist. In addition, there is disunity within empirical literature among the approaches taken to address anti-racism across the various disciplines (Legha & Miranda, 2020; Niemonen, 2007). Despite this distinction, there is a collective interest across disciplines in engaging anti-racist practices.

Addressing these critical gaps in the literature, the purpose of this edited book is to provide examples of theories, practices, strategies, interventions, and actions that dismantle racism through an anti-racist approach and paradigm across various helping professions. As further addressed in by authors Vajda, Belcher, Borden & Rivas in Chap. 2, an anti-racist approach is rooted in a deep exploration and reflection of existing practices, strategies, and paradigms and their role in further perpetrating systems of oppression. To address this need, this book provides helping professionals an interdisciplinary structure to critique existing approaches that have failed to eradicate systemic inequalities across helping professions. This timely interdisciplinary contribution across helping professions offer providers resources to improve their practice, their pedagogical stance, and their interdisciplinary knowledge as it relates to anti-racism and anti-racist approaches. Anti-racism also requires helping professionals to translate research and theory into practice that will lead to actions that dismantle racism within helping professions. The chapters that follow answer the anti-racist call to action by providing strategies for helping professions and professionals to become anti-racist. This presentation of anti-racist research, theory and practice responds to Kendi's (2019) call to action to examine and revise institutional policies and practices to become anti-racist.

Finally, as previously noted, the current edited book also takes a unique approach to connect a number of disciplines including counseling, social work, education, psychology and health care under the umbrella of helping professionals. Individual professions such as counseling, social work, education and health care are rarely understood as a collective because they each address divergent aspects of anti-racism. Current research has attempted to examine anti-racism across disciplines from one or more aspects such as theory (Holst, 2020); Pedagogy (Baker-Bell, 2020); Research (Knowles & Hawkman, 2020); or practice (Legha & Miranda, 2020). However, while such insights offer valuable strategies for engaging in anti-racist strategies, they are fragmented in their focus on either educational pedagogy, practice, or policy; and thus, fall short of providing a holistic approach for engaging in anti-racism. Consequently, our book offers a holistic resource that simultaneously examines history, policy, practice, pedagogy, and research. This book also utilizes the innovative approach of offering a critical examination of anti-racism within disciplinary education, professional standards, and practice protocols that espouse anti-racism in multifaceted ways. Collectively this book contributes to existing literature by providing interdisciplinary strategies for helping professionals to engage in anti-racism through critical evaluation of research, practice, and policies. Doing so empowers helping professionals across disciplines to employ anti-racist strategies that deconstruct and dismantle racism embedded within the foundational origins, professional standards, and disciplinary practices of helping professions while simultaneously merging research, practice, and advocacy that adapts anti-racist practices.

Structure and Outline

We have organized this textbook into three distinct sections: section I is focused on anti-racist theoretical perspectives, section II is focused on engaging in anti-racist pedagogy, and section III addresses anti-racist practices helping professionals. These sections explore various helping fields and provide evidenced-based perspectives on shaping a more anti-racist narrative as a profession and a professional.

Section I, which focuses on the theoretical underpinnings necessary for anti-racist helping professions, begins with Chap. 2 which not only further expands on the key terms introduced in the introduction, but situated them within an anti-racist paradigm more broadly. Additionally, this introductory chapter will serve to provide an overview of key paradigms relevant, across professions, to anti-racism. The subsequent chapters delve into specific theoretical frameworks and topics specific to certain helping professions, although special attention will be given to the generalizability of the proposed topics more broadly as a means of facilitating interprofessionalism. Chapter 3 seeks to decenter counseling, which has traditionally focused on Eurocentric models of care, to emphasize the need to include Afrocentric Models necessary for counselors to meet the needs of the Black community. Chapter 4 emphasizes how linguicism grows out of racist ideologies and is reinforced by it, and utilizes the Sobrato Early Academic Language (SEAL) to showcase an Antilinguicist approach that facilitates critical consciousness, exploration of professional identity, and intersectionality among school staff. Chapter 5 expands on the concept of allyship, introducing the problematic role that "performative allyship" can have on dismantling systems. In contrast, it provides a framework for how individuals can move towards being anti-racist co-conspirators. Finally, Chap. 6 deconstructs the implications of the benevolent racism and anti-Blackness that permeate the 'helper' identity and identifies strategies for interrupting and dismantling the savior complex through anti-racist pedagogy and other techniques. Collectively, this section provides several theoretical frameworks by which helping professionals can draw on in their work towards dismantling systems of oppression.

Recognizing the critical need to ensure that the way we train and educate the next generation of helping professionals is aligned with anti-racist practices, the subsequent section focuses on anti-racist pedagogy. Specifically, Section II begins with Chap. 7 that provides an overview of pedagogy within various disciplines, and how each is needed to advance anti-racist pedagogy for the collective interprofessional helping field. The next six chapters offer specific aspects of pedagogy that instructors should understand to engage in anti-racist pedagogical practices. Chapter 8 illustrates the impact of educators' anti-racist language. This approach asserts that anti-racist instructional techniques require intentional and strategic uses of anti-racist language. The next three chapters offer critical steps for revising traditional instructional content and practices into anti-racist pedagogy. Chapter 9 highlights the need to decenter Whiteness by engaging in anti-racist practices that utilize culturally-informed curriculum. While teaching psychopathology, a fundamental course for various disciplines such as counseling and clinical psychology, this chapter asserts that anti-racist pedagogy requires a committed refusal to reiterate White supremacy to emerging professionals through instructional content and practices. In an expanded way, Chap. 10 asserts that anti-racist pedagogy must displace Whiteness as the standard through the inclusion of critical pedagogy that utilizes critical race theory, feminist thought and the civil rights movement. Chapter 11 continues this notion by offering an illustration of how anti-racist pedagogy that emphasizes Black experiences can be utilized to challenge students to engage in critical self-reflection. The inclusion of culturally responsive content into graduate programs will position emerging practitioners to engage in culturally relevant practices of intervention, prevention, and advocacy. Chapter 12 acknowledges the current progress within curriculums reflected by multicultural competencies, while arguing anti-racist strategies are necessary for pushing emerging professionals to take the steps necessary for meeting the needs of marginalized populations. Finally, Chap. 13 concludes this section by providing an illustration of how helping professionals can develop and train emerging professionals from an anti-racist perspective by critically reexamining the content of disciplinary specific textbooks. Collectively, this section offers strategies for how educators can engage in anti-racist pedagogy.

Finally, the last section, Section III, focuses on identifying anti-racist perspective towards the direct application of working within a variety helping professions. Specifically, Section III provides concrete examples of how anti-racist perspectives are applied in helping professions. It begins with Chap. 14 which provides an overview of the application of anti-racist theory and pedagogy within practice. It also centers the tenets of interprofessional practice within helping professions by noting the impact helping professionals can have on populations they serve if they engage in understanding the work of other fields of practice. Chapters 15 and 16 focus on school counseling settings. Chapter 15 notes the importance of promoting anti-racism within school settings and the role of school systems in addressing oppression. Chapter 16 is an actual case study of how anti-racism can be done in school settings. It provides specific strategies and the impact those strategies have on the environment. Chapters 17 and 18 focus on mental health settings in both counseling and clinical psychology. Chapter 17 focuses on anti-racist best practices for mental health professionals being knowledgeable and skilled in working with populations impacted by antisemitism and Islamphobia. Chapter 18 critiques DEI training and proposes anti- racists perspectives in clinical psychology training programs. This section closes out with Chap. 19 provides a discussion of health care settings and the infusion of anti-racist perspectives. The chapter proposes an action plan that addresses health disparities among minority populations through an anti-racist lens. Chapter 20 explores telehealth anti-racist experiences within nursing and social work. Finally, this section closes out with Chap. 21 which focuses on equipping educators with culturally responsive anti-racist practices for educating and working with multiracial people by exploring ways to assess personal anti-racist identity, pedagogy, and change language and interactions. In sum, Section III provides examples of how to apply anti-racist strategies and perspectives and the impact of those applications in various fields of study across helping professions.

Although this edited collection should by no means be considered as an exhaustive endpoint, as we outline within our Epilogue, it serves as a critical stepping stone for dismantling systemic racism and oppression within helping professions. This edited book is significant in its specific focus on anti-racist theory, pedagogy, and practice within several related but distinct helping fields, such as psychology, social work, and professional counseling. For helping professionals, it is our expectation that this collected body of work will serve as a critical foundation for guiding anti-racist practices across various helping professions. In academic settings, not only will the theoretical and practical chapters provide rich knowledge centered on anti-racist theory and practice within helping professions, potentially leading to future research, but the chapters on anti-racist pedagogy can also be utilize for re-conceptualizing the training and education programs for helping professions.

References

Abedi, V., Olulana, O., Avula, V., Chaudhary, D., Khan, A., Shahjouei, S., Li, J., & Zand, R. (2021). Racial, economic, and health inequality and COVID-19 infection in the United States. *Journal of Racial and Ethnic Health Disparities, 8*, 732–742. https://doi.org/10.1007/s40615-020-00833-4

Alegria, M., Vallas, M., & Pumariega, A. J. (2010). Racial and ethnic disparities in pediatric mental health. *Child and Adolescent Psychiatric Clinics of North America, 19*(4), 759–774. https://doi.org/10.1016/j.chc.2010.07.001

American Medical Association. (2020, June 7). *AMA Board of Trustees pledges action against racism, police brutality*. https://www.ama-assn.org/press-center/press-releases/ama-board-trustees-pledges-action-against-racism-police-brutality

American Psychological Association. (2020, June 2). *APA's action plan for addressing inequality*. http://www.apa.org/news/apa/2020/action-addressing-inequality

American Public Health Association. (2020, May 29). *Racism is an ongoing public health crisis that needs our attention now*. https://www.apha.org/News-and-Media/News-Releases/APHA-News-Releases/2020/Racism-is-a-public-health-crisis

American School Counselor Association. (2021). *The school counselor and anti-racist practices.* https://www.schoolcounselor.org/Standards-Positions/Position-Statements/ASCA-Position-Statements/The-School-Counselor-and-Anti-Racist-Practices

Arroyo, M., & Gasman, A. T. (2014). An HBCU-based educational approach for Black college student success: Toward a framework with implications for all institutions. *American Journal of Education, 121*(1), 57–85.

Baker-Bell, A. (2020). *Linguistic justice Black language, literacy, identity, and pedagogy.* Routledge.

Benner, A. D., Wang, Y., Shen, Y., Boyle, A. E., Polk, R., & Cheng, Y. P. (2018). Racial/ethnic discrimination and well-being during adolescence: A meta-analytic review. *The American Psychologist, 73*(7), 855–883. https://doi.org/10.1037/amp0000204

Blitz, L. V., Greene, M. P., Bernabei, S., & Shah, V. P. (2014). Think creatively and act decisively: Creating a antiracist alliance of social workers. *Social Work, 59*(4), 347–350. https://doi.org/10.1093/sw/swu031

Carter, R. T., Johnson, V. E., Kirkinis, K., Roberson, K., Muchow, C., & Galgay, C. (2019). A meta-analytic review of racial discrimination: Relationships to health and culture. *Race and Social Problems, 11*, 15–32. https://doi.org/10.1007/s12552-018-9256-y

Chung, R. C.-Y., & Bemak, F. P. (2012). *Social justice counseling: The next steps beyond multiculturalism.* Sage Publications, Inc.

Hall, W. J., Chapman, M. V., Lee, K. M., Merino, Y. M., Thomas, T. W., Payne, B. K., Eng, E., Day, S. H., & Coyne-Beasley, T. (2015). Implicit racial/ethnic bias among health care professionals and its influence on health care outcomes: A systematic review. *American Journal of Public Health, 105*(12), e60–e76. https://doi.org/10.2105/AJPH.2015.302903

Holst, J. D. (2020). Toward a theory of race, change, and antiracist education. *Adult Education Quarterly, 70*(2), 175–192. https://doi.org/10.1177/0741713619884580

Kaholokula, J. K. (2016). Racism and physical health disparities. In A. N. Alvarez, C. T. H. Liang, & H. A. Neville (Eds.), *The cost of racism for people of color: Contextualizing experiences of discrimination* (pp. 163–188). American Psychological Association. https://doi.org/10.1037/14852-008

Kendi, I. X. (2019). How to be an antiracist – Book club kit. *One World.*

Khazanchi, R., Evans, C. T., & Marcelin, J. R. (2020). Racism, not race, drives inequity across the COVID-19 continuum. *JAMA Network Open, 3*(9), e2019933. https://doi.org/10.1001/jamanetworkopen.2020.19933

Knowles, R. T., & Hawkman, A. M. (2020). Anti-racist quantitative research: Developing, validating, and implementing racialized teaching efficacy and racial fragility scales. *Urban Review, 52*, 238–262. https://doi.org/10.1007/s11256-019-00526-1

Kohli, R., Pizzaro, M., & Nevárez, A. (2017). The "new racism" of K–12 schools: Centering critical research on racism. *Review of Research in Education, 41*, 182–202.

Legha, R. K., & Miranda, J. (2020). An anti-racist approach to achieving mental health equity in clinical care. *The Psychiatric Clinics of North America, 43*(3), 451–469. https://doi.org/10.1016/j.psc.2020.05.002

Liese, K. L., Mogos, M., Abboud, S., Decocker, K., Koch, A. R., & Geller, S. E. (2019). Racial and ethnic disparities in severe maternal morbidity in the United States. *Journal of Racial and Ethnic Health Disparities, 6*, 790–798. https://doi.org/10.1007/s40615-019-00577-w

Myrdal, G. (2001). An American dilemma: The negro problem and modern democracy. In E. Cashmore & J. Jennings (Eds.), *Racism: Essential readings* (pp. 35–48). SAGE Publications Ltd. https://doi.org/10.4135/9781446220986.n5

Niemonen, J. (2007). Antiracist education in theory and practice: A critical assessment. *The American Sociologist, 38*, 159–177. https://doi.org/10.1007/s12108-007-9006-x

Paradies, Y., Ben, J., Denson, N., Elias, A., Priest, N., Pieterse, A., Gupta, A., Kelaher, M., & Gee, G. (2015). Racism as a determinant of health: A systematic review and meta- analysis. *PLoS One, 10*(9), e0138511. https://doi.org/10.1371/journal.pone.0138511

Pascoe, E. A., & Smart Richman, L. (2009). Perceived discrimination and health: A meta- analytic review. *Psychological Bulletin, 135*(4), 531–554. https://doi.org/10.1037/a0016059

Posner, S. (2017, August 13). After Charlottesville Rally ends in violence, Alt-Right vows to return. *Rolling Stone.* https://www.rollingstone.com/politics/politics-news/after-charlottesville-rally-ends-in-violence-alt-right-vows-to-return-117471/

Sandifer, M. C., Gibson, E. M., & Brant-Rajahn, S. N. (2021). WOKE: Advocacy for African American students. In M. A. Rausch & L. L. Gallo (Eds.), *Strengthening school counselor advocacy and practice for important populations and difficult topics* (pp. 19–40). IGI Global. https://doi.org/10.4018/978-1-7998-7319-8.ch002

Spanakis, E. K., & Golden, S. H. (2013). Race/ethnic difference in diabetes and diabetic complications. *Current Diabetes Reports, 13*(6), 814–823. https://doi.org/10.1007/s11892-013-0421-9

Section I

Antiracist Helping Professions Theoretical Underpinnings

2

Introduction to Anti-Racist Theories

Anthony J. Vajda, T'Airra Belcher, Ne'Shaun Borden, and Francisca Rivas

Introduction

A foundational knowledge and understanding of an anti-racist paradigm is necessary across helping professions to serve as a foundation by which we critically evaluate theoretical and practice perspectives. Awareness, knowledge, and skills are three pillars that assist in deepening

A. J. Vajda (✉)
University of Oklahoma, Norman, OK, USA
e-mail: vajda@ou.edu

T. Belcher
Loyola University, New Orleans, LA, USA
e-mail: tcbelche@loyno.edu

N. Borden
Jacksonville University, Jacksonville, FL, USA
e-mail: nborden@ju.edu

F. Rivas
Old Dominion University, Norfolk, VA, USA
e-mail: Friva002@odu.edu

© The Author(s), under exclusive license to Springer Nature Switzerland AG 2022
K. Johnson et al. (eds.), *Developing Anti-Racist Practices in the Helping Professions: Inclusive Theory, Pedagogy, and Application*,
https://doi.org/10.1007/978-3-030-95451-2_2

understanding of systems of power, privilege, and oppression in society (Sue & Sue, 2015). Essential to a better understanding of these is necessitates maintaining an active role in gaining insight and awareness of one's role in perpetuating oppression and marginalization, pursuing knowledge of how to actively navigate systems of power and privilege at individual, institutional, and societal levels, and developing skills to advocate for minoritized individuals and groups through professional work in the helping fields (Sue & Sue, 2015). The utilization of awareness, knowledge, and skills, are at the center of working toward being an antiracist individual and helping professionals. Privilege is the presence of innate factors—finances, shelter, familial support, networking—which increase a person's access to stability. Generally, privilege is not a negative concept, and all people have some form of privilege. Privilege creates power for some groups or individuals through systemic advantages (Lenski, 1966). Power can provide control when wielded against others to maintain an advantage, which illustrates the concerns about systems of power and privilege. The use of power to maintain systems of power and privilege—utilizing your privilege to determine the trajectory of another group of people—can be seen in racism (Anderson & Collins, 2020b).

Racism, sexism, and ableism are examples of phenomena maintained by systems of power and oppression that impact a person's quality of life and existence in society (Anderson & Collins, 2020b; Hooker, 2016; Jones, 2014; Sue & Sue, 2015). Depending on a person's intersecting identities, the contextual and systemic barriers faced due to these identities impact access to adequate healthcare, education, financial support, and familial support. When specific identities or group affiliations do not have a negative impact on the individual in terms of access to resources or social determinants of health and wellbeing (i.e. able bodied individuals with healthcare), it is a likely indication that a person has identity-based privilege. While an equitable society wherein all individuals were able to achieve the same access to resources would be ideal, the achievement of such an ideal would only be possible through hard work at all levels of the system to dismantle deep-rooted biases and prejudices which fuel the injustices faced by many in our society. The increase in death rate, incarceration, and violent acts, in addition to the widening of the educational gap, provide a grimmer experience of the systems of power and privilege often faced by minoritized groups based on their race, ethnicity, gender, socioeconomic status, ability, and sexual and affectional orientation (Anderson & Collins, 2020a; Anderson & Collins, 2020b; Borden et al., 2019; Hooker, 2016).

The Matrix of Domination is a paradigm which discusses multiple systems of power and privilege and provides a conceptualization of how these layers of oppressive forces significantly impact a person's life trajectory. The paradigm is useful to convey the social oppression experienced by individuals oppressed based on the status of their gender, race, and class and provides us with language to discuss the interplay of these complex dynamics (Collins, 2002). Those with direct or easy access to the systems of power and privilege often have social locations that are heterosexual, white, educated, male, able-bodied, and wealthy. Anti-Racist paradigms such as those discussed in this chapter aim to support helping professionals to deconstruct systems of power and privilege by gaining a better understanding of their role in the system. Beyond understanding one's role in the system is to take an active stance in becoming an antiracist helping professional through practice and advocacy. Critical race theory, critical consciousness, and intersectionality provide foundational knowledge for helping professionals to move toward an antiracist vantage point in their individual lives and professional work.

Antiracist Paradigms

Critical Race Theory

Critical Race Theory (CRT), born as a result of the civil rights movement of the 1960s, stresses the interplay of race, racism, and power and aims to transform these relationships by considering them in a broad perspective which includes the consideration of historical context, economics, and the dynamics of group and self. While having begun as a movement in law, it has now spread to many disciplines and has evolved to consider issues across systems and institutions including education and inequities in social determinants of health (Ansell, 2008; Crenshaw et al., 1995).

To better understand CRT and its application to the helping professions, it is essential to have knowledge of five themes that are woven throughout the theory: ordinariness, material determinism, social constructionism, differential racialization, and intersectionality (Delgado & Stefancic, 2017). Ordinariness refers to the idea that racism is common and deeply rooted in our society which makes it so difficult to address. Material determinism is a means by which society allocates privilege and racial hierarchies determining who gets tangible benefits such as jobs, access to schools, and resources. It describes that privilege benefits the dominant group and continues to oppress the minoritized. Social constructionism, a term that many helping professionals are likely familiar with, refers to the notion that we create our social realities and the meaning we attribute to them. As such, race is a product of social thought and not a biological feature, used to group individuals together by traits that are superficial rather than valuing individuals for their morality, intelligence, and/or personality. Differential racialization refers to the changing depiction of minoritized racial groups dependent on the needs of the dominant group. And lastly, another familiar concept is intersectionality. Intersectionality describes the notion that no one has one single isolated identity, that each piece of identity is an aspect which contributes to a more complex whole, influencing the way one experiences the world around them, navigates through systems, and faces systemic and structural barriers (Delgado & Stefancic, 2017).

CRT provides a framework for helping professionals to build upon the awareness of their own implicit biases and to continue to seek knowledge regarding the myriad of ways that systemic oppression impacts the clients we work with. Being an antiracist helping professional requires us to go beyond knowledge of theory and terms, and to advocate in such a way that challenges the dominant discourse through our practice and our daily lives. Helping professionals, as part of their obligation to their ethical code and duty to their communities, must utilize knowledge learned to ensure consistent reflection on their own social location and privilege associated with it. By reflecting on these privileges, and discovering one's own implicit biases and prejudices, helping professionals can use this heightened awareness to build better and stronger relationships with communities they serve. Today, we see CRT as an application to many of our social justice issues such as poverty, policing and criminal justice, school curricula, hate speech, color blindness, immigration, globalization, and voting rights (Delgado & Stefancic, 2017). Helping professionals are well-positioned in society to work with individuals to address health disparities and to work within institutions at the systemic level to be a part of an ever-evolving force of change, dismantling structures of power and injustice to support continued structural change.

Critical Consciousness

Critical Consciousness has been defined as "the ability to recognize and analyze systems of inequality and the commitment to take action against these systems" (El-Amin et al., 2017). Paulo Freire, a Brazilian born adult educator, is credited with developing this theoretical and pedagogical framework. Freire published *Pedagogy of the Oppressed* in 1970 and *Education for Critical Consciousness* in 1973. Although Freire published many works throughout his lifetime that examined his educational practices and the influence of oppression on education, *Pedagogy of the Oppressed,* has often been hailed as his most important work (Smith, 2021). Freire's' theory of Critical Consciousness is largely influenced by his experiences and social context which include growing up in post-colonial Brazil, losing his father at an early age, leaving elementary school to help provide financially for his family, and later campaigning for and teaching in adult literacy programs in Brazil (Smith, 2021). From Freire's experiences, he developed concepts for the classroom to promote critical consciousness as educators.

Freire believed that traditional education was largely a banking model by which teachers deposited information into students. In the banking model, there is a clear hierarchy with the teacher being the sole owner of knowledge and the student being the recipient (Jemal, 2017). Freire (2005) theorized that this style of teaching would not allow for students to engage in critical reflection. Critical reflection is a process that allows learners and educators to identify inequity. Freire believed that learners could not become free with the banking model of education as it largely served to reinforce systems of inequity and oppression (Jemal, 2017). Freire (2005) theorized that for critical reflection to occur that the relationships between teachers and students needed to be more democratic and that students must be actively engaged in and aware of societies ill such as oppression and inequity. Freire believed that critical consciousness involved social analysis and social engagement and action (Jemal, 2017).

Freire also developed the idea of "Conscientização." The term conscientização refers to "learning to perceive social, political, and economic contradictions, and to take action against the oppressive elements of reality" (Freire, 2005, p. 35). According to Jemal (2017) this term is often used interchangeably with critical consciousness; however, they are not the same. Conscientização is more accurately the action by which critical consciousness is achieved. Although, Freire's theory is highly regarded and has also been applied across many disciplines such as public health, psychology, and social work (Jemal, 2017) it has also been criticized because Freire does not outline a route by which to implement his theory in the classroom. Scholars have stated the theory is one dimensional and only focuses on thinking of social change without providing action steps for educators (Jemal, 2017). Freire writing has also been criticized as inaccessible to the average person. Ways for educators to promote critical consciousness in the classroom, past what Freire has posited, will be discussed in depth in Chap. 4 as well as ways in which individuals can engage in critical consciousness on their own.

Intersectionality

Kimberlé Williams Crenshaw is a full-time law professor at Columbia University, a distinguished law professor at University of California, Los Angeles (UCLA), and a pioneering scholar for social justice and human rights, Black feminist legal theory, and critical race theory, which has led to her coining the term *intersectionality* in 1989 (The trustees of Columbia University, 2021). Through Crenshaw's work in identity politics and violence against women, the term intersectionality was born. Identity politics are helpful in that they are able to highlight group differences in terms of power and social justice, providing a source of strength, community, and intellectual development (Crenshaw et al., 1995; Crenshaw,

1989). However, Crenshaw identifies that it fails by ignoring intragroup differences that occur in these marginalized groups.

When the intragroup differences are ignored, this can create tension and stress within the group (Crenshaw et al., 1995). What this means is having an either/or practice of identity, such as "women" or "people of color" which does not consider those experiences of women of color as well as women of color who hold other identities such as education status or ability status. With intersectionality, these experiences held by intragroup members are not invalidated and the stress on the group is lessened by validating each member's whole self and their experiences.

Crenshaw originally described intersectionality as a way to view bias and discrimination against black women (1989) but the term has since been expanded on by Crenshaw and others to incorporate more than gender and racial identities in terms of power and discrimination. Intersectionality is a framework that incorporates the interconnected identities that an individual or group may hold that impact the social inequalities and discrimination that they may experience (Crenshaw, 1989, 1991; Crenshaw et al., 1995; Cooper, 2016). By incorporating intersectionality, the individual is seen as a whole, including all identities of privilege and marginalization they hold, which can increase better outcomes for treatment and understanding systemic injustices that occur for individuals and groups. For example, while a White, queer, differently abled male may hold privilege in his status of being White and male, he also holds marginalized statuses as that he is LGBT+ and differently-able bodied. Holding these privileged statuses does not negate his marginalized experiences he may have due to his ability status or sexual orientation, just like those marginalized statuses do not void the privilege that that individual also holds. Keeping in mind that these identities also are a spectrum, depending on where you fall on the line, can increase the amount of oppression or privilege that identity holds. Being able to incorporate all identities an individual may hold can aid in better understanding systems of power and prejudice as well as lessening the intragroup stress that occurs when viewing individual group memberships as black and white.

Conclusion

Creating a foundational knowledge and understanding of an anti-racist paradigm is necessary across helping professions to critically evaluate theoretical and practice perspectives, understand individuals and their social situations, and know the systems that create power and discrimination for individuals and groups. In understanding power and privilege, individuals can critically evaluate their roles in perpetuating oppression and discrimination as well as foster ways to dismantle systemic injustices. The chapter has provided a brief overview of the antiracist paradigm and covered key theoretical paradigms central to creating an antiracist theoretical framework. The key paradigms discussed were critical race theory, critical consciousness, identity development, and intersectionality.

References

Anderson, M. L., & Collins, P. H. (2020a). *Why race, class, and gender still matter. Race, class, and gender: Intersections and inequities* (10th ed.). Cengage.

Anderson, M. L., & Collins, P. H. (2020b). *Systems of power and inequity. Race, class, and gender: Intersections and inequities* (10th ed.). Cengage.

Ansell, A. (2008). Critical race theory. In R. T. Schaefer (Ed.), *Encyclopedia of race, ethnicity, and society, volume 1* (pp. 344–346). SAGE Publications.

Borden, N., Belcher, T., Rivas, F., & Ricks, S. A. (2019). Bringing social movements into human services classrooms: Movements and human services education. *Journal of Human Services, 38*.

Collins, P. H. (2002). *Black feminist thought: Knowledge, consciousness, and the politics of empowerment* (1st ed.). Routledge.

Cooper, B. (2016). Intersectionality. In L. Disch & M. Hawkesworth (Eds.), *The Oxford handbook of feminist theory*. https://doi.org/10.1093/oxfordhb/9780199328581.013.20

Crenshaw, K. (1989). Demarginalizing the intersection of race and sex: A black feminist critique of antidiscrimination doctrine, feminist theory and antiracist politics. *University of Chicago Legal Forum, 1989*(1), 139–167.

Crenshaw, K. (1991). Mapping the margins: Intersectionality, identity politics, and violence against women of color. *Stanford Law Review, 43*(6), 1241–1299. https://doi.org/10.2307/1229039

Crenshaw, K., Gotanda, N., Peller, G., & Thomas, K. (1995). *Critical race theory: The key writings that formed the movement.* The New Press.

Delgado, R., & Stefancic, J. (2017). *Critical race theory: An introduction* (3rd ed.). University Press.

El-Amin, A., Seider, S., Graves, D., Tamerat, J., Clark, S., Soutter, M., Johannsen, J., & Malhotra, S. (2017). Critical consciousness: A key to student achievement.

Freire, P. (2005). *Pedagogy of the oppressed: 30th anniversary edition.* The Continuum International Publishing Group Inc.

Hooker, J. (2016). Black lives matter and the paradoxes of U.S. Black politics: From democratic sacrifice to democratic repair. *Political Theory, 44*(4), 448–469.

Jemal, A. (2017). Critical consciousness: A critique and critical analysis of the literature. *The Urban Review, 49*(4), 602–626. https://doi.org/10.1007/s11256-017-0411-3

Jones, C. P. (2014). Systems of power, axes of inequity: Parallels, intersections, braiding the strands. *Medical Care, 52*(10), 71–75. https://doi.org/10.1097/MLR.0000000000000216

Lenski, G. (1966). *Power and privilege: A theory of social stratification.* McGraw-Hill.

Smith, P. (2021). *Paulo Friere.* Salem Press. Encyclopedia.

Sue, D. W., & Sue, D. (2015). *Counseling the culturally diverse: Theory and practice.* Wiley.

3

The Importance of Culturally Responsive and Afrocentric Theoretical Frameworks-A Call for More Inclusive Curriculum in Counselor Education

Erin Durrah, Andrea Hampton Hall, and Anthony J. Vajda

Introduction

Every Counselor Education program requires master's students to take a foundational theories class. While in this class, students are expected to explore and conceptualize the theory of counseling best fitting their worldview which serves as a framework to conceptualize and guide treatment. Although the structure of the theory course varies from program to program, the content must meet specific standards set by the Council for Accreditation of Counseling and Related Programs (CACREP). Counseling theory textbooks often mention names familiar to most

E. Durrah (✉) • A. H. Hall • A. J. Vajda
University of Arkansas, Fayetteville, AR, USA

University of Oklahoma, Norman, OK, USA
e-mail: vajda@ou.edu

© The Author(s), under exclusive license to Springer Nature Switzerland AG 2022

K. Johnson et al. (eds.), *Developing Anti-Racist Practices in the Helping Professions: Inclusive Theory, Pedagogy, and Application*,
https://doi.org/10.1007/978-3-030-95451-2_3

counseling professionals; Adler, Rogers, Beck, and Freud just to name a few. The philosophical conflicts between these frameworks and their founders are studied emphasizing the importance of developing a practice consistent with the needs of specific populations. While some of the frameworks are structured and have distinguishable phases and steps, others are more abstract in nature.

Giving students a foundation and theoretical framework is essential for the education of counselors in training and gives students a way to understand human behavior and the intrinsic motivations behind those behaviors. However, each of the models incorporated in introductory and even advanced theory courses, present the perspectives of a predominately male group of psychiatrists and psychologists of European descent, without any mention of contributions to the field by non-White practitioners (Whitten, 1993). The prioritization of Eurocentric counseling models has resulted in a narrow and inflexible view of minoritized client's behaviors (Sommers-Flanagan & Sommers-Flanagan, 2004). Clients who have marginalized identities are often seen through a Western Eurocentric lens that ignores the systemic barriers in our diverse society (Jamison, 2009).

Counselor Education programs have attempted to integrate the Multicultural Counseling Competencies since they were proposed by Sue & Sue in 1999 and then endorsed by the American Counseling Association (ACA) and the American Psychology Association (APA). This increased recognition is an admittance that these competencies are needed to reframe and redesign "ethnocentric monocultural counselor preparation" (Arredondo & Arciniega, 2001, p. 265). An examination of information from the United States (U.S.) Census Bureau regarding the future of demographics in the U.S. further illustrates the need for culturally responsive counselors. According to the U.S. Census Bureau's projections, "beyond the year 2030 the U.S. population is projected to grow slowly, to age considerably, and to become more racially and ethnically diverse" (2015). A 2020 Census report goes on to state that the non-Hispanic White population will shrink from 199 million in 2020 to 179 million in 2060 (Vespa et al., 2020). The Hispanic population will have a projected growth from 253 million in 2020 to 275 million in 2060. The population of people who identify two or more races is projected to have the fastest growth followed by the Asian population. The U.S.'s foreign born population is projected to rise from 44 million to 69 million by

2060 (Vespa et al., 2020). Counselor Education programs are being challenged in 2021 to think past current traditions and decolonize their programs, syllabi, and way of thinking. Counselors must be prepared to serve the continually diversifying population of the U.S.

In furtherance of the need for culturally responsive interventions, the Ratts et al. (2015) updated and endorsed the Multicultural and Social Justice competencies in order to better address the gap in counselors' cultural awareness. These competencies were originally presented by Sue & Sue in 1999. The Association for Multicultural Counseling and Development (a division of the ACA) revised the competencies to offer a better framework that informs counseling theories, practices, and research (Ratts et al., 2015). In this newly revised format, counselors are given a visual map of the relationship between constructs and competencies. The quadrants are used to illustrate the intersections of identities and dynamics of power, privilege, and oppression. The 2015 MSJCC also adds the domain of the counseling relationship to prompt counselors to be aware of how the positions of privilege and power impact the counseling relationship.

The Prioritization of Eurocentric Models in Counseling Theory Instruction

Eurocentrism is the tendency to interpret the history and cultures of non-European societies from a European or Western perspective. There are some common features of Eurocentric thought (Schiele, 1994). These generally include undervaluing non-European societies and viewing those societies as inferior. Eurocentrism commonly refers to the history and culture of other societies in European terms and erases the details of those cultures when Europe expanded and engulfed these societies. This time is often referred to in history books as the "European Expansion" that brought about "civility" to these otherwise "uncivil people" of other cultures (Bowden, 2005). Eurocentrism is not a new or modern idea. In the fifth century, Greek historian Herodotus writes of the "barbaric" hordes in Asia. Eurocentrism can be seen throughout history, but it is not constant. There are particular times that Eurocentrism is noted as more pronounced including during the age of Imperialism and Colonialism in the nineteenth and twentieth centuries (Hostettler, 2012).

There are many beliefs that lead to Eurocentric thinking, which in turn results in undervaluing or judging non-Eurocentric societies. These include the belief that non-European societies are despotic and servile which conflicts with the West's value of individualism. Non- European societies are pagan or believe in strange religions which are inferior to Christianity. Non-European societies are poor, weird, or underdeveloped, whereas European/Western societies are progressive, rich, and value industrialization (DeGruy Leary, 2005). European settlers came to America and brought with them viewpoints and ideals. As America dominated the world economy, dominance of the educational curriculum soon followed. The result of the American domination meant that universities throughout the world began to model American ideals which were based on a predominately White male experience (Alvares, 2011).

Eurocentrism is observed specifically in academia and is prioritized in research. According to the United Nations Educational Scientific Cultural Organization's (UNESCO) World Science Report (2010) social science research outside of the non-European world is considered insignificant in quality and is rarely cited. The report goes on to say that North American research cited zero research from both Asia and Africa. Students are not oblivious to the centralization of European theorists and research. In a qualitative study by Hays and colleagues (2007) wherein counselors were asked to discuss their experiences in their programs, they cited Eurocentric theories as one of the reasons they were uncomfortable and underprepared for addressing issues of privilege and oppression. The participants stated that only Eurocentric theories were taught in their programs and it was their impression that those theories were most valued by the faculty. These same participants reported that the teachings of racist psychologists were referenced in class, but little attention was paid to their oppressive views (Hays et al., 2007). Eurocentric theories have privileged White, middle/upper class, heterosexual male experiences as the basis by which others are compared. These theories use individualism, independence, and autonomy as markers of mental health and do not allow for the processes in which individuals with multiple oppressed identities can fully develop an overall sense of healing and cultural identity (Constantine, 2002; Williams, 2005). If students are aware of the burgeoning need to increase their knowledge of multicultural issues and are aware that the traditional theories have value but are Eurocentric, why then do Counselor Education programs continue to prioritize these theories and theorists?

Cultural Competencies and Demographics of Counselors in Training

Cultural competence and multicultural competence are the two terms most commonly seen in Counselor Education literature when referring to expertise in the field. Sue (1998) defined cultural competence as "the belief that people should not only appreciate and recognize other cultural groups but also be able to work effectively with them" (p. 440). Multicultural counseling competence generally refers to the counselor's views/beliefs, knowledge, and skills that relate to working with culturally diverse groups (D.W. Sue et al., 1998). For counseling to be effective it must acknowledge the cultural nuances that exist in every counseling relationship. Multicultural competence is more than basic counseling techniques (i.e., empathy, positive regard, paraphrasing) but those techniques are needed in order to fully engage the client and utilize multicultural competencies. Many counselors in training mistakenly think that the mastery of basic skills means that they can work with any client regardless of race, age, socioeconomic status, etc. Some researchers argue that counseling and multicultural counseling are two separate things when in fact they are intertwined (Goh, 2005). It can be argued that the consequence of not developing cultural competency skills is not only neglectful, but harmful.

Since the civil rights movement, there has been discourse around potentially harming clients by using theories and interventions that ignore the systemic racism that exists in America. The multicultural counseling and psychotherapy movement (MCP) has frequently highlighted the potential harm of culturally insensitive or even oppressive therapy practices for diverse individuals (APA, 2003; Wendt et al., 2014). The interventions utilized by counselors are often based on the Eurocentric theories taught in Counselor Education programs. Considering that many students and faculty in Counselor Education programs identify as

White, the emphasis on cultural competency is crucial in order to serve a population that will continue to be more diverse as time goes on. The Council for Accreditation of Counseling and Related Educational Programs (CACREP) 2017 Vital Statistics Report states that 71% of full-time faculty in Counselor Education programs are White versus 14% of faculty who identified as Black. In 2017 59% of master's students in Counselor Education programs identified as White versus 18.39% who identified as African American/Black (pg. 6). The demographics of counselor educators and counselors in training clearly demonstrate that multicultural competency is essential in order to achieve competence and expertise in the field.

Health Disparities and Mistrust

There is a plethora of research and statistics that demonstrate the health disparities that exist in the U.S. for people of color. A quick search of government health resources brings forth a list of health issues that are seen more in communities of color. There is also a gap in access to treatment for these illnesses in these same communities. The need for culturally aware education and clinical practice is supported by the health disparities affecting the African American/Black community including accessibility to proper medical and mental health care and higher rates of hypertension (U.S. Department of Health and Human Services Office of Minority Health, 2021b), diabetes, and stroke (Center for Disease Control, 2017; U.S. Department of Health and Human Services Office of Minority Health, 2021a). Unfortunately, minority communities have experienced mistreatment and misdiagnosis by mental health professionals and the medical community. Furthermore, researchers have repeatedly documented dissatisfaction with treatment and mistrust of clinicians among racial minorities (Chang & Berk, 2009; U.S. Surgeon General, 2001). MCP literature has documented racism and discrimination by individual mental health practitioners. Ridley's 2005 study referenced 132 peer-reviewed journal articles that exposed racism in the American mental health care delivery system. The racism described in these articles were experienced by Black clients who worked with non-Latino White practitioners. Racism manifested itself through overly pathologized diagnosis and the tendency to recommend shorter and less intensive interventions. It was also noted that the interventions usually suggested were of lower quality. Schizophrenia and other psychotic disorders were over diagnosed in Black clients (Metzl, 2010; Pavkov et al., 1989). A common reason given for overdiagnosis of racial minorities was that the clinicians were imposing Eurocentric standards when assessing what was "normal" and what was not (Metzl, 2010). These serious diagnoses have long lasting implications for people and their families. Not only do diagnoses follow the client for the rest of their life, but treatment plans based on misdiagnosis can lead to mental, emotional, and financial strain. White/Caucasian counselors need to be aware of the experiences and disparities in order to better understand non- White clients. Harmful practices can traumatize clients and send them further away from the counseling space. As the Covid 19 pandemic exposes these already vulnerable communities to more stress, unemployment, financial strain, and illness, more people of color will seek counseling.

Black Psychology Theory and Afrocentric Paradigms

The aforementioned Eurocentrism present in counseling education and practice has contributed to the erasure of scholarship centering the counseling needs of diverse populations. While some students may be aware of this gap in the curriculum, it could lead some helping professionals in training to believe that there are no relevant theories available to address the specific needs of communities of color, such as the Black community (Whitten, 1993). The purpose of the following discussion is to provide an overview of Afrocentric paradigms, highlighting not only their existence but also establishing the importance of integrating Black Psychology theories into our Counselor Education curriculum. A critical redevelopment of our pedagogies is especially important during this pivotal moment in history (McGoldrick & Hardy, 2008). As we re-examine the insidious impact of racism on our public policies and systems of care, thanks in large part to the Black Lives Matter movement, we must also dedicate ourselves to the removal of oppressive structures and processes that undermine equitable access to culturally responsive care and learning opportunities.

Black Psychology is defined by many scholars as a theoretical approach rooted in the knowledge of African history and principles, which acknowledges the unique struggles, achievements, and cultures of individuals of African descent (Akbar, 1999). In practical terms, it prioritizes the complexity of the Black experience and positions the examination of psychological processes to include the impact of sociopolitical, economic, and systemic factors erased or unacknowledged by the dominant culture (Jones, 1972). The composite Afrocentric philosophies represent the antithesis of the Eurocentric philosophies, as the theoretical focus shifts from individual ego drives that may inform behavior, to an analysis of the relationship between the mind, body, and spirit, along with its effect on community and the individual (Akbar, 1999).

The goal of the Black Psychology movement, beginning in the early twentieth century, was to honor the true experiences of African descendants by developing and amplifying psychological theories and practices reflective of authentic African cultural processes (Piper-Mandy & Rowe, 2010). The movement emerged in part as a response to the cultural encapsulation evident in general psychology theories (Nobles, 1986). An example of problematic European American perspectives regarding the mental states of black people in America is evident in Samuel Cartwright's assessment and assignment of mental disorders to non-compliant slaves who sought freedom or resisted the oppressive strongholds of their masters (DeGruy Leary, 2005; McGoldrick & Hardy, 2008). The pathologizing of Black trauma responses and the resilience of Black people in the face of brutal dehumanization was emboldened by racist narratives and spurred the development of additional invalid scientific assessments of Black intelligence and physical ability (McGoldrick & Hardy, 2008).

Given the racially hostile sociopolitical climate established in early American history, the necessity of an Afrocentric approach and theoretical base was clear (Jamison, 2009). The initial formulations of Black psychology focused intently on the restoration of African integrity by removing the hegemonic misperceptions presented by Eurocentric theories in favor of factual conceptualizations emanating directly from the

Black community. The development of an African centered scholarly body of work has been described by many academics within the Africana intellectual community. Much like the psychodynamic, cognitive, and behavioral theoretical constructs formalized within the European psychology tradition, Maulana Karenga (1992) has identified the traditional, reformist, and radical schools of thought present within the Black psychology paradigm.

The traditional school consists of work by several psychologists including the late Kenneth and Mamie-Phipps Clark, authors of the groundbreaking doll study which clarified the ways in which anti-black narratives are internalized by children (Jamison, 2008). Clinicians linked to the traditional school, considered some elements of the prevailing models to be relevant to the Black experience but rejected the damaging misconceptions offered by Eurocentric models. Jamison (2008) highlighted the complexities of the traditional school of thought, specifically concerning the emphasis placed on addressing the misperceptions of White psychologists and adapting existing Eurocentric frameworks. However, the contributions to society made by the Clarks, along with the issues examined by the traditionalist group of researchers, are clear (Jamison, 2008).

The reformist school of thought advanced the work of the traditionalists, by adopting a social justice and equity informed approach to research, clarifying the psychological processing and development of African descendants (Karenga, 1992). From the reformist perspective, the work endeavored represented an adaptation of Eurocentric models benefitting all people and confronting the history of racism in America (Jamison, 2008). Joseph White, considered by many to be the "father of Black psychology", championed the establishment of distinct Afrocentric frameworks (Jamison, 2014), and supported the formation of the Association of Black Psychologists in 1968. Examining the shortcomings inherent in Eurocentric philosophies and stressing the importance of countering the misconceptions of Black inferiority by developing culture specific theoretical frameworks and tools (White, 1970), are the hallmarks of the reformist school. However, critics of the reformist approach decry the continued alignment with aspects of the Eurocentric models (Jamison, 2008).

The third approach identified by Karenga, is the radical school of thought which includes the pioneering works of Nobles, Akbar, Kambon, Myers, Welsing, and Wright, among others (Jamison, 2008). The radical school scholarship focuses intently on the African worldview, as the elemental source of information necessary to accurately evaluate and conceptualize the needs of African descendants (Jamison, 2008). Under the umbrella of the radical school, are scholars whose theories are considered philosophically radical and others who subscribed to a politically radical theoretical approach (Clark et al., 1975). Nonetheless, both camps prioritized the authentic discovery of African philosophies, ideals, and ways of being that have been lost due to oppression, through a variety of proposed theoretical frameworks entirely disconnected from the European perspective (Jamison, 2008).

The body of African centered scholarship produced by many sentient practitioners has solidified the relationship between the forced divestment of African culture experienced by Black people, and the resultant presence of culturally specific psychological dysfunction. Scholars such as Joy DeGruy and Kenneth Hardy have contributed greatly to the research that has further clarified the etiology and impact of racial trauma, repudiating the persistent cognitive dissonance held by the dominant culture around the residual effects of slavery on African descendants. Their work has provided practical intervention tools accessible to helping professionals, lay organizations, and other stakeholders seeking healing and education. Yet, the vital discourse offered through the vast Afrocentric pedagogy remains unintegrated in mainstream public and academic spaces.

The philosophies produced by Black psychology theorists have created guiding principles reconnecting Black people to liberatory and uplifting narratives of blackness and African culture, promoting re-education and respect for African identities (Akbar, 1999). The therapeutic promotion of self-love, empowerment, and reprogramming through an Afrocentric lens, presents a model for black people to explore but is also informative to members of other cultural groups. It serves to dismantle centuries of anti-black racism and stereotypes while highlighting the documented evidence of African centrality in the establishment of human civilization. Myers asserts that Africa's status as the source of all humanity renders the Afrocentric approach to counseling amenable to an understanding of the human condition more broadly (Jamison, 2008). Therefore, greater empathy for African descendants and clarity regarding their strengths and needs can facilitate a deeper appreciation for members of other groups marginalized by systemic racism, White supremacy, and other forms of oppression.

Without proper inclusion into general psychology and counseling curriculum, counselors-in-training, marriage and family therapists, social workers or psychologists, and other helping professionals are limited to Eurocentric models of practice and care, despite the availability of a robust array of Afrocentric models. Counselor educators and other helping professionals are relegated to a default Eurocentric model while teaching and engaging in therapeutic or clinical work, which increases the likelihood of assuming the abnormality or deficiency that Jamison (2009) warns is inherent when treating Black people through the European worldview and theoretical framework.

Just as clinicians are currently able to acknowledge training in a preferred Eurocentric model of psychotherapy such as the cognitive behavioral or person-centered approaches, they should also have sufficient training and support to claim a preference for clinical practice through a Black psychology paradigm. Whether practitioners prefer the traditional, reformist or radical schools of thought, clinicians with access to counseling curriculum inclusive of these theories would be able to cite specific Black psychology theorists whose philosophies they use to ground their culturally responsive counseling interventions confidently. The failure to include Black Psychology in counseling curriculum, also infringes upon the ability of institutions to ensure the production of culturally responsive, antiracist practitioners with training to meet the industry standards regarding competence in this area of practice.

Relevance to Counselor Educators

Despite the reactionary nature of recent systemic, departmental, and programmatic changes in Counselor Education in the general field and across institutions stemming from the murders of George Floyd, Breonna Taylor, and other Black people, movement toward more inclusive curricula, resources, and coursework remains necessary regardless of the stimulus for these changes. It has become increasingly important for counselor educators as leaders in the counseling field to directly address culturally encapsulated frameworks and ideologies in order to promote the development of antiracist, competent counselors as well as future leaders and counselor educators.

Recommendations for an Antiracist Curriculum

To train culturally competent counselors and future counselor educators, it is simply not enough to address multiculturalism, plurality, and diversity. Curriculum in Counselor Education must dive beyond addressing diversity to focus on equity, inclusion, and antiracism. Part of this process should involve the intentional inclusion of diverse perspectives in the coursework through readings, multimedia, case studies, textbooks, guest speakers, and other resources. Coursework should engage students in critical perspectives, theories and frameworks proposed by members of minoritized groups. However, including diverse perspectives is only a piece of the work that must be done.

Solely including a diversity of perspectives is not enough. This action once again merely addresses the issue of plurality. Instead of stopping at this step, counselor educators should be active agents of change by engaging students in critical reflection both of themselves as individuals but also contextually as professionals. This means that counselor educators should include as part of their course discussions the historical context of the information disseminated as well as critical discussion of the current state of affairs of the societies we live and work in. While it is essential for counselors-in-training to be aware of and know about Black psychology and Afrocentric models of treatment in counseling and psychology, it is equally as important that students understand that knowledge is only a part of the journey. It is what they do with the knowledge, the application of knowledge, which is the most important component. It is critical for students to understand how Whiteness has functioned as a norm and to dismantle this ideology that has pervaded our society, including the field of counseling. Critical analysis and reflection of counseling theory and approaches to treatment must occur in order to support continued efforts toward a more equitable society.

Neutrality, or inaction, is a function of upholding systemic racism in our society as well as in the profession of counseling. This occurs both systemically and institutionally. For this to change, counselor educators must model antiracist thinking and behavior by actively engaging in dismantling the systems of racism and bias in the classroom, in the program, and at the organizational and professional level. Counselor Education programs would benefit from more focused efforts on discussing the relevance of White supremacy, its historical context, and how policies and practices of the profession have been influenced by this systemic ideology. Part of these efforts toward addressing White supremacy should also include developing an understanding of the lived experiences of students, clients, and colleagues. Texts such as *Why Are All Black Kids Sitting Together in the Cafeteria?* (Tatum, 2017) and *White Rage* (Anderson, 2016) are resources that faculty members could use to initiate deeper analysis of the functions of White supremacy and its impact on worldview as well as relationships with clients and peers. These texts provide cultural and historical context of White supremacy and discuss ideas such as the complexity of racial and ethnic identity including racial identity development models. Rather than providing students with the aforementioned information in diversity classes, this information should be threaded through all core curriculum in some form or fashion, with the diversity in counseling or multicultural counseling course utilized as a space for deeper, more critical reflection of oneself in relation to others. The examination of Whiteness in the counseling profession should aim to encourage the understanding of the forces of power, privilege, and oppression. Whitten (1993) emphasizes that the exposure to race and culture should enhance the quality of students' experiences by providing a new context for understanding race. Additionally, this curriculum provides a lens through which faculty can address how oppression has impacted other disenfranchised and minoritized groups such as LGBTQ+ individuals, immigrants, persons with disabilities, and individuals living at these intersections of identity.

Chapter Summary

Giving students a foundation and theoretical framework is essential for the education of counselors in training and gives students a way to understand human behavior and the intrinsic motivations behind those behaviors. However, each of the models incorporated in introductory and even advanced theory courses, present the perspectives of a predominately male group of psychiatrists and psychologists of European descent, without any mention of contributions to the field by non-White practitioners. Just as clinicians are currently able to acknowledge training in a preferred Eurocentric model of psychotherapy such as the cognitive behavioral or person- centered approaches, they should also have sufficient training and support to claim a preference for clinical practice through a Black psychology paradigm. Whether practitioners prefer the traditional, reformist or radical schools of thought, clinicians with access to counseling curriculum inclusive of these theories would be able to cite specific Black psychology theorists whose philosophies they use to ground their culturally responsive counseling interventions confidently. The failure to include Black Psychology in counseling curriculum also infringes upon the ability of institutions to ensure the production of culturally responsive, antiracist practitioners with training to meet the industry standards regarding competence in this area of practice. Counselor Education programs would benefit from more focused efforts on discussing the relevance of White supremacy, its historical context, and how policies and practices of the profession have been influenced by this systemic ideology. Part of these efforts toward addressing White supremacy should also include developing an understanding of the lived experiences of students, clients, and colleagues.

Conclusion

As helping professionals, counselor educators, and supervisors we engage in reflective practices that allow us to acknowledge our many identities and positionality, while also considering the impact of our experiences on the students we teach, the populations that we serve, and the participants of our research initiatives. It is important for culturally responsive practitioners across disciplines to understand where we lack information and education about specific cultural group experiences and why that gap in our knowledge exists. Once these deficits have been identified, it is incumbent upon us to develop plans of action in order to remediate any cultural and educational blind spots that we may have. Doing so prevents bias from entering our practices and undermining the integrity of our professional work, our industry ethical standards, and our relationships with clients.

The chapter highlights the issue of cultural encapsulation in counseling curriculum as a vehicle to stimulate further critical reflection regarding the prioritization of Eurocentric foundational counseling theories to the exclusion of Afrocentric and other multicultural frameworks. Updating our teaching curriculum and practices to address these instructional gaps requires the infusion of Black psychology and other inclusive paradigms within our educational repertoires. It is also important to note that including more culturally responsive materials may also require advocacy in the form of increased demand for access to Afrocentric educational materials and resources. At the administrative level, this entails counselor educators and helping professionals alerting university libraries and other stakeholders to the absence of Black psychology literature such as journal subscriptions and books from their databases and advocating for greater access. As we position ourselves as antiracist practitioners, supervisors, mentors, scholars, and researchers we must continue to question the influence of our educational traditions and commit to improving them in ways that reflect the diversity, humanity, and beauty of marginalized cultures and identities frequently erased from scholarly discourse and counseling practice.

Guiding Questions

1. Imagine a counseling student approaches you and shares that they do not identify with the dominant theories in counseling curriculum, because they do not center the experiences of minoritized groups and in their case specifically Black clients/individuals. How would you approach this conversation?

2. Consider materials used in your current curriculum. What are you currently using that might challenge your students to examine scholarship that exists beyond the traditional Eurocentric theoretical frameworks? What could you include in your curriculum to be more inclusive?
3. Compile a list of scholarly resources (academic journals, research databases, libraries, etc...) that allow you to deepen your exploration of Afrocentric and other multicultural theoretical paradigms of counseling.

Quiz Questions

1. Eurocentrism is defined as_______________:

    a. The tendency to interpret the history and cultures of non-European societies from an African perspective.
    b. The tendency to interpret the history and cultures of non-European societies from a European or Western perspective.
    c. The tendency to interpret the history and cultures of non-European societies from a multicultural lens infused with European or Western perspectives.
    d. Both b and c.

2. Multicultural competence requires_______________:

    a. The prioritization of one specific group as the standard for understanding the experiences of others.
    b. The recognition and appreciation of diverse cultural groups and identities.
    c. The mastery of specific knowledge related to diverse cultural group experiences.
    d. Both a and c.

3. A byproduct of applying Eurocentric counseling standards to clients of color may be the presence of_______________:

    a. misdiagnosis or pathologizing of clients of color.
    b. client reports of mistreatment and discrimination while accessing services.
    c. Both a and b.
    d. None of the above.

4. The goal of the Black Psychology Theory Movement was_______________:
   a. To honor the experiences of African descendants.
   b. To center more accurate psychological theories and reflections of the African experience.
   c. To counter the Eurocentrism evident in mainstream general psychological theories typically promoted.
   d. All of the above.
5. Theorists commonly associated with the "traditionalist school" of Black psychology theory are:
   a. Sigmund Freud
   b. Kenneth Clark and Mamie Phipps Clark
   c. Maulana Karenga
   d. Insoo Kim Berg
6. Theorists commonly associated with the "reformist school" of Black psychology theory are:
   a. Albert Ellis
   b. Fritz Perls
   c. Joseph White
   d. Kobi K.K. Kambon
7. Theorists commonly associated with the "reformist school" of Black psychology theory are:
   a. Wade Nobles
   b. Na'im Akbar
   c. Linda James Myers
   d. All of the above

References

Akbar, N. (1999). *Know thyself.* Mind Productions & Associates.

Alvares, C. (2011). Steeped in Eurocentrism. Economic and Political Weekly, 77–79.

American Psychological Association. (2003). Guidelines on multicultural education, training, research, practice, and organizational change for psychologists. *American Psychologist, 58*, 377–402. https://doi.org/10.1037/0003-066X.58.5.377

Anderson, C. E. (2016). *White rage: The unspoken truth of our racial divide*. Bloomsbury USA.

Arredondo, P., & Arciniega, G. M. (2001). Strategies and techniques for counselor training based on the multicultural counseling competencies. *Journal of Multicultural Counseling and Development, 29*(4), 263–273.

Bowden, B. (2005). The colonial origins of international law. European expansion and the classical standard of civilization. *Journal of the History of International Law/Revue d'histoire du droit international, 7*(1), 1–24. https://doi.org/10.1163/1571805054545145

Centers for Disease Control. (2017). *African American Health*. Retrieved January 3, 2020, from https://www.cdc.gov/vitalsigns/aahealth/index.html

Chang, D. F., & Berk, A. (2009). Making cross-racial therapy work: A phenomenological study of clients' experiences of cross-racial therapy. *Journal of Counseling Psychology, 56*, 521–536. https://doi.org/10.1037/a0016905

Clark (X), C., McGee, D. P., Nobles, W., & Weems (X), L. (1975). Voodoo or IX: An introduction to African psychology. *Journal of Black Psychology, 1*(2), 9–29.

Constantine, M. G. (2002). The intersection of race, ethnicity, gender, and social class in counseling: Examining selves in cultural contexts. *Journal of Multicultural Counseling and Development, 30*, 210–215.

DeGruy Leary, J. (2005). *Post-traumatic slave syndrome: America's legacy of enduring injury and healing*. Uptone Press.

Goh, M. (2005). Cultural competence and master therapists: An inextricable relationship. *Journal of Mental Health Counseling, 27*(1), 71–81. Retrieved from https://search.proquest.com/scholarly-journals/cultural-competence-master-therapists/docview/198796594/se-2?accountid=8361

Hays, G. D., Dean, J. K., & Chang, C. Y. (2007). Addressing privilege and oppression in counselor training and practice: A qualitative analysis. *Journal of Counseling and Development, 85*, 317–324. https://doi.org/10.1002/j.1556-6678.2007.tb00480.x

Hostettler, N. (2012). *Eurocentrism: A Marxian critical realist critique*. Routledge.

Jamison, D. (2008). Through the prism of Black Psychology: A critical review of conceptual and methodological issues in Africology as seen through the paradigmatic lens of Black Psychology. *The Journal of Pan African Studies, 2*(2), 96–117.

Jamison, D. (2009). Returning to the source: An archeology and critical analysis of the intellectual foundations of contemporary Black psychology. *Journal of African American Studies, 13*, 348–360. https://doi.org/10.1007/s12111-009-9092-7

Jamison, D. (2014). Daudi Azibo: Defining and developing Africana psychological theory, research and practice. *The Journal of Pan African Studies, 7*(5), 2+.

Jones, R. (Ed.). (1972). *Black psychology*. Harper & Row.

Karenga, M. (1992). *Introduction to black studies*. University of Sankore.

McGoldrick, M. & Hardy, K. (Eds.). (2008). Re-visioning family therapy: Race, culture, and gender in clinical practice. The Guilford Press

Metzl, J. M. (2010). *The protest psychosis: How schizophrenia became a Black disease*. Beacon Press.

Nobles, W. (1986). Bibliographic essay: African (Black) psychology: Transformed and transforming. *Sage Race Relations Abstracts, 11*(1).

Pavkov, T. W., Lewis, D. A., & Lyons, J. S. (1989). Psychiatric diagnosis and racial bias: An empirical investigation. *Professional Psychology: Research and Practice, 20*, 364–368. https://doi.org/10.1037/0735-7028.20.6.364

Piper-Mandy, E., & Rowe, T. D. (2010). Educating African-centered psychologists: Towards a comprehensive paradigm. *Journal of Pan African Studies, 3*(8), 5+. https://link.gale.com/apps/doc/A306596720/LitRC?u=faye28748&sid=LitRC&xid=4b7f999a

Ratts, M. J., Singh, A. A., Nassar-McMillan, S., Butler, S. K., & McCullough, J. R. (2015, June 29). *Multicultural and Social Justice Counseling Competencies Revisions*. Counseling.Org. Retrieved May 3, 2020, from https://www.counseling.org/docs/default-source/competencies/multicultural-and-social-justice-counseling-competencies.pdf?sfvrsn=20

Schiele, J. H. (1994). Afrocentricity: Implications for higher education. *Journal of Black Studies, 25*(2), 150–169. https://doi.org/10.1177/002193479402500202

Sommers-Flanagan, J., & Sommers-Flanagan, R. (2004). *Counseling and psychotherapy theories in context and practice: Skills, strategies, and techniques*. Wiley.

Sue, D. W., Carter, R. T., Casas, J. M., Fouad, N. A., Ivey, A. E., & Jensen, M. (1998). *Multicultural counseling competencies: Individual and organizational development*. Sage.

Sue, S. (1998). In search of cultural competence in psychotherapy and counseling. *American Psychologist, 53*, 440–448.

Tatum, B. D. (2017). *Why are all the black kids sitting together in the cafeteria? And other conversations about race*. Basic Books.

U.S. Census Bureau. (2015). *Projections of the size and composition of the U.S. population: 2014–2060.* https://www.census.gov/content/dam/Census/library/publications/2015/demo/p25-1143.pdf
U.S. Department of Health and Human Services Office of Minority Health. (2021a). *Health Diabetes and African Americans.* Retrieved January 3, 2021, from https://www.minorityhealth.hhs.gov/omh/browse.aspx?lvl=4&lvlid=18
U.S. Department of Health and Human Services Office of Minority Health. (2021b). *Heart Disease and African Americans.* Retrieved January 3, 2021, from https://www.minorityhealth.hhs.gov/omh/browse.aspx?lvl=4&lvlid=19
U.S. Surgeon General. (2001). *Mental health: Culture, race, and ethnicity. A supplement to mental health—A report of the surgeon general.* U.S. Department of Health and Human Services. https://pubmed.ncbi.nlm.nih.gov/20669516/
United Nations Educational Scientific and Cultural Organization. (2010) *World social science report 2010; Knowledge divides.* https://unesdoc.unesco.org/ark:/48223/pf0000188395?posInSet=3&queryId=d62d2256-9176-4b9e-be00-34e0389888e0
Vespa, J., Medina, L., & Armstrong, D. M. (2020, February). Demographic Turning Points for the United States: Population Projections for 2020 to 2060 (No. P25-1144). https://www.census.gov/content/dam/Census/library/publications/2020/demo/p25-1144.pdf
Wendt, D. C., Gone, J. P., & Nagata, D. K. (2014). Potentially harmful therapy and multicultural counseling: Bridging two disciplinary discourses. *The Counseling Psychologist, 1*(25). Sage Publications.
White, J. (1970). Guidelines for Black psychologists. *The Black Scholar, 1*(5), 52–57. https://doi.org/10.1080/00064246.1970.11644160
Whitten, L. A. (1993). Infusing black psychology into the introductory psychology course. *Teaching of Psychology, 20*(1), 13–21. https://doi.org/10.1207/s15328023top2001_3
Williams, C. B. (2005). Counseling African American women: Multiple identities-multiple constraints. *Journal of Counseling and Development, 83*, 278–282.

4

Antilinguicist Schools, Antilinguicist Systems

Joanna Meadvin, Adriana Díaz, Guadalupe Díaz, Anya Hurwitz, Martha I. Martinez, Corina Sapien, and Cory Weschler

Introduction

Sobrato Early Academic Language (SEAL) was founded in 2008 in California to improve educational outcomes for Dual Language Learners / English Learners (DLLs/ELs). SEAL is a research-based systems change model grounded in teachers' professional development and focused on preschool through 6th grade. The model coalesces around four pillars: academic language, the creation of rich and affirming environments, alignment of the preschool and elementary systems and articulation across grades, and partnerships between families and schools. The intention is to demonstrate what teaching and learning can look like when the needs of DLLs/ELs are centralized and addressed at every level from

J. Meadvin (✉) • A. Díaz • G. Díaz • A. Hurwitz • M. I. Martinez • C. Sapien • C. Weschler
Sobrato Early Academic Language, Oakland, CA, USA
e-mail: joanna@seal.org; Adriana@seal.org; gdiaz-lara@fullerton.edu; Anya@seal.org; Martha@seal.org; Corina@seal.org; Cory@seal.org

© The Author(s), under exclusive license to Springer Nature Switzerland AG 2022

K. Johnson et al. (eds.), *Developing Anti-Racist Practices in the Helping Professions: Inclusive Theory, Pedagogy, and Application*,
https://doi.org/10.1007/978-3-030-95451-2_4

classroom practice to state policy. Core to SEAL's mission—to prepare all English Learners in the state of California to learn, thrive and lead—is the conviction that children's home languages are an enormous asset.

Carrying out this mission means acknowledging that while schools are key to social change, they are also primary reproducers of racism, inequity, and language loss. California has a particularly pernicious history of linguistic discrimination. In 1998, Proposition 227, the culmination of years of anti-immigrant and anti-Latinx sentiment, effectively made bilingual education illegal in the state. In 2016, Proposition 58 repealed the restrictions of 227, but almost twenty years of English-only policy have taken a toll that has surely contributed to the conditions confronting English Learners in California. Among these longstanding challenges are inequitable access to appropriately trained teachers, inequitable access to appropriate assessment, inadequate instructional time, inequitable access to instructional materials and curriculum, and extensive segregation into schools that place them at high risk for education failure (Gándara et al., 2003). Perhaps, the most damaging legacy is a school system that continuously fails to recognize home language as an asset. Not only are many DLLs/ELs not given the opportunity to fully develop academic language in English, but in English-only school environments, many of them also lose their home language. These conditions result in major inequities. As a whole, DLLs/ELs are twice as likely to drop out of high school as their native English-speaking peers (Callahan, 2005).

California's DLLs/ELs, 80% of whom are Spanish speakers, are subject to linguicism, a set of ideologies, structures and practices that are used to legitimate and reproduce inequities between groups on the basis of language.[1] Linguicism is not merely the linguistic equivalent of racism, but rather, linguicism both grows out of racist ideologies and is also reinforced by them. In other words, California's DLLs/ELs suffer inadequate access to power and resources on the basis of language because damaging "English Only" rhetoric and policies are simultaneously the result of and provide cover for racist beliefs. The effects of linguicism are further

[1] While the overwhelming majority of California's DLLs/ELs have a home language of Spanish, over 70 different language groups are represented in the school-age population (California Department of Education, 2020a).

amplified by racism, when, for example, a teacher sees her Brown students from Mexico as entering the classroom with "no language."

Ibram X. Kendi (2019) argues that it is not enough to simply be passively "not racist," rather, we must actively work to dismantle racist ideology, systems, policies and practices; we must be antiracist. In this vein, SEAL is not committed merely to improving outcomes for DLLs/ELs, but rather to being an antilinguicist organization, dedicated to creating antilinguicist schools in antilinguicist school systems. We are unique in that our well-elaborated professional development model and our 12 years of experience on the ground in schools enable us to be a powerful antilinguicist presence at the levels of both practice and policy.[2] SEAL schools serve as proof of practice for antilinguicist pedagogy at the same time that SEAL as an organization fosters antilinguicist state and local policies. SEAL works simultaneously at the levels of ideology, systems, policies and practices.

This chapter will first discuss why language is central to the SEAL model. It will then discuss the definition of linguicism and elaborate what is meant by "antilinguicist" practice. Next, the chapter will elaborate SEAL's antilinguicist work in its Elementary and Preschool models, as well as work with administrators, and policy efforts. The chapter will conclude by sketching next steps along with SEAL's vision for the future.

Why Language?

SEAL was born out of (and into) a political context that dictated which educational policies and practices were permissible for students learning English. The modern history of bilingual education in the state of California can be traced back to *Lau v. Nichols (1974)* in which the United States Supreme Court ruled that students, primarily Chinese-speakers, were being denied access to equal educational opportunity because they lacked the English skills to understand and participate in educational programs (Hurwitz & Olsen, 2018). In the decades since, EL education has been required nationally by all K-12 systems, including

[2] To date we have reached 50,000 students and trained 1600 teachers.

those in California. However, in order to understand and operate in a post-Lau California (and understand the trajectory that multilingual education has taken in the state), SEAL operates with the longer historical understanding that as a nation of immigrants, language in the United States has always been related to power, social control, and race. Historically there have been vast differences in how certain ethnicities have been treated with regards to language (Wiley & Wright, 2004). Language was used to systematically oppress and disempower both native populations and Africans brought as slaves. Meanwhile, multilingualism was tolerated and even promoted in certain communities of European descent. Wiley and Wright (2004) suggest that during World War I, nativist sentiments became mainstream and English as a key tool of assimilation became more widely promoted within communities of European descent.

California has a long history of linguicism tied to racism. Indeed, a key legal precedent that preceded the *Brown v. Board of Education* decision was *Westminster v. Mendez* (1947), a federal case designed to address segregated (language-based) Mexican remedial schools in Orange County, California. When the *Lau* case created the legal basis for bilingual education in California (Olsen, 2009), the Office of Civil Rights then drafted the Lau Remedies which essentially mandated bilingual education for ELs, but this was met with considerable backlash and was never formalized into law (Wiley & Wright, 2004). Still, California passed legislation supporting bilingual education. This led to yet more backlash: in 1998, the passage of Proposition 227 virtually eliminated bilingual education and led to two decades of English-only policies.

Several scholars (Flores & Murillo, 2001; Johnson & Martinez, 2000) have linked the passage of this proposition to anti-immigrant, anti-Mexican public sentiment in California. Johnson and Martinez (2000) have argued that the wording of Proposition 227, known as "English for the Children," used language as a proxy for national origin, and specifically discriminated against people of Mexican ancestry. They further argue that given the proposition's frequent mention of the word "immigrant," in a state in which the vast majority of immigrants are from Mexico and Latin America, there is "little doubt that a motivating factor behind its passage was to attack educational opportunities for

Spanish-speaking Latinas/os, especially Mexican immigrants" (p. 1252). Given California's history of anti-Mexican racism (which continues to show itself in massive underfunding of schools that serve Mexican immigrant and Mexican American students) it is clear that White backlash against increased immigration from Latin America throughout the latter part of the 20th century contributed to anti-immigrant propositions—among them, Proposition 227—that passed in the 1990s. In 2008, when SEAL was founded, Proposition 227 was still in effect. When Proposition 58 passed in 2016, the English-only requirements of 227 were repealed, opening up new horizons for English Learner and bilingual education. However, two decades of English-only education have taken a toll, not only on California's teaching force, but also on a generation of ELs who were denied access to both best practices in the teaching of English and full literacy in their home language.

What Does It Mean to Be Antilinguicist?

Tove Sknutnabb-Kangas (2015) defines linguicism as, "ideologies, structures, and practices which are used to legitimate, effectuate, regulate and reproduce an unequal division of power and resources (both material and immaterial) between groups which are defined on the basis of language" (p. 310). Similar to Ibram X. Kendi's definition of racism, key to the definition of linguicism is an acknowledgment that social inequities are the product of unequal and discriminatory distribution of power and resources. And while linguicism is clearly linked to and intertwined with racism, it also exists in its own right as an explicit ideology and set of structures and policies that have real, material effects on the lives of millions of children across the United States.

SEAL's antilinguicist work exists on a spectrum. ELs have been grossly underserved in California schools for many years. They have been taught in deficit-based environments (Pettit, 2011), are concentrated in under-resourced schools (Gándara et al., 2003), and, despite legal requirements to the contrary, are frequently denied access to grade-level content and effective English language development (Olsen, 2010; Santibañez & Umanksy, 2018). SEAL addresses some of these inequities by prioritizing the needs of DLLs/ELs through sound research-based pedagogy. SEAL has always advocated for bilingual education in a school system in which home language, and its multiple attendant cognitive, cultural, and economic benefits, are often ignored and denied. Further, from its inception, SEAL has promoted culturally and linguistically responsive education grounded in assets-based pedagogy. All of these core practices are antilinguicist, but they are also aimed at elevating the needs of DLLs/ELs within existing systems. As an organization, our understanding of the entanglement of race, power, and language has deepened, and we have begun to infuse critical consciousness among educators, particularly bilingual educators (Alfaro & Bartolomé, 2017; Cervantes-Soon et al., 2017), into our practice and policy. This means that in addition to researching, enacting, and advocating for best- practices for multilingual education and effective systems change, we have begun to explore—at the levels of classroom practice, school administration, local and state policy—the intersections of language, race, and power. This includes explicitly addressing with students, teachers, administrators, and policy makers the legacies of institutional racism and language as sites of conflict.

Teacher Practice

SEAL began as a PK-3rd grade systems change model, simultaneously training all teachers in specified grade spans (PK/TK[3]-1, 2-3) at partner schools. However, because the preschool system largely functions separately from the elementary school system, and because the needs of preschool children are unique, in the past 5 years, as will be discussed below, SEAL has refined and elaborated its preschool specific practices. Additionally, in response to our elementary school partners' requests that their entire teaching staff (TK-6) be SEAL-trained, as well as our concern over the persistent issue of Long-Term English Learners, we have

[3]TK stands for Transitional Kindergarten, which is the first year of a two-year kindergarten program that uses a modified kindergarten curriculum. California's TK program was established in 2010 (California Department of Education, 2020b). In a few of our partner school districts, preschool (PK) and TK classes are offered; however, all school districts that offer kindergarten, must also offer a TK program.

expanded our elementary school offerings to include a 4-6th grade component.[4]

Elementary School

Elementary school teachers receive six days of training during the school year for two years, participate in grade-level planning days, can choose to participate in a summer intensive teaching experience, and are supported by a SEAL-trained coach facilitator.[5] In conjunction with teacher training, SEAL works with school and district leaders to address instructional delivery, curriculum planning, and systems alignment.[6] Teachers, administrators, and coaches all receive training on creating a school culture in which school and home contexts are integrated, and family partnership is nurtured. This level of intensive involvement allows SEAL to participate in the shift of school culture towards assets-based pedagogy grounded in best practices for DLLs/ELs, and antiracist and antilinguicist practices.

Underlying our professional development model is a commitment to shifting teacher practice towards putting the academic needs of English Learners first, thinking about every minute of the day as an opportunity to develop student language, and seeing DLLs/ELs as wholly competent and deserving of high quality, rigorous and rich instruction. Research shows that teacher beliefs about DLLs/ELs in general, and second language acquisition in particular, influence both teaching practices and also teachers' expectations about students' academic potential (National Academies, 2017). In addition to explicit and intensive professional development on high-leverage instructional strategies for DLLs/ELs, this work includes training teachers to use the tools of Anti-Bias education (Derman-Sparks & Olsen Edwards, 2010) and the Teaching Tolerance

[4] A Long-Term English Learner is a student who has been enrolled in school in the United States for more than six years and has not attained sufficient proficiency in English to be reclassified. These students incur major academic deficiencies.

[5] This is what the model looked like pre-pandemic. We have shifted to virtual trainings for the time-being and are building out our infrastructure to permanently deliver our model through blended methods.

[6] For an in-depth description of the SEAL model, including foundations, pillars and practices, see our publications: Preschool, TK-3, 4-6.

Social Justice Standards. We have trained over 1,600 teachers, who have been at various points of engagement with and understanding of linguicism and racism. Some of the teachers we work with are just beginning to dismantle negative implicit beliefs about the academic capabilities of students who speak a language other than English at home. Others are ready to do deep work with students around the politics of race and language through community meetings and social action projects. Beginning in the youngest grades, in the context of a training module titled, "World in the Classroom," teachers are given strategies to dismantle "colorblind" ideologies by speaking frankly with students about issues of race, gender, sexuality, family structure, language, religion and ability. This work includes using rubrics developed by SEAL to critically analyze classroom materials in order to be certain that the worlds of all students are reflected, welcomed, and celebrated. Other rubrics help teachers analyze who speaks within their classrooms to ensure equity of participation which is critical for ELLs/DLs.

Support for home language is a key, constantly evolving, component of the model. While research shows that access to home language helps students' English language development, for SEAL, full access to and development of the home language is a human right. Not only does multilingualism provide cognitive and economic benefits, but it also powerfully connects children to their families and cultures (Arriagada, 2005; Oh & Fuligni, 2009). Our research, as well as numerous studies in the field, have proven time and time again that bilingual education provides students with the best outcomes (in both English and home language) (National Academies, 2017). However, bilingual education is currently not possible for every DLL/EL given systemic capacity. Thus, SEAL trains teachers in both bilingual and Structured English Immersion classrooms in a variety of strategies that support home language.[7] These strategies include Pathway to Biliteracy displays and activities, home language interviews, student language biographies and poems, language portfolios, multilingual resources, community language studies, multilingual team

[7] Structured English Immersion is a classroom setting for English learners in which nearly all classroom instruction is provided in English but with a curriculum and presentation designed for pupils who are learning English.

names and chants, home-school connections, and multilingual celebrations. Students across grade levels are encouraged to set their sights on earning the California Seal of Biliteracy.[8] Teachers are also provided with training on key issues of language transfer between English and students' home languages. Increasingly, and especially for older students, teachers are equipped with strategies to talk with students about the connections between language and power, analyzing why and how language is deployed in their school, their community, and in the larger world.

Our work with bilingual teachers goes further. During convenings designed specifically to meet the needs of bilingual teachers, SEAL takes up the spirit of two questions posed by García (2020): "How can I teach the English language as a site of conflict and a result of colonialism and global capitalism, rather than the solution" and "How can I teach the difficult history of Spanish language imperialism and the effects it has had in Latin America, as well as those who have crossed the line into the imperial North?" These conversations help teachers move from the important work of best practices for language learning into critical consciousness and reflective practice. To this end, participants write bilingual autobiographies, and reflect on the connection between their personal relationship with language and their persona in the classroom. Texts and videos are used to launch discussions about the power of English in their own schools and classrooms. Teachers make specific plans for how they will make space for Spanish and other languages in their classrooms. These activities help teachers attend to issues of language and power in their school, as well as form networks of support.[9] SEAL has also begun to offer a series of webinars about California's history of bilingual education and EL policy as a means of helping teachers and administrators best support students and families to advocate for their linguistic and educational rights.

---

[8] In 2012, California became the first state in the nation to establish a Seal of Biliteracy award to students who have attained proficiency in two or more languages at high school graduation.

[9] Because of their greater baseline awareness of issues related to language and power, bilingual teachers tend to be excited about this work. However, while this work is perhaps even more crucial for Structured English Immersion (SEI) classrooms (where the vast majority of our DLLs/ELs are educated), that population of teachers tends to be a bit more resistant—or at least in greater need of background information and education. SEAL is in the process of building out these kinds of trainings for teachers of classrooms that are officially English Only.

Increasingly, in addition to addressing attitude and practice, SEAL provides elementary school teachers with curriculum content as a means of helping to ensure that the curriculum delivered to students is culturally responsive/sustaining, and to supplement state curriculum standards that implicitly promote both white supremacy and English dominance. One example of this was a set of resources created for the opening of the 2020–21 school year to help partner educators respond to the emergency created by the pandemic. These "Back to School Toolkits" were fully elaborated mini-units for TK through sixth grade designed to establish antiracist, antilinguicist (virtual) classroom communities, and help students and teachers process trauma and grief related not only to the pandemic but also to the epidemic of police violence and the outpouring of public protest. Focused on the theme of community, the units expose students to a range of age-appropriate concepts from intersectional identity to community-based action. Students explore topics such as segregation, privilege, racism, hunger, the effects of the pandemic, protest, and student activism through video, art, story, and writing.

A growing aspect of SEAL's antilinguicist approach is family-school partnerships. Family-school partnerships benefit all children; however, they are especially crucial for DLLs/ELs because school language and cultural environments often differ vastly from that of their home. SEAL teachers seek to understand the cultures and communities of their students and out of this understanding, create an environment that fosters connection and integration. This means, at minimum, knowing which languages are spoken by students in the classroom (this is accomplished through home language surveys) and sending home material in all languages. Additionally, teachers create multilingual letters sharing the unit's theme, share weekly communication, create "bridging school to family projects" and "home-school connections" that invite families to work with their students on small, meaningful projects connected to the unit's theme in their home language. Families are also invited to Gallery Walks, which are end of unit celebrations in which students serve as docents and guide their families on a tour of their learning in the language of their choice. Teachers and coaches run special topic and strategy workshops in which families are invited to learn various SEAL strategies (which they can practice at home) or come together and discuss topics such as raising bilingual children.

Family partnership strategies have always been central to SEAL; however, as the model grows and changes, we have begun to provide our school partners with strategies grounded in social justice practices that critique systemic inequity, address trauma, and craft counter narratives that can help students and families thrive. This includes helping teachers and administrators acknowledge the fear that students and families may feel about increased anti- immigrant rhetoric, and the burden borne by families of color due to the race and poverty-based effects of the global pandemic. SEAL teachers set student-centered goals in collaboration with families and conduct family interviews. Many teachers have been trained to create and share *testimonios* with students and families, guide students to write their own *testimonios* in class and run workshops in which caregivers create *testimonios* to share with their children.[10] These activities are designed not only to build safe and inclusive classrooms, but also to encourage students to see themselves, their families, their communities and their languages, as sources of wisdom and knowledge. In the context of distance learning, teachers are creating Family Cohorts—small groups of families initially convened by teachers or staff to, for example, discuss their children's learning, or discuss multilingual strategies and the benefits of bilingualism and biliteracy. Once these groups are established, they can be an ongoing way for families who have been isolated by economic stress, social distancing and racial injustice to connect and share assets.

Preschool

Because the preschool years are a sensitive period for language development, adequate training for teachers is crucial. These early years both set the foundation for lifelong health and success and are also the years in which children enter the school system and home language loss usually

[10] "There are various definitions for "Testimonio," a research methodology developed in Latin America, including a witness or first-person account created by someone who has faced instances of oppression or marginalization (Passos DeNicola et al., 2015).

begins (Durán et al., 2010; Fillmore, 1991). Attending high quality preschools has shown to have positive impacts on academic, cognitive, socio-emotional and language development, with DLLs benefiting as much or more than their non-DLLs counterparts (Yoshikawa et al., 2013). Additionally, research indicates that preschool programs that integrate intentional language instruction in both the home language and English, or implement dual language education, promote bilingualism and achievement in both languages and prevent language loss (Barnett et al., 2007; Durán et al., 2010; Yoshikawa et al., 2013).

Despite the vital importance of these years, preschool teachers on the whole receive less training, especially training that focuses on supporting DLLs. They also receive less prep time, and far lower salaries than their K-12 counterparts. This is predictable in a racist and sexist society that devalues the work of educating our youngest children. A larger proportion of California preschool teachers are multilingual women of color than their elementary counterparts (Austin et al., 2019), and the preschool teaching force, largely made up of women who are a huge linguistic and cultural resource for California's children, is undervalued and underserved. High quality professional development focused on the language needs of DLLs is both antiracist and antilinguicist in that it channels resources towards the goal of creating racial and linguistic equity for both teachers and students. Because many of the preschool teachers we work with are Spanish dominant, SEAL has begun to create materials in Spanish. This shift enacts our commitment to linguistic equity in the training space. Rather than simply speaking (in English) about the importance of home language, SEAL's Spanish preschool trainings offer teachers the opportunity to learn in Spanish. Teachers respond quite powerfully to this practice, which is an important antidote to linguicism that demands that even training spaces dedicated to multilingualism conduct their business in English.

Just as the foundation of the TK-6 model is high-leverage, research-based pedagogical strategies designed for DLLs/ELs, the preschool model is anchored in research-based developmentally appropriate strategies for DLLs. SEAL trains preschool teachers to ground learning in intellectually engaging content that gives children access to rich, deep learning experiences that build a foundation for their academic trajectory. This includes modeling precise vocabulary to talk about curriculum content and emotions. Learning centers, think-pair-share and other strategies provide students with the opportunity to practice oral language. Structured read alouds, chants, songs, and libraries that include rich literature in the home language and English provide students opportunities to engage with both languages orally and in text. Dramatic play and hands-on activities encourage children to learn through play. Unique to the preschool model are Persona Dolls.[11] These dolls are not playthings, rather they are members of the class with fully fleshed out identities who, through interactive storytelling, help children be empathetic and explore differences. They also can be used to reduce classroom conflict and make space to deal with the effects of trauma, separation and loss. Preschool teachers use Persona Dolls for age- appropriate exploration of topics such as race, class, gender, socioeconomic status, family structure, language and nationality. A persona doll might, for example, express fear that their family will be deported, pride over their growing ability to speak two languages, or passion about attending a Black Lives Matter protest with their mother.

Perhaps most importantly, at the preschool level, teachers partner with families as a means of assuring that thematic, language-rich units are relevant to children's lives. Teachers and staff conduct "Language & Interests" interviews in order to best celebrate each child's language and culture in the classroom. Each month, a different language is highlighted. "Language Presence in the Classroom" planning templates help teachers ensure that all student languages are represented in the classroom with books, songs and chants, key words and phrases, numbers and colors. Students and family members who speak these languages, not teachers, are the experts. This means that children's language knowledge is an explicit resource in the classroom and family members are invited to read books, sing songs, or make presentations in their language. This is important on two levels. One, it is unlikely that California preschool teachers will know all of the

[11] Persona Dolls were created by the Pacific Oaks Anti-Bias Curriculum early childhood education project. This anti-bias curriculum has grown into an international movement—teachers in South Africa, for example, used persona dolls to help young children talk about race in the aftermath of apartheid. The dolls themselves are modeled after real children, and as such have a variety of skin colors, hair types and facial features that reflect a large variety of ethnicities.

languages spoken by children in their classes. In some of SEAL's partner school districts, over 65 languages are spoken by children. Although there is less linguistic diversity at the individual classroom level, serving more than five language groups in a single classroom isn't uncommon (Hurwitz & Olsen, 2018). In this context, families are a particularly invaluable resource for expertise on their own children's languages. Further, this practice encourages children to see family knowledge as valid, expansive and equal to that of the teacher. This sets them on the path to value their own language and culture. As with the elementary school model, teachers and staff also convene family cohorts who come together to build connection and support, gain a deeper understanding of the strategies and techniques teachers are implementing to aid in their children's growth and development, as well as develop their capacity to lead in community spaces. The goal is that families increasingly take ownership of the group's time, process, and agenda.

Administrator Practice

As mentioned above, in tandem with teacher training, administrators receive their own training cycles, largely focused on creating equity for DLLs/ELs. At the beginning of their SEAL journey, administrators are asked to assess where their schools stand in terms of understanding and acting upon research-based best practices for DLLs/ELs. They are also asked to assess their own understanding of the historical context and policies that have contributed to schooling that fails ELs/DLLs. For administrative purposes, chief among these goals is alignment and articulation within and across systems. In other words, administrators are tasked with assuring that students have a consistent, well-articulated and comprehensive educational experience. Administrators are supported to achieve this goal through leadership convenings, instructional rounds (reflection on SEAL implementation in the classroom with the support of SEAL staff), check-ins, bilingual program design meetings, attendance at teacher training modules, pre- and post-module communication, technical assistance and family-school partnership modules.

During convenings, administrators delve into research on best practices for DLLs/ELs, reflect on SEAL implementation in their school, and explore historical and current state and national policy implications. Perhaps more importantly, as this work is being done, administrators become part of a network of peer SEAL education leaders. This means that through training, in addition to becoming experts in SEAL implementation, administrators develop an understanding of larger educational and political contexts, and SEAL's impact as a practice-based model that affects the field at large. For example, SEAL staff have guided administrators to plan for strategic leveraging of the opportunities presented by state policy and accountability guidelines. Principals were asked to reflect upon how they might make use of the state's request for "non-academic" indicators and "whole-child outcomes," as a means of reassessing school values and shifting teacher practice—and all-important student assessment—towards non-traditional measures. These measures might include family and language pride, curiosity, collaboration, joy in diversity, caring and human connectedness, or the ability to act with others or alone against prejudice and discrimination. As will be discussed below, SEAL has also worked extensively with administrators to enact California's English Learner Roadmap policy. As these changes come to fruition, SEAL gathers data on student impact and disseminates this data to the field. Administrators then use these data to become powerful advocates for the implementation of state policy that centers the experiences and needs of DLLs/ELs. In other words, the SEAL network actively seeks to interpret and implement state policy for antiracist and antilinguicist systems and practices, and then use the results of that implementation to advocate for further antiracist and antilinguicist policies.

SEAL also offers schools bilingual program support and consultation. Leading up to (and since) the passage of Proposition 58 in 2016, there has been a surge of interest in bilingual programing, with particular force from middle- and upper-class families interested in the benefits of bilingualism for their children. Given that bilingual programing provides the best outcomes for ELs, SEAL welcomes this growing interest, while acknowledging the potential for inequitable implementation of new programs. A growing body of literature (Cervantes-Soon et al., 2017; Morales & Rao, 2015; Palmer, 2009; Valdés, 1997) has highlighted how the inclusion of English dominant students in two-way bilingual programs can create inequities for ELs and other linguistically minoritized students when there is not a strong commitment to prioritizing their needs. The SEAL bilingual consulting team guides schools to create and expand effective research-based bilingual programs (sometimes these are referred to as dual language programs) that centralize ELs. This includes needs assessment, partnership in the creation of action plans, and school board and community presentations, guidance with steering committees and workgroups, and a cache of resources on bilingual programs.

Because bilingual programming was largely absent for a generation, California also faces a severe shortage of bilingual teachers. SEAL supported a partnership of 10 districts that collaboratively applied for and won a grant from the California Department of Education to increase the number of teachers who attain bilingual certification. SEAL's Bilingual Teacher Professional Development Program (BTPDP) has increased the number of authorized bilingual teachers in consortium districts, placed these teachers in bilingual settings, and provided these new bilingual teachers with high-quality professional development focused on the needs of English Learners. Participating teachers receive training in academic Spanish, free university- level course work, test preparation, waived bilingual authorization fees, and mentoring and coaching. The BTPDP has helped nudge, financially assist, and mentor teachers who speak Spanish to obtain their bilingual authorization and to move them into bilingual classrooms. Many of these teachers are native-Spanish speakers who might not have obtained their bilingual authorization without the resources provided by the grant project. This not only helps to create the next generation of diverse and effective bilingual teachers, but it also provides students with all important role-models that are representative of a diverse student population.

Policy

Because linguicism, like racism, exists at every level, from the smallest interaction between a student and teacher, to state and federal policies, SEAL uses lessons learned through practice and research to advocate for local and state policy change. Thus, SEAL responds to state policy, turning it into effective practice, and then partners with advocacy organizations across the state as a means of influencing the creation of equity-minded policies. This work is strengthened through strategic partnership with other non-profit organizations such as EdTrust West, Early Edge, Californians Together, California Association for Bilingual Education and Advancement Project California. This consortium of organizations has advocated for antilinguicist policies in open letters to then President Elect Biden, the State Superintendent, legislators, the California Department of Education, and the California State Board of Education. It has also attended meetings with Governor Newsom's staff, given testimony at State Board of Education meetings, and put forth numerous other advocacy efforts. SEAL's founder, Dr. Laurie Olsen, chaired the committee that created California's English Learner Roadmap, which was adopted as State policy in 2017. The EL Roadmap is fully aligned with SEAL's mission, vision and research base. It represents a huge policy shift, transitioning California's official stance towards English Learners to one that is equity and assets based. Further, the California Department of Education now uses SEAL resources as an illustrative example of implementation of the EL Roadmap.

While SEAL does work at the state level, much of the organization's focus is actually on local policy. SEAL works with district and school leaders who both implement regional, state and national policies and also create local policy in their sites and across their districts. SEAL helps these leaders understand that past patterns of practices, such as English only and deficit approaches, tracking, scattered and disconnected interventions, have led to the creation of a generation of Long-Term English Learners. SEAL helps leaders prioritize and centralize the needs of DLLs/ELs, by calling on them to critically examine funding allocation practices and enact research on best practices such as home language development and benefits of bilingualism/biliteracy. SEAL's stance is that DLLs/ELs deserve joyful, engaging, language rich learning across the day, with intentional planning spent in all aspects of their learning. Leaders are asked to build systems and policies that support this equity-minded comprehensive approach. SEAL also coordinates districts to do work connected to the larger policy context.

Where Do We Go from Here?

All helping professionals and helping institutions must grapple with their own positionality with regards to linguicism. While many of us have taken up Dr. Kendi's exhortation to actively work to dismantle racist ideology, systems, policies and practices, our own linguicism often goes unrecognized. As noted above, linguicism is not merely the linguistic equivalent of racism, but rather, linguicism both grows out of racist ideologies and is also reinforced by them. Thus, as helping professionals work to dismantle racism, we must also turn our attention to ideologies, structures and practices that are used to legitimate and reproduce inequities between groups on the basis of language. While SEAL is actively engaged in dismantling linguicism within school systems, all helping professionals benefit from recognizing that all ways of speaking, inclusive of standard and non-standard dialects of English, are worthy of respect, affirmation and celebration.

At SEAL, our understanding of our role in working towards transformative, antilinguicist schools continues to grow and deepen. As noted above, our work exists on a spectrum. On one end, we centralize the needs of DLLs/ELs in a system that has historically failed them. This is an approach that seeks to advance the interests of DLLs/ELs within the system *as it currently exists*; our goal is for students to have command of the academic English and Spanish (or other home languages) that will allow them to succeed and thrive. It is a realistic, incremental approach that, our research shows, improves outcomes for the children that we serve. However, it is also true, as García (2020) argues, that the very concept of a standard language that everyone must conform to erases the richness and variety of languages that students speak. As an organization, we know that the concept of standard language has historically been used as a disciplinary tool (McWhorter, 2001). Moving away from the concept of standard language certainly represents a more radical approach. We have begun to expand work that helps teachers and students to become critical interlocutors of language and the systems of power within which it is embedded. This work is challenging and ongoing.

We also know that although fighting linguicism is our mission, we cannot focus on linguicism without also confronting the amplifying effects that racism has on linguicism. It is an oversimplification to describe the population that we focus on as DLLs/ELs: they are also children of color, subject to the life-denying effects of racism. This means that we must be committed not only to antilinguicist schools, but also to explicitly antiracist schools. This is especially urgent given that language has historically been used as a tool to divide Latinx and Black communities. A more just future requires intersectional solidarity. Nurturing these solidarities is central to our mission.

Bettina Love (2019) writes:

> Abolitionist teaching asks educators to acknowledge and accept America and its policies as anti-Black, racist, discriminatory, and unjust and to be in solidarity with dark folx and poor folx fighting for their humanity . . . to learn the sociopolitical landscape of their students' communities through a historical, intersectional justice lens . . . [educators] must recognize America and its schools as spaces of Whiteness, White rage, and White supremacy. (p. 12)

While we do not identify ourselves as an abolitionist organization, Love calls us to think about what it means for the teachers and administrators with all of their structural, economic and institutional privilege, to be in solidarity with children who are fighting for their humanity. Love calls us, at SEAL, to turn inward and think about how we, as an education non-profit, with all of our structural, economic and institutional privilege also contribute to the problems of systemic racism and linguicism even as we fight for justice. This work is both aspirational and ongoing.

Guiding Questions

1. What is "linguicism" and what are its historical impacts on California's school population?
2. How are antilinguicism and antiracism related?
3. Why is it crucial to support students' home language?
4. How can teachers, administrators and policy-makers support home language?

Content Questions

1. What is SEAL's approach to supporting English Learners?
2. What have been some of the impacts of historical English Only policies on California's student population?
3. What is the significance of the *Lau v. Nichols* decision?
4. How does SEAL train Elementary teachers to support home language?
5. How does SEAL train Preschool teachers to support home language?

References

Alfaro, C., & Bartolomé, L. (2017). Preparing ideologically clear bilingual teachers. *Issues in Teacher Education, 26*(2), 11–34.

Arriagada, P. A. (2005). Family context and Spanish-language use: A study of Latino children in the United States. *Social Science Quarterly, 86*(3), 599–619.

Austin, L., Edwards, B., Chávez, R., & Whitebook, M. (2019). *Racial wage gaps in early education employment.* Center for the Study of Child Care Employment. Retrieved from https://cscce.berkeley.edu/racial-wage-gaps-in-early-education-employment/

Barnett, W., Yarosz, D., Thomas, J., Jung, K., & Blanco, D. (2007). Two-way and monolingual immersion in preschool education: An experimental comparison. *Early Childhood Research Quarterly, 22*(3), 277–293.

California Department of Education. (2020a). *English learner students by language and grade: State of California, 2019–20.* Retrieved from https://dq.cde.ca.gov/dataquest/dataquest.asp

California Department of Education. (2020b). *Transitional Kindergarten FAQs.* Retrieved from https://www.cde.ca.gov/ci/gs/em/kinderfaq.asp#program

Callahan, R. M. (2005). Tracking and high school English learners: Limiting opportunity to learn. *American Educational Research Journal, 42*(2), 305–328.

Cervantes-Soon, C. G., Dorner, L., Palmer, D., Heiman, D., Schwerdtfeger, R., & Choi, J. (2017). Combating inequalities in two-way language immersion programs: Toward critical consciousness in bilingual education spaces. *Review of Research in Education, 41*, 403–427. https://doi.org/10.3102/0091732X17690120

Derman-Sparks, L., & Olsen Edwards, J. (2010). *Anti-bias education for young children and ourselves.* National Association for the Education of Young Children.

Durán, L. K., Roseth, C. J., & Hoffman, P. (2010). An experimental study comparing English- only and transitional bilingual education on Spanish-speaking preschoolers' early literacy development. *Early Childhood Research Quarterly, 25*(2), 207–217. https://doi.org/10.1016/j.ecresq.2009.10.002

Fillmore, L. W. (1991). When learning a second language means losing the first. *Early Childhood Research Quarterly, 6*, 323–346.

Flores, S. Y., & Murillo, E. G. (2001). Power, language, and ideology: Historical and contemporary notes on the dismantling of bilingual education. *The Urban Review, 33*(2), 183–206. https://doi.org/10.1023/A:1010361803811

Gándara, P., Rumberger, R., Maxwell-Jolly, J., & Callahan, R. (2003). English learners in California schools: Unequal resources, unequal outcomes. *Education Policy Analysis Archives, 11*(36).

García, O. (2020). The education of Latinx bilingual children in times of isolation: Unlearning and relearning. *MinneTESOL Journal, 36*(1).

Hurwitz, A., & Olsen, L. (2018). *Supporting dual language learner success in Superdiverse PreK-3 classrooms: The Sobrato early academic language model.* The Migration Policy Institute.

Johnson, K. R., & Martinez, G. A. (2000). Forging our identity: Transformative resistance in the areas of work, class, and the law: Discrimination by proxy: The case of proposition 227 and the ban on bilingual education. *UC Davis Law Review, 33*(4).

Kendi, I. X. (2019). *How to be an antiracist.* One World.

Love, B. (2019). *We want to do more than survive: Abolitionist teaching and the pursuit of educational freedom.* Beacon Press Books.

McWhorter, J. (2001). *The power of Babel: A natural history of language.* Harper Collins.

Morales, P. Z., & Rao, A. B. (2015). How ideology and cultural capital shape the distribution of Illinois' bilingual education programs. *Teachers College Record.* Retrieved from https://www.tcrecord.org

National Academies of Sciences, Engineering and Medicine. (2017). *Promoting the educational success of children and youth learning English: Promising futures.* The National Academies Press. https://doi.org/10.17226/24677

Oh, J. S., & Fuligni, A. (2009). The role of heritage language development in the ethnic identity and family relationships of adolescents from immigrant backgrounds. *Social Development, 19*(1), 202–220. https://doi.org/10.1111/j.1467-9507.2008.00530.x

Olsen, L. (2009). The role of advocacy in shaping immigrant education: A California case study. *Teachers College Record, 111*(3), 817–850. Retrieved from https://www.tcrecord.org/content.asp?contentid=15345

Olsen, L. (2010). *Reparable Harm*. Californians Together.
Palmer, D. (2009). Middle-class English speakers in a two-way immersion bilingual classroom: "Everybody should be listening to Jonathan right now…". *TESOL Quarterly, 43*(2), 177–202.
Passos DeNicola, C., González, M., Morales, S., & Romaní, L. (2015). Teaching through *testimonio*: Accessing community cultural wealth in school. *Journal of Latinos and Education, 1*(16), 228–243.
Pettit, S. K. (2011). Teachers' beliefs about English language learners in the mainstream classroom: A review of the literature. *International Multilingual Research Journal, 5*(2), 123–147.
Santibañez, L., & Umanksy, I. (2018). English learners: Charting their experiences and mapping their futures in California schools. *PACE Research Brief.* Retrieved from https://gettingdowntofacts.com/sites/default/files/2018-09/GDTFII_Brief_EnglishLearners.pdf
Skutnabb-Kangas, T. (2015). *Linguicism. The encyclopedia of applied linguistics.* Blackwell.
Valdés, G. (1997). Dual-language immersion programs: A cautionary note concerning the education of language-minority children. *Harvard Educational Review, 67*(3), 391–425. https://doi.org/10.17763/haer.67.3.n5q175qp86120948
Wiley, T. G., & Wright, W. E. (2004). Against the undertow: Language-minority education policy and politics in the "Age of Accountability". *Educational Policy, 18*(1), 142–168.
Yoshikawa, H., Weiland, C., Brooks-Gunn, J., Burchinal, M., Espinosa, L., Gormley, W. T., Ludwig, J., Magnuson, K., Phillips, D., & Zaslow, M. (2013). *Investing in our future: The evidence on preschool.* Society for Research in Child Development.

5

Moving Beyond Performative Allyship: A Conceptual Framework for Anti-racist Co-conspirators

Leslie Ekpe and Sarah Toutant

Introduction

It is a precarious time to be engaging in anti-racist work given the extreme sociopolitical polarization our society is living in. In 2017, we witnessed white supremacists flood the streets of Charlottesville, Virginia, holding Tiki torches, swastikas, and semi-automatic rifles chanting "white lives matter" and "Jews will not replace us" (McEldowney, 2018, n.p.). In response to this bigotry, the 45th President of the United States (U.S.) stated there were "very fine people on both sides" (McEldowney, 2018, n.p.), further validating that our commander and chief at the time, did not condemn white supremacy. This protection of Whiteness from the

L. Ekpe (✉)
Texas Christian University, Fort Worth, TX, USA
e-mail: l.ekpe@tcu.edu

S. Toutant
University of Southern California, Los Angeles, CA, USA
e-mail: toutant@usc.edu

© The Author(s), under exclusive license to Springer Nature Switzerland AG 2022

K. Johnson et al. (eds.), *Developing Anti-Racist Practices in the Helping Professions: Inclusive Theory, Pedagogy, and Application*,
https://doi.org/10.1007/978-3-030-95451-2_5

President himself, coupled with the state-sanctioned police violence against Black people, caused protests across the nation to erupt in the summer of 2020. Hundreds of thousands of people from different races and ethnicities began to awaken to the anti-Black racism plaguing the U.S. as they marched and proclaimed the famous slogan created by three Black women, "Black Lives Matter" (Garza, 2014). The Black Lives Matter (BLM) movement has even been referred to as the "new civil rights era" (Freelon et al., 2016).

In response to such necessary protests, colleges and universities across the nation issued public statements detailing their stances on racism in America. Given the historically White patriarchal structures of higher education institutions (Haynes et al., 2020), many college and university presidents struggled to condemn anti-Blackness and racism in their campus-wide statements intentionally. However, some presidents and other critical institutional leaders were particular and continuously pushed their students, faculty, and staff to think critically about how they could show up as allies. Many academics have identified others who use their power to stand in solidarity with oppressed people as "allies." However well-intentioned these campus-wide calls for allyship were, we argue it led to a watered-down understanding of what genuinely being an anti-racist ally means.

This chapter urges higher education professionals to critically think about the limited ways allyship serves us. Specifically, we provide a conceptual framework in which we refer to as I-ARC, an intersectional, anti-racist co-conspirator framework. This chapter pushes education leaders and thinkers to resist rudimentary understandings of race and racism through traditional understandings of allyship. Instead, we argue the need for co-conspirators who adopt anti-racist practices. The objectives of this chapter are for readers to thoroughly understand the difference between allyship and co-conspirators, adopt anti-racist practices, and learn how to apply an I- ARC framework.

It is not enough solely to be an ally. However, one must be a co-conspirator—this requires risk-taking and rule-breaking—the term "ally" does not capture this radical embodiment (Clemens, 2017). To frame our study, we define co-conspirator using Love's (2019b) definition. Love (2019b) states,

> A co-conspirator says, 'I know the terms; I know what white privilege and white supremacy mean; now, what risks am I willing to take?' It's saying, 'I'm going to put my privilege on the line for somebody.

We use this definition as the basis for our work. Co-conspirators ought to be anti-racist, committed to hearing and understanding, and able to relinquish authority by using the right to call others to lead (Kendi, 2019a). Moving beyond ally-ship involves countering bigotry and injustice, not only helping the people impacted by it. The term co-conspirator is one who advocates an anti-racist agenda or expresses an anti-racist concept by their actions.

The concept of anti-racism is critical when discussing co-conspirators. Anti-racism means exercising optimism, undermining systems of injustice, freedom activities, and telling the truth. The art of regeneration is the practice of anti-racists; it is a practice of compassion. Kendi explains, "The only remedy to racist discrimination is anti-racist discrimination" (Kendi, 2019a, 2019b). Anti-racist practices are the best cure for racial discrimination. In this, racial discrimination has long been rooted in the traditions of Whiteness. We define Whiteness using Frankenberg's (1993) definition as it relates to full access of privilege,

> Whiteness signals the production and reproduction of dominance rather than subordination, normativity rather than marginality, and privilege rather than disadvantage.

'Whiteness' is used in this context as a condition and practice of racial differentiation achieved through the enactment of privilege as normative (Fine et al., 1997).

Lastly, anti-racism also requires that one be intersectional in their activism, which is why we include intersectionality in our framework. Coined by legal scholar, Kimberlé Crenshaw, intersectionality is an analytic concept grounded in Black feminist and critical race theories to illustrate how:

> Women of color are differently situated in economic, social, and political worlds. When reform efforts undertaken on behalf of women neglect this

fact, women of color are less likely to have their needs met than women who are racially privileged (Crenshaw, 1990, p. 1250).

An intersectional lens allows us to grapple with the ways in which historical systems of racism and sexism influence women. Since Black women are so often nudged to the margins of exclusive antiracist and feminist efforts, it is important to explicitly state that intersectionality is a theory centered around Black feminists. Therefore, we utilize intersectionality to highlight, as Harris and Patton (2019) explain, intersectionality demonstrates how "discourses of resistance, such as feminism and anti-racism, often frame identities as isolated and mutually exclusive, resulting in the 'theoretical erasure' of Black women who hold multiple minoritized identities" (Harris & Patton, p. 347). To combat this erasure, we pull from the works of women of color scholars who discuss critical race feminism, which we detail later in the chapter.

Due to allyship not intentionally adopting ant-racist practices, we are still bristling at the term "ally" because we have witnessed people practicing allyship in performative ways. In this way, they have not participated in taking actionable steps to establish substantive ties with racially minoritized people. We posit that "performative allyship" is the practice of citing buzzwords, creating social posts to perform allyship with rudimentary understandings of race and racism, and gestures that promote the significant moral compass of an individual, as opposed to dismantling oppressive systems.

The chapter intentionally encourages moving away from performative allyship. In it, we discuss anti-racism and co-conspirators in academia by ultimately proposing an intersectional, anti-racist co-conspirator (I-ARC) conceptual framework. First, we will provide a more detailed overview of the problem and illustrate how an anti-racist educator actively aims to abolish the mechanisms, rules, procedures, and structures that establish inequality and perpetuate the race- based inequities among people of color (POC). Next, we refer to previous theoretical perspectives regarding allyship. We then follow this with a discussion on the need for change and why higher education must move towards an I-ARC conceptual framework. Next, we explain our proposed framework and conclude with a reflection on its effectiveness in practice. Finally, we finish this chapter with recommendations for higher education researchers and practitioners.

Purpose of Chapter

"I Can't Breathe!" "Hands Up Don't Shoot!" "Black Lives Matter!"

While the challenges that Black people face have been widely discredited by the assumption that society has progressed past racism and slavery, the recent murders of Jacob Blake, Ahmad Arbery, Breonna Taylor, and George Floyd—to name a few—have brought to light the magnitude of racial inequality in the U.S. and beyond. More precisely, what does it entail to move past allyship and become a co-conspirator in the movement towards equity? These problems have repercussions for White academics in the university who aim to shift the discourse about social inequality and eventually dismantle injustice mechanisms. Publicized racism against the Black community is always extensive. For decades, the dominant influence of bigotry, and its adverse impact on mental and physical health, has become an undeniable fact for Black people. Although the toll that institutionalized injustice has on Black people is apparent to some, more and more people are becoming aware, thus fueling more people into allyship roles.

The BLM organization emerged in 2012 following the murder of Trayvon Martin in 2012. Garza (2014) explains BLM was created in response to the anti-Black bigotry that permeates our culture and indeed, sadly, our movements. The campaign has changed the way the world is talking about race and fairness. So, when White community members increasingly entered the social justice struggle, the ally's position shifted. Allyship is mutually beneficial and mutually supportive; however, one protestor suggests that the Black community is not obliged to support the White community. In this, amid ethnic abuse, we call for co-conspirators, not allies. We encourage groups of all races to collaborate for a shared purpose rooted in co-conspiracy: equity.

The BLM protests have been described as the biggest protests in the U.S. since the Civil Rights Movement saw protests in every state—including all the U.S. territories—over several weeks (Clayton, 2018). Recent developments have increasingly shown the need for non-Black people to act in tackling bigotry in all its dimensions. The act of an ally is, nonetheless, rooted in Whiteness. This chapter is a call for White people in the academy and non-Black POC who participate in Whiteness to recognize their position in the anti-White supremacy movement.

Through drawing on critical race scholarship, we strive to push people in higher education positions towards co-conspiratorship, thus ultimately analyzing their participation in White supremacy traditions.

This chapter presents a conceptual framework that argues against allyship and calls for co-conspirators. We created our framework of what it means to be an anti-racist co-conspirator, theorist and educator, by centering key concepts of critical scholars who have come before us. Framed by ideas of anti-racism, co-conspirators, and Critical Race Feminism (CRF), this chapter analyzes the reflections and the literature on White loyalty in an attempt to problematize the role of White intellectuals and those who participate in Whiteness. We do this by advocating for an alternate position: a co-conspirator.

Allyship Literature

The terms ally, allies, and allyship have commonly been used to apply to any person who supports a marginalized identity that they are not a part of (Ramsey, 2014). Ramsey (2014) further describes the ally as a verb; it is about persons with privilege using their advantages to disrupt inequality and engage alongside people who are part of marginalized communities to promote equity. Fundamentally, those who wish to exercise allyship should bring others up by "advocating; not seeing venting as a personal attack; acknowledging systemic inequality and understanding the effect of microaggressions; believing underrepresented people's experiences; and hearing, encouraging, self-reflecting and modifying" (Ally and action, n.d.).

Such racial allyship might look like reading about anti-racism, listening to racially minoritized people's experiences, knowing when to speak up and when to listen, and more. Such well-intentioned discourse has swept the nation as calls for more "allies" can be seen in academic literature, social media, news outlets, and more. Carlson et al. (2019) state that there is push back around the use of 'allyship' claiming "urging for an evolution of our collective thinking about what is needed from people privileged by or benefiting from inequalities" (Carlson et al., 2019, p. 890). Despite these warranted critiques, to move forward with reimagining a conceptual framework that moves away from an allyship lens to an intersectional, anti-racist co-conspirator lens, it is first essential to address previous theoretical framings of allyship.

Many of the theoretical models and literature exploring allyship emerged in the 1990s and early 2000s. For example, Washington and Evans (1991) work on allies to the LGBTQ+ community explored actionable steps to allyship. They explained that allies first need to become aware to find knowledge and educate themselves to equip them with the skills to act. Years later, Bishop (2002) created a model for becoming an ally based on her personal insider experiences as an adult educator, workshop leader, community developer, and activist. In her work, she pushes allies to partake in the following:

- Understanding the systemic nature of oppression
- Understanding the different types of oppressions
- Developing consciousness and healing
- Becoming a worker in one's liberation
- Ultimately becoming an ally

Much of Bishop's (2002) argument is that allies must grapple with how oppression came about, what holds oppression in its place, and how there must be a level of consciousness-raising as well as healing on a macro and micro level.

In addition to Bishop's (2002) work, Broido's (2000) study explored social justice allyship in student affairs literature. Broido (2000) conducted a grounded theory study to understand how straight, White male college students became allies. They found that "increased information in social justice issues, engagement in meaning-making processes, and self-confidence" were integral in participants' development as allies (Broido,

2000, p. 7). Whereas Broido's (2000) study focused on precursors to action rather than operationalizing allyship, Edwards (2006) conceptualized social justice allyship by creating a model. Edwards (2006) used White racial identity development to inform their model. They argue that there are three statuses allies navigate through: an ally for self-interest, an ally for altruism, and an ally for social justice. To further explain, an ally for self-interest is "primarily motivated to protect those they care about from being hurt" and may only confront oppressive behavior when the individual they care about is present (Edwards, 2006, pg. 46). Feelings of guilt frequently drive an ally motivated by altruism instead of understanding that they also perpetuate oppression systems. Lastly, an ally for social justice is the status that Edwards (2006) illustrates as aspirational in which allies work in collaboration with oppressed groups to dismantle systemic racism.

Washington and Evans (1991), Bishop (2002), Broido (2000), and Edwards' (2006) models of allyship shaped the ways higher education researchers and practitioners thought about allyship. Although all such literature was popularized, these models posed dangerous rhetoric; they relied on a binary version of race (Patel, 2011). Patel (2011) argued that some of these models essentialized POC by lumping them into one category. Essentialization is problematic because it is critical to disaggregate racial groups. In other words, Black, Latinx, Asian, South Asian, Pacific Islanders, and Native American/Indigenous people all have their histories that have been affected by systems of oppression. Such binary allyship models do not account for these critical differences nor explain the importance of being anti-racist.

Additional criticisms against allyship discuss how individuals lack engagement and activism within allyship (Carlson et al., 2019, p. 889). Related to our previous argument of "performative allyship," activism must be intentional and not performative. Relatedly, Davis III et al. (2019) made clear that if one is genuinely dedicated to activism, they "should be grounded in the work of activism and organizing for transformative change rather than simply the words" (p. 100). Overall, allyship literature does not apply to our current socio- political climate. Racially minoritized peoples and other historically marginalized populations no longer need allies. Instead, they need co-conspirators (Love, 2019b).

Times are changing, and how we conceptualize allyship must involve critique, action, and an intentional reimagining of what it means to actively do activist, anti-racist and co-conspirator work. Although allyship includes standing in unity with oppressed people, being a co-conspirator requires putting oneself on the line, operationalizing one's privilege—all at the expense of giving up the protection of such privilege.

The main distinctions between becoming an ally and becoming a co-conspirator are that co-conspirators take personal risks by endangering their comfort, endangering their livelihoods, sacrificing their physical security, and in certain situations, gambling for their freedom—all in favor of the most minoritized. Whereas the ally model ideologically places those with privilege in support roles that are safe and not too risky, thus preserving racial hierarchies. Whether represented as a performative ally, an optical ally, or clicktivism, allyship preserves White individuals' conscience.

Problematic Anti-racist Teacher Education Practice(s) and Implementation

Our engagement and service as higher education professionals working with students and community members of all races is imbued with ethics. Yet, avoiding the spiritual implications of our practice risks perpetuating immoral regimes of control and inequality. Unless there is a fundamental and radical shift in the degree of Black representation in political roles, the undeniably inequitable and discriminatory impact on all racialized communities will continue. Nothing less than drastic reform is needed to switch from dazzling progressive street actions to a lasting and sustainable new commitment in real power-sharing with Black, Indigenous and People of Color (BIPOC). In this section, we discuss the importance of higher education being anti-racist and the need for such change. We also highlight social movements and the strong impacts they have had on higher education. Lastly, we frame co-conspiratorship further before delving into our conceptual framework.

Higher Education

Encouraging equitable education environments requires more than sensitivity and representation of all pupils, teachers, and staff; it is also about removing institutional and cultural obstacles in the way of services and opportunities. Thus, in order to address equity in higher education, we must also understand how oppression functions in our society. Moreover, oppressive structures embedded into economic systems, treatment services, environmental policies, and the criminal justice system discriminate against historically minoritized groups.

Young (2000) argued in the statement below that, while there is a history of oppression among socially subordinate groups, such history is made up of different legacies and implications for each group:

> In the most general sense, all oppressed people share some inhibition of their ability to develop and exercise their capacities and express their needs, thoughts, and feelings. (p. 271).

It is also important to remember that individuals coming from socially subordinate groups are not immediately born with an awareness of their racial origin (Bettencourt, 2020). Ayers (2010) argues the importance of "working the gap." To achieve this, faculty must help students consider and identify mechanisms of dominance and inequality while at the same time finding ways to challenge the current social order. White educators, as co-conspirators, should challenge themselves with questions such as:

- "What does it mean to take risks and initiative to challenge the status quo through our curriculum and pedagogy?" (Powell & Kelly, 2017).
- "How do we move our white students beyond fear and guilt, or worse, the role of a benevolent savior?" (Powell & Kelly, 2017).

Patel (2011) explains this binary allyship model as a top-down vision of prejudice based on a set of assumptions:

> Engaging in discussion about the shortcomings of a binary model in which people are split into White/Non-White categories and acknowledging that

> subordinated people also engage in the process of racial identity exploration, the need for a new term to address subordinated racial group members who work in the interests of racial groups outside of their own becomes clear. (pg. 79)

Patel (2011) implies that grandeur in teaching holds one foot in truth while the other reaches what should be. One of the most critical locations to be a co-conspirator is in our education system. Faculty teach students to "work" by instruction and pedagogical decisions. The differences: the void between the world as it is and the world as we wish it to be (Ayers, 2010, p. 137).

Need for Change

The concept of White saviorism refers to the belief that a White person, or a White community, saves POC (Maurantonio, 2017). Well-meaning White people are likely—even expected—to slip into the paternalistic pit of thinking they are supporting or protecting POC. The idea that White people are culturally superior can lead to apathy in the face of inequities for POC and can also make and justify dehumanization and abuse. In this, before White individuals recognize the effect of modern and past prejudice on persons of color and themselves, we will continue to default on saviors. Saviorism and allyship coincide significantly. As a result, allyship can express itself as a mistaken benevolence towards POC. Dr. Joy DeGruy explains the misguided benevolence foundation,

> [People in the U.S.] have hundreds of years of being traumatized. Human beings learn how to survive despite the trauma. My sense is you [white people] have a pathology associated with how [white] people were able to deal with unearned privilege... the self had to legitimize what was going on [through] dehumanizing [Black] people: It's their fault... they, in some way, brought this upon themselves...they are inherently inferior. This then makes [white people] 'benevolent' because [they're] simply trying to 'help.' (Albert & Cover, 2019)

Although there might be perceived or actual danger of behaving or speaking out, it is the co-conspirator's job to handle anxieties and sit in frustration in both large and small moments that are an unavoidable part of social reform.

Various papers have been written to encourage cultural sensitivity and practice-oriented modesty, such as self-reflection, knowledge building, and reiterating ethical responsibilities of collaborating with clients of diverse backgrounds (Dennison et al., 2019; Wright, 2019). However, the core tenet targets White practitioners. Both allies and contributions to structural oppression, particularly in the sense of inequality and the discrimination towards Black people, are not limited to White individuals. Systemic racism is a large-scale and unavoidable hierarchical system of discrimination built by White people and primarily aimed at minority racial and ethnic communities (Feagin, 2006). Solidarity is open acts that criticize (and, in some cases, punish) pre-existing racial views, model anti-racist verbal conduct, and show equivalence between injustices faced by Black and non-Black persons of color. Antiracism is not the lack of discriminatory attitudes, but rather thoughts and actions that consciously encourage racial equity (Kendi, 2019a, 2019b).

Social Movements

The fight for real equity in the academy is influenced by the fight for fundamental human rights outside academia, so we find it critical to also discuss such social movements and their effects on the academy. One of such pivotal movements is the Civil Rights Movement. This movement brought about a revolution in public education through school desegregation mandates (Clayton, 2018). In retrospect, of course, we can see that the enduring impact of the Civil Rights Movement on American education has been mixed, as have recent revolutions, such as the conservative restoration of the 1980s (Apple, 2001). The Civil Rights Movement reversed numerous policies by pursuing alternative social, political, and educational concepts and objectives. The legacy of the Civil Rights Movement continues to flourish in U.S. colleges and universities. For example, there is a revived demand that has echoed through television and social media to improve how and when students think about bias in colleges and universities. Professionals in higher education tend to take the initiative now and work more actively and jointly to revise our endeavors so that they are intellectually inclusive, focused, and utterly transferable so that genuine justice can be reached for minoritized populations.

Today, social movements have found themselves interwoven in all our practices in social media. Social revolutions start, after all, with people. Thus, one can see that social media can drastically convert how people participate. This recently happened in the BLM campaign. This development gradually grew to coalesce as the movement became nationally known during the U.S. presidential election of 2016 for its street protests (Drakulich et al., 2020). According to Snow and Benford (1999), a frame convergence mechanism happens as social movements connect their agendas to other social movements' interests and converge into a single community, an ongoing and systematic way to attract members to the cause.

Indeed, social movements themselves serve as educators, engaging people in informal schooling through participating in campaign events, non-formal education through movement education programs, and even, often, quasi-formal education through special schools within movements (Niesz et al., 2018). Given the relevance of social movements to activism and education for social movements, we articulate the immediate need to increase understanding of such agitation by involving educational researchers across a wide variety of fields to co-conspirators.

Co-conspirator Is a Verb

Calling oneself a co-conspirator is insufficient; there is work tied to the word (Bettencourt, 2020). Co-conspirators must be alert and present and display dedication to activism, regardless of how they might feel (Jackson et al., 2020). It takes a great deal of critical self-reflection and action to move for authentic activism. These people must treat co- conspiracy with modesty, understanding that one cannot be responsive to input and criticism (Michael & Conger, 2009). There are some main factors to ensure that allies/accomplices are in line with equity to be a successful co-conspirator. One should note that activism is a long- standing allegiance.

Indeed, when exercising co-conspiratorship, there are degrees and heights of sacrifice. This continuing dedication involves transparency and accountability to ensure that co- conspirators treat their newfound path towards steadfast support of equity. This path requires the desire to accept and be conscious of the risks and compromises that are consistent. A co-conspirator's job is challenging, but diligence means knowing that activism is for the common good. Being a co-conspirator entails accepting the risk of enduring harm. Our scholarship as educational researchers should embody our genuine ambition for cultural evolution to cultivate a solicitous and cooperative approach to racial equality.

A Conceptual Framework for Anti-racist Co-Conspirators

Given the need to reconceptualize allyship, we present an I-ARC or intersectional, anti- racist co-conspirator conceptual framework for higher education professionals to utilize in their research and practice. First, we provide an overview of anti-racism as defined by Dr. Ibram X. Kendi (2019b). Second, we discuss what it means to be a co-conspirator utilizing Dr. Bettina Love's (2020) work. Third, we engage Critical Race Feminism (CRF) and its tenants. Lastly, utilizing the concepts mentioned above, we provide four assumptions of an I-ARC conceptual framework and explain how we envision operationalizing such a framework.

Anti-Racism

In their acclaimed book, Kendi (2019a, 2019b) presents the theory of anti-racism, which they define as a system of ideas and policies that reject racial inequity. Kendi (2019a, 2019b) is explicit that people are either racist or actively anti-racist; there is no in-between. Anti-racism is essentially policies that lead to racial equity. As Kendi (2019a, 2019b) explains, we live in a society where racial inequity is the norm, and when people do nothing to address such norms, the norm persists, which is racist. Thus, to be anti-racist is to be actively challenging such racist norms; anti-racism cannot occur without action. Such action must undo racist policies. Further, some believe that Kendi (2019a, 2019b) states Black people and other POC cannot be racist—a long-standing argument. However, in his 2019 interview at the University of Michigan, he explains the conversation is more complicated than arguing about racism versus personal prejudices and biases. He explains that if Black people or other POC do not "go after" racist policies and only focus their efforts on individual racist people, they contribute to harm against Black people and POC. Hence, not attacking, critiquing, and addressing racist policies is a harmful act, which inherently is not anti- racist.

Co-conspirators

The need for co-conspirators is increasingly being highlighted in current literature (Love, 2019b). When asked the difference between an ally and a co-conspirator, Love (2019a) explained that "Allies know all the language, they read all the books, they come to the meeting with all the terms…" (n.p.). In other words, allies perform, and they check off boxes to show they care. However, a co-conspirator "puts something on the line for somebody" (Love, 2019a, n.p.). In Love's (2019b) book, she provides a powerful example of what this looks like. In 2015, a young Black woman, Bree Newsome, climbed a flagpole at the South Carolina State Capitol and took down a confederate flag. She did this ten days after a White supremacist killed eight Black parishioners and their pastor at Emanuel African Methodist Episcopal Church in Charleston. She knew she would be arrested. While police officers attempted to get her down from the flagpole by threatening to tase the flagpole, she was climbing. A White man, James Tyson, who did not know Bree, stepped in and put his hand on the pole to prevent police from harming her. James is a co-conspirator.

Critical Race Feminism

In order to be an anti-racist co-conspirator, one must also recognize the importance of intersectionality. Although Kendi's (2019a, 2019b) conceptualization of anti-racism addresses intersectionality, we argue that Critical Race Feminism is also needed to ensure this framework addresses gender and its nuances. CRF is an analytical tool and a branch of Critical Race Theory (CRT). Thus, CRF often intersects with tenets of CRT but is distinctly differentiated by actively resisting centering men's voices and conflating White women's experiences with the experiences of women of color (Evans-Winters & Esposito, 2010). For our conceptual framework, we draw from the following principles of CRF in particular: (1) critical race feminism focuses on the lives of women of color who face multiple forms of discrimination due to the intersections of race, class, and gender within a system of White male patriarchy and racist oppression; (2) critical race feminism centers the multiple identities and consciousness of women of color (i.e., anti- essentialist); and (3) critical race feminism requires an interdisciplinary approach to research that incorporates theories and concepts from a variety of academic fields (Evans-Winters & Esposito, 2010).

We use CRF (Wing, 2020) to bring to our examination of co- conspiracy the specificities of injustice of identity to women of color. Recognizing these individual problems can contribute to the development of appropriate solutions aimed at the communities in question, whether they are students, faculty or employees. In order to properly appreciate the plight of women of color, it is important not only to look at their cultural identity and gender identity, but also to examine the convergence of these identities (Wing, 2020).

Towards an I-ARC Conceptual Framework

By pulling from anti-racist, co-conspirator, and CRF literature, we can use aspects of all concepts to create an I-ARC conceptual framework. To further specify, we argue an I-ARC conceptual framework believes the following principles to be valid:

1. All POC and women of color do not have the same experiences, and disaggregating their identities is essential in policymaking, activism, and rhetoric.
2. Anti-racism also requires one to be anti-patriarchy, anti-homophobia, and anti- transphobia.
3. Co-conspirators must fight against both racist people and policies and be willing to put their lives, privilege, bodies, financial assets, and more on the line in the name of racial equity.
4. Partaking in performative practices without acting against racist policies participates in racism and causing further harm.

We utilize the I-ARC Conceptual Framework as a foundation towards increasing solidarity. We agree with Powell and Kelly (2017) as they state anticipating, "continued uprising and messy dialogues around what it means actively work for and demand racial justice" (p. 58). As scholars in education, we agree that scholar advocates must operate in a cross-disciplinary alliance.

Principle 1 Experiences differ within marginalized communities. As a co-conspirator, it is critical to be aware that experiences influence advocacy. Co-conspirators must be aware that racialized experiences are not a "one size fits all" type of scenario (e.g., not all Black people have the same experiences). Additionally, co-conspirators also recognize they do not have the lived experiences to speak for BIPOC. For this reason, a co-conspirator must invest and support those who have lived and experienced marginalization. Principle 2 If one is to practice anti-racism, be aware that this includes holistic practice. Moreover, racism, homophobia and sexism are intrinsically connected. While it can be uncomfortable to evaluate one's privilege, we must understand that many Lesbians, Gay, Bisexual, Transgender, Queer, Intersexed, and Asexual (LGBTQIA+) people are victims of double or triple marginalization in terms of gender identity, sexual orientation, and race. Homophobia and transphobia are also related to aspects of systemic racism; we must respond compassionately and equitably. Principle 3 Being a co-conspirator is a lifelong commitment. We understand that there are multiple facets of how we are consciously fighting institutional racism and continuous injustice. Co-conspirators are mindful of the sacrifices they make to promote social justice. They ask themselves these questions, "Who benefits from this purpose? What is the support of society? What is the interest in this community that dominates the story of outsiders, and a salvific tale of outsiders?" Social justice movements will turn quickly into cultural and/or financial ownership unless we are aware of the gains, who holds influence. Principle 4 Lil Wayne, also known as Dwayne Michael Carter, Jr., once stated, "Real G's move in silence like lasagna" (Genius, 2010). This quote should be the co-conspirator's model. In no way should co-conspirators be looking for a pat on the back. If everything is done for a response or praise, then one can assume that they are performative in their activism. In this way, co-conspirators must commit to performing necessary ordinary acts, which nobody can ever see. They must accept that a co-conspirator membership does not come with a medal of honor as being a co-conspirator rejects anything reminiscent of a savior model.

Reflection on the Effectiveness of Practice(s)

We know that with current times, it does not hurt to try to implement new conceptual frameworks. We have new fights and trials we are battling. We cannot solely rely on older frameworks to attack new problems in our society. The co- conspirator aims not only to re-allocate authority but also to abolish our country's culture of White supremacy. However, this can contribute to cognitive dissonance and frustration for many allies who benefit from these processes in ways they do not appreciate until their privilege and benefits are disrupted (Powell & Kelly, 2017). There is not one proper manner to move from co- conspirator action in opposition to White supremacy. It is messy, hard, however, the need to take motion is urgent. Nevertheless, to build a more just world, it is going to take change and uncomfortability.

Co-conspiracy is what one does, not in words alone. Many people who suggest a change from ally vocabulary also note that the issue with an ally is not so much in the first sense of the term; it is how people who wish to declare themselves supportive of oppressed groups have diluted it and misused it without genuinely disrupting injustice. A desire to fight racist practices and beliefs is the main trait of co-conspirators. To co-conspire implies to be constantly and regularly active. Critical contemplation and group formation are a vital step in the creation of identification as a co-conspirator.

Moving Forward

Despite the fact that the protests were explicitly described as Black-centered spaces by the organizers, much of the discourse resulting was based on White individuals, White philosophies, and discussions that White intellectuals might or may not have had. Whiteness is currently characterized by what it's not: Blackness. The authors agree that the process of engaging in constructive discourse on anti-racism-both personal and systemic change-begins with self- reflection and a link to why this work is important to us individually. Our framework calls for White intellectuals and activists to serve as accomplices, acting in unity with POC in social justice and anti-racist movements.

Co- conspirators must take action without waiting for an invitation from POC. Allies remain on the sidelines until they are called to action for fear of overstepping. Consequently, this positions the burden of planning and educating primarily on POC. There is no right way to switch from an ally to a real co-conspirator against White supremacy. We understand that this could be different based on the job environment and the groups one represents. It is complicated, hard, and we might not always get it right, but the need for action is urgent.

Conclusion

Racism is as prevalent in the twenty-first century in the whole of America as ever. This must immediately end. To do that, White people must take action themselves. Rather than allies, they must be co-conspirators. Further, this framework also applies to non-Black POC, as some do not entirely grasp the extent of race and racism; they must make a deliberate attempt to listen and partake in conduct that does not perpetuate their prejudice on a day-to-day basis.

The role of a co-conspirator is to also fight when those most marginalized can fight no more. This extreme fatigue of fighting against racial injustice is referred to as racial battle fatigue prompted by "the protracted inability and/or unwillingness of the U.S. nation-state to alter conditions of racial justice fundamentally" (Itagaki, 2016, p. 6). As we trek towards a new democracy, we acknowledge that the road will not be easy; however, we hope for a new tomorrow. We utilize frameworks such as I-ARC that serve as a foundation for choosing to engage in the action's implications.

Co-conspiratorship ensures people are committed to the cause, despite the risks. Being a co-conspirator means being fierce and taking steps to lift the state of our democracy. Promoting fair educational systems is also about eradicating institutional and systemic barriers to equitable access for all racially and ethnically marginalized peoples. Finally, it disrupts the often-racist patriarchal mechanisms (Sanborn et al., 2019) of authority that continues to (re)create inequities in our colleges and universities.

Reflection/Discussion Questions

1. **No room for Whiteness in co-conspiratorship:** Because the system is based on Whiteness, oftentimes BIPOC communities are not considered. In essence, White educators must be openly anti-racist, dedicated to listening and learning, and prepared to leveraging privilege to empower others.
2. **Co-conspiratorship is not about you:** Co-conspirators recognize that ending all kinds of tyranny, including those from which they may profit, is in their own best interests. Co- conspirators pledge to take themselves out of situations that deal with the oppression of marginalized groups, and further educate themselves on racial justice matters. Co-conspirators do not seek remuneration for doing the right thing.
3. **A lifetime commitment to social justice:** Dismantle systems built for Whites in order to achieve power by making room for POC. Working against racism is a marathon, not a sprint. Every person deserves an equal chance at success, and race should never be an

impediment to that achievement. Anti-racist practices must be actively embodied in all the labor, of co-conspirators, in order to dismantle systematic racism.

Guiding Questions

1. Anti-racism practices as a co-conspirator means:
2. The **I-ARC Conceptual Framework** serves as a foundation for change within systems that have traditionally been exclusive towards historically marginalized communities. How does one dismantle power structures that could possibly interfere with applying the **I-ARC Framework**?
3. The term intersectionality coined in 1989 by Kimberlé Crenshaw, academic and civil rights activist, describes the phenomena of numerous, intersective, and often conflicting identities that may exist inside a single individual (Harris & Patton, 2019). How does intersectionality play an integral part in understanding one's role as a co-conspirator?
4. The murder of George Floyd in May of 2020 sparked national outraged. So much so, that businesses, organizations, and educational entities took part through action to show solidarity with communities who continue to be oppressed. However, the spark in action was perceived as performative for many since the death of George Floyd was not the first time a Black man was killed as a result of police brutality. Co-conspirators are those who are actively working against the White supremacist system and the advantages that come with it. How might the **I-ARC Framework** be implemented to ensure that performative co-conspiratorship does not occur?
5. Allyship allows individuals to be passive or decide to opt-out when it becomes too uncomfortable while co-conspiratorship empowers those to become bold and fight against the inequalities, atrocities, and violence against BIPOC communities. In what ways can co- conspiratorship show up in teacher practices?

References

Albert, D., & Cover, L. (2019). From Saviorism to Co-Conspiring. Retrieved from https://www.promise54.org/from-saviorism-to-co-conspiring/

Ally and action. (n.d.). *Ally and Action | Rio Salado College*. Available at: https://www.riosalado.edu/about/deib/ally-and-action

Apple, M. W. (2001). *Educating the "right" way: Markets, standards, god, and inequality*. Routledge.

Ayers, W. (2010). *To teach: The journey of a teacher*. Teachers College Press.

Bettencourt, G. M. (2020). "You can't be a class ally if you're an upper-class person because you don't understand": Working-class students' definitions and perceptions of social class allyship. *The Review of Higher Education, 44*(2), 265–291. https://doi.org/10.1353/rhe.2020.0041

Bishop, A. (2002). *Becoming an ally: Breaking the cycle of oppression in people*. Zed Books.

Broido, E. M. (2000). The development of social justice allies during college: A phenomenological investigation. *Journal of College Student Development, 41*(1), 3–18.

Carlson, J., Leek, C., Casey, E., Tolman, R., & Allen, C. (2019). What's in a name? A synthesis of "allyship" elements from academic and activist literature. *Journal of Family Violence*, 1–10.

Clayton, D. M. (2018). Black lives matter and the civil rights movement: A comparative analysis of two social movements in the United States. *Journal of Black Studies, 49*(5), 448–480. https://doi.org/10.1177/0021934718764099

Clemens, C. (2017). *Ally or accomplice? The language of activism*. Retrieved from https://www.tolerance.org/magazine/ally-oraccomplice-the-language-of-activism

Crenshaw, K. (1990). Mapping the margins: Intersectionality, identity politics, and violence against women of color. *Stanford Law Review, 43*, 1241.

Davis, C. H., III, Harris, J. C., Stokes, S., & Harper, S. R. (2019). But is it activist?: Interpretive criteria for activist scholarship in higher education. *The Review of Higher Education, 42*(5), 85–108. https://doi.org/10.1353/rhe.2019.0046

Dennison, A., Lund, E., Brodhead, M., Mejia, L., Armenta, A., & Leal, J. (2019). Delivering home-supported applied behavior analysis therapies to culturally and linguistically diverse families. *Behavior Analysis in Practice*, OnlineFirst, 1–12.

Drakulich, K., Wozniak, K. H., Hagan, J., & Johnson, D. (2020). Race and policing in the 2016 presidential election: Black lives matter, the police, and dog whistle politics. *Criminology, 58*(2), 370–402. https://doi.org/10.1111/1745-9125.12239

Edwards, K. E. (2006). Aspiring social justice ally identity development: A conceptual model. *NASPA Journal, 43*(4), 39–60.

Evans-Winters, V. E., & Esposito, J. (2010). Other People's daughters: Critical race feminism and black girls' education. *Educational Foundations, 24*, 11–24.

Feagin, J. R. (2006). *Systemic racism: A theory of oppression.* Routledge/Taylor & Francis Group.

Fine, M., Weis, L., Powell, L., & Wong, M. (Eds.). (1997). *Off white: Readings on race, power and society.* Routledge.

Frankenberg, R. (1993). *White women, race matters: The social construction of whiteness.* Routledge.

Freelon, D., McIlwain, C. D., & Clark, M. (2016). *Beyond the hashtags: #Ferguson, #Blacklivesmatter, and the online struggle for offline justice.* Center for Media & Social Impact, American University, Forthcoming.

Garza, A. (2014). A herstory of the #blacklivesmatter movement by alicia garza. *The Feminist Wire.* https://thefeministwire.com/2014/10/blacklivesmatter-2/

Genius. (2010, December). *Lil Wayne (Ft. Cory Gunz)—6 foot 7 foot.* Retrieved from inter https://genius.com/Lil-wayne-6-foot-7-foot-lyrics

Harris, J. C., & Patton, L. D. (2019). Un/doing intersectionality through higher education research. *The Journal of Higher Education, 90*(3), 347–372.

Haynes, N., Cooper, L. A., Albert, M. A., & Association of Black Cardiologists. (2020). At the heart of the matter: Unmasking and addressing the toll of COVID-19 on diverse populations. *Circulation, 142*(2), 105–107.

Itagaki, L. (2016). *Civil racism: The 1992 Los Angeles rebellion and the crisis of racial burnout.* University of Minnesota Press.

Jackson, R. G., Huskins, K., Skelton, S. M., & Thorius, K. A. K. (2020). *Allyship & accomplice: Two sides of the same coin. Equity dispatch.* Midwest & Plains Equity Assistance Center (MAP EAC).

Kendi, I. X. (2019a). *How to be an anti-racist* (1st ed.). One World.

Kendi, I. X. (2019b). *How to be an anti-racist: A conversation with Ibram X. Kendi* [Interview by Z. Warfield]. https://www.yesmagazine.org/social-justice/2019/10/25/racist-policy-antiracism-resist/

Love, B. (2019a). *Ally vs. Co-Conspirator: What it means to be an abolitionist teacher*. Lecture presented at We Want to Do More Than Survive. Retrieved 2019, from https://www.c-span.org/video/?c4844082/user-clip-ally-vs-conspirator-means-abolitionist-teacher

Love, B. L. (2019b). *We want to do more than survive: Abolitionist teaching and the pursuit of educational freedom*. Beacon Press.

Love, B. L. (2020). Teachers, we cannot go back to the way things were. Education Week.

Maurantonio, N. (2017). "Reason to hope?": The white savior myth and progress in "post-racial" America. *Journalism & Mass Communication Quarterly, 94*(4), 1130–1145.

McEldowney, M. (2018). *What Charlottesville changed*. Retrieved from https://www.politico.com/magazine/story/2018/08/12/charlottesville-anniversary-supremacists-protests-dc-virginia-219353

Michael, A., & Conger, M. C. (2009). Becoming an anti-racist White ally: How a White affinity group can help. *Perspectives on Urban Education, 6*(1), 56–60.

Niesz, T., Korora, A. M., Walkuski, C. B., & Foot, R. E. (2018). Social movements and educational research: Toward a united field of scholarship. *Teachers College Record, 120*(030308), 1–41.

Patel, V. S. (2011). Moving toward an inclusive model of allyship for racial justice. *The Vermont Connection, 32*(1), 9.

Powell, J., & Kelly, A. (2017). Accomplices in the academy in the age of black lives matter. *Journal of Critical Thought and Praxis, 6*(2). https://doi.org/10.31274/jctp-180810-73

Ramsey, F. (2014, November 22). *5 tips for being an ally*. [Video File]. Retrieved from https://www.youtube.com/watch?time_continue=97&v=_dg86g-QlM0&feature=emb_logo

Sanborn, E. K., Jackson, R. G., Moore, T. S., Skelton, S. M., & Thorius, K. A. K. (2019). *Developing authentic socially just spaces at the systemic level. Equity dispatch*. Midwest & Plains Equity Assistance Center (MAP EAC).

Snow, D. A., & Benford, R. D. (1999). Alternative types of cross-national diffusion in the social movement arena. See della Porta et al. 1999, pp. 23–49.

Washington, J., & Evans, N. J. (1991). Becoming an ally. In *Beyond tolerance: Gays, lesbians, and bisexuals on campus* (pp. 195–204).

Wing, A. (2020). Critical race feminism. In M. David & M. Amey (Eds.), *The SAGE encyclopedia of higher education* (Vol. 1, pp. 319–321). SAGE Publications. https://doi.org/10.4135/9781529714395.n127

Wright, P. I. (2019). Cultural humility in the practice of applied behavior analysis. *Behavior Analysis in Practice, 12*, 805–809. https://doi.org/10.1007/s40617-019-00343-8

Young, I. M. (2000). Five faces of oppression. In M. Adams, W. J. Blumenfeld, R. Castaneda, H. W. Hackman, M. L. Peters, & X. Zuniga (Eds.), *Readings for diversity and social justice: An anthology on racism, antisemitism, heterosexism, ableism, and classism* (2nd ed., pp. 35–44). Routledge.

6

Service or Saviorism: Deconstructing Benevolent Racism in the Helping Professions

Brittany M. Wake

The term 'helping professional' elicits connotations of altruism and humanitarianism attributable to individuals who have established careers supporting the health and/or development of others. It is observable through even the most inconsequential or casual conversations that these professionals integrate the aforementioned connotations into their own self-concept and personal identity, often citing an aptitude for helping as the impetus for their occupational endeavors. For evidence of this phenomenon we need go no further than the classrooms of helpers-in-training. Early in my own experience of graduate training to become a professional clinical mental health counselor, a professor asked the students in the class to introduce ourselves by explaining our attraction to the counseling field. As the first student motioned to introduce themselves and express their passion for the field, the professor added the caveat—"and please, something other than your service to your friends as

B. M. Wake (✉)
North Carolina State University, Raleigh, NC, USA
e-mail: bwake@ncsu.edu

© The Author(s), under exclusive license to Springer Nature Switzerland AG 2022

K. Johnson et al. (eds.), *Developing Anti-Racist Practices in the Helping Professions: Inclusive Theory, Pedagogy, and Application*,
https://doi.org/10.1007/978-3-030-95451-2_6

the resident counselor." The exasperation evident in the professor's comment communicated the extent to which early conceptualizations of one's professional identity can be painfully trite or cliché. Both impressed by the accuracy of the professor's prediction, evidenced by my classmates' reevaluation of their responses, and self-conscious about my own reasons for pursuing a counseling degree, I became more observant of conceptualizations of professional identity across settings.

In addition to narratives about one's personal history indicating a proclivity for service- oriented work (counseling, teaching, nursing, etc.), it is notable that conversations about helping identity typically include some allusion to the professional's specific desire or inclination to serve "under-resourced" or otherwise marginalized communities including Black, Indigenous, and other People of Color (BIPOC). More thorough and sophisticated articulations of this drive include the contextualization of disparities in representation and wellness outcomes as well as other repercussions of systemic oppression. So what possible threat could be posed by burgeoning professionals expressing an intention to improve the lives of marginalized communities? In pursuit of their goals, however well-intentioned, both BIPOC and White professionals risk perpetuating saviorism and disempowering the communities they strive to serve when these goals are devoid of adequate problematization of conceptualizations of help and service. Absent this interrogation, saviorism is identifiable in these conceptualizations marked by paternalistic practices derivative of pro-racist ideology and White Supremacy Culture where people of color, particularly Black people, are simultaneously infantilized and adultified. These practices are reflective of benevolent racism which is defined by Esposito and Romano (2016) as "a seemingly race-conscious frame that acknowledges and ostensibly condemns a system of White privilege and racial inequity, but does so in ways that legitimize and reinforce racist attitudes, policies, and practices" (p. 161). This chapter deconstructs 'helping' behavior imbued with benevolent racism through an examination of oppression, identity development, and suggestions for potential pedagogical approaches and techniques that address microaggressive tendencies.

Contextualizing Systemic Racism and Related Oppression in the Helping Professions

Despite our enduring, collective insistence that oppression is antithetical to our professions, an honest reckoning with the current and historical context of oppression within systems of education, medicine, mental health support, and others can immediately sober us of such a delusion. Not only is oppression endemic to our professions, it is foundationally so. The cursory consideration of existing racial disparities in each of our fields can exemplify the gravity and pervasiveness of systemic oppression.

School suspensions and expulsions that generate the nexus of the school-to-prison pipeline; maternal and infant mortality rates gone unremedied by preventive measures; and diagnoses of severe and persistent mental health challenges that seemingly justify institutionalization are but three specific consequences of systemic oppression that derive from historical and continued practices of institutional racism in helping professions. These practices are rooted in White supremacy, and specifically anti-Black conceptualizations of Black people as criminals who are immune to pain and prone to pathology. I center the experiences of Black people in my specification of anti-Blackness because it precisely contextualizes the racial caste system of the United States (U.S.), which not only positions Whiteness at the apex of the hierarchy, but relegates proximity to Blackness to the lowest point. The aforementioned conceptualization and caste system rely on the belief, implicit or otherwise, in the subordinate humanity of BIPOC communities relative to White people. Belief in the subordinate humanity of BIPOC communities in the context of professional helping may appear hyperbolic at first glance given the common thought that suggests such beliefs are reserved for people who espouse conscious hate toward BIPOC communities. Upon closer inspection, however, it is evident that some compulsory 'helping' behaviors are also dehumanizing given their paternalistic connotations. Consider, for example, the history of discourse on benevolent sexism. Undermining the autonomy and agency of women by assuming they are incapable of completing a task, physical or intellectual, and attempting to 'rescue' them from the event without provocation is a socialized practice among cisgender men. This practice is typically regarded as an extension of kindness though it may communicate an indignity or perception of inferiority to the woman receiving the 'help'. Framed by Sue et al. (2007) as *micro-insults*, this form of dehumanization is a common occurrence across various experiences of marginalization from ableism to xenophobia. Of course our professions *should* be sites of liberation from and resistance to oppression, and perhaps that is what we intend to convey when we take positions of moral authority relevant to our respective personal and professional identities. The reality of our existence within a society bound by cis-hetero Patriarchy and White Supremacy, however, requires a critical assessment of our own complicity in systems of oppression—even when we believe our actions are a form of kindness.

White Supremacy Culture and Saviorism

Popular discourse, and often academic discourse, routinely fails to adequately and accurately contextualize White Supremacy. Common rhetoric typically ignores or minimizes the structural and cultural pervasiveness of racism by relegating it to acts of extreme violence committed by individuals who choose to identify as Nazis, KKK members, Proud Boys, and other white nationalists (Sondel et al., 2019). This rhetoric suggests that consciously espousing hate for racially marginalized people is elemental to White Supremacy and thus absolves White people who do not knowingly express racist vitriol. Critical examination of this phenomenon, however, situates White Supremacy within its proper sociopolitical context beyond its more virulent iterations. Sondel et al. (2019) describe White Supremacy as:

> Not only the extreme political movement of hateful racists but also the everyday, mundane social practices that position White perspectives at center stage and protect the interest of White People at the expense of people of color (Delgado & Stefancic, 1997)… That is, White supremacy is not only about individuals' identities but also about ideologies and institutions, much as Dyson (1996) argues about Whiteness itself. Similarly, hooks (1989) challenges us to see supremacy in not merely individual actions, but in the "very structure of racist domination and oppression"

> (p. 113) that permeates society and is resistant to so-called liberal attempts to challenge racism. (pp. 5–6)

Relying solely on the most egregious and overt forms of White supremacist behavior and implying that malicious intent is a requisite component of White Supremacy serves only to obfuscate its ubiquity and perpetuate its cultural insidiousness. It is precisely the cultural prevalence of White Supremacy that Okun (n.d.) exposes in their description of the characteristics of White Supremacy Culture within professional organizations: *perfectionism, sense of urgency, defensiveness, quantity over quality, worship of the written word, only one right way, paternalism, either/or thinking, power hoarding, fear of open conflict, individualism, I'm the only one, progress is bigger – more, objectivity*, and *right to comfort*. Within this contextual framework, saviorism can be understood as a composite of each of these characteristics, specifically emphasizing *only one right way, paternalism*, and *objectivity*. According to Okun (n.d.), hierarchical thinking or the belief that there is "only one right way" (p. 4) is a manifestation of White dominance that perpetuates the recursive belief in the omniscience of Whiteness evolving from such supremacist ideologies as Manifest Destiny. In Okun's (n.d.) own words, this is:

> The belief [that] there is one right way to do things and once people are introduced to the right way, they will see the light and adopt it. When they do not adapt or change, then something is wrong with them (the other, those not changing), not with us (those who 'know' the right way.) [It is] similar to the missionary who does not see value in the culture of other communities, [but] sees only value in their beliefs about what is good. (p. 4)

Even more incendiary than sheer egocentrism and controlling behavior that might repel others in interpersonal relationships, the only-one-right-way rhetoric deployed in institutional settings and as a societal principle has deleterious effects on entire communities of people, particularly in combination with paternalism and perceived objectivity. By examining the relationship between hierarchical thinking, the sociopolitical power to impose these ideas through paternalism, and the justification of this power based on positivist or objective ontological and epistemological beliefs, we can more readily identify the oppression of the marginalized communities subject to claims of 'better' knowledge (Okun, n.d.). When enacted by helping professionals, these behaviors, considered to be benign or benevolent, are the embodiment of saviorism. Belying the notion that the U.S. has unearthed the last vestiges of what Bonilla-Silva (2015) refers to as "racial domination projects (e.g., colonialism, slavery, labor migration, etc.)" (p. 1359), the saviorism inherent in helping institutions continues the tradition of cultural practices that position Whiteness as the normative standard of human progress by which all others are to be measured.

So what exactly *is* saviorism and how do we make the distinction between that and advocacy for and/or service to racially minoritized communities whose needs have been grossly undermined and neglected, currently and historically? In a seven-part series of tweets from his Twitter account, memorialized in his article from The Atlantic, author Teju Cole (2012) provided an acerbic and poetic depiction of what he has coined the "White Savior Industrial Complex" (para 1) that supports a clear distinction. According to Cole (2012):

> The White savior supports brutal policies in the morning, funds charities in the afternoon, and receives awards in the evening. The banality of evil transmutes into the banality of sentimentality. The world is nothing but a problem to be solved by enthusiasm. This world exists simply to satisfy the needs – including, importantly, the sentimental needs – of White people and Oprah. The White Savior Industrial Complex is not about justice. It is about having a big emotional experience that validates privilege. (paras. 3–5)

Based on this depiction, the distinction between serving and saving lies in discernment of whose thoughts and feelings are being prioritized in supposed acts of altruism. It is dependent upon which voices are being amplified when considering what constitutes helpful behavior. Arguably the most important distinction that can be gleaned from Cole's (2012) description is that service and advocacy are politically dense with the constant work of obstructing oppression while saviorism is opportunistic, pursuing "justice" that is leisurely and convenient. Consistent with the previous discussion of the ways in which White Supremacy Culture permeates all of our lives, People of Color and White people, it follows that People of Color can perpetuate saviorism along with their White peers. It is the differential sociopolitical power, race-based or otherwise, between helping professionals and the communities we seek to support that is the foundation for saviorism. Because they experience different vantage points of Whiteness, however, White helping professionals and helping professionals of color have disparate access to power and wield it differently, operating two sides of the same coin: the former relying on internalized superiority while the latter emphasizes exceptionalism and respectability politics.

Internalized Superiority

In the U.S. system founded upon ideals of racial Capitalism, sociopolitical hierarchies are fundamental. The stratification of race, specifically, positions White people as the dominant and supreme beings at the apex of the hierarchy. Beyond the vital political and economic power this stratification affords White people in terms of material advantages directly at the expense of Black, Indigenous, and other People of Color, there are also salient cultural implications. Among the most prominent of the cultural implications are those that suggest that the advantages of Whiteness are justifiable. This suggestion is derived from the internalized belief of White people that they are indeed more evolved and innately human than their peers. As previously mentioned, this assertion may appear to be hyperbolic or feel unfair, particularly to those that vehemently deny any personal support of White supremacy. To reiterate my earlier sentiments, however, thorough engagement with critical race studies demonstrates that it is both naïve and even disingenuous to expect that the enveloping culture of White Supremacy is easily avoided at the individual level and could possibly leave some White people unscathed by ingrained superiority (DiAngelo, 2011). DiAngelo (2011) frames this phenomenon as one resulting from White people being well, if not excessively, represented in all facets of life with neutral to positive depictions. It is the defensiveness or *fragility* (DiAngelo, 2011) regarding this cultural truth that makes its continuation possible, thus perpetuating outcomes such as saviorism. If White people are led to believe throughout their lives that they are superior to people of color- and they are led to believe this- there is a high potential of them imposing themselves onto others. In the helping professions, this can be manifested in the way White people approach the people they serve from a deficit perspective, seeking to provide a charitable effort to BIPOC communities supposedly deprived of the same quality character as the helper.

Exceptionalism and Respectability Politics

Despite not possessing the power of Whiteness, People of Color in the U.S. are inculcated by its principles and are capable of enforcing it amongst their peers. In an American Psychological Association conference award address, Comas-Díaz (2000) used the term *horizontal hostility* to refer to this phenomenon in which "people of color project their self-hate onto other people of color with horizontal hostility that cannot be expressed directly to the ones in power" (p. 1320). Akin to the defense mechanisms of displacement and projection outlined in psychoanalytic theory, Comas-Díaz (2000) conceptualizes horizontal hostility as a result of *Post- Colonization Stress Disorder*, a non-pathological and adaptive response to colonial oppression. In the helping professions, horizontal hostility is not necessarily enacted through the use of slurs, insults, pejoratives, or other forms of derogation that may typically occur within and between communities of color. In the context of helping, horizontal hostility is much more likely to include the enforcement of respectability politics and exceptionalism which direct Black, Indigenous, and other People of Color to conform to the demands of Whiteness by assimilating to the cultural norms of White people that supposedly represent the standard of behavior.

Cole's (2012) aforementioned reflections on the White Saviorism Industrial Complex include a contemptuous mention of Oprah Winfrey. It is tempting to dismiss this comment as simple sneering humor directed at the billionaire class who hoard wealth and assuage their guilt with charitable efforts or as a convenient reference to the lore associated with Oprah herself as a transcendental figure who transforms the lives of communities across the globe, particularly in African nations. Cole's (2012) inclusion of Oprah as an arbiter of the White Saviorism Industrial Complex, however, speaks profoundly to the influence Black, Indigenous, and other People of Color can have when they are positioned in proximity to Whiteness and power through Capitalism. A critical aspect of Oprah's transcendental identity is the celebration of her as a prominent emblem of upward mobility or what is colloquially referred to as a "rags-to-riches" story. It is a story that is exploited as the *exceptional* effort of a person experiencing intersectional oppressions deriving from race, class, and gender domination; a story that is abused to assume some legitimacy to the myth of meritocracy (Sue et al., 2007). When Black, Indigenous, and other People of Color are exceptionalized and subsequently internalize the rhetoric that mark them as distinct from and superior to other People of Color, they are prone to inflicting that ideology onto their peers through elitist notions of rugged individualism. As another example, we can refer to former U.S. President Barack Obama and former First Lady Michelle Obama for a case study. President Obama's election in 2008 was a monumental and historic victory for the U.S. as he became the first, and thus far the only, Black, Indigenous, or other Person of Color to be elected to the office along with his Black wife and children. Consistent with their role as the verifiable exception, the Obamas offer a version of help by weaponizing respectability politics evidenced in their admonishment of young Black people during their respective addresses at Historically Black College and University (HBCU) commencement ceremonies. Potentially perceived by the Obamas as preparation to thrive in a racist system, their comments, in line with the rhetoric of "when they go low...", rightfully drew ire from critics who note that it is erroneous to believe that compliance with oppression begets liberation or that oppressed peoples bear individual culpability for their experiences of systemic racism. This misguided adoption of exceptionalism and its translation into the imposition of respectability politics illustrates how these concepts coincide with saviorism exhibited by helping professionals of color. Without thorough investigation of our authority, validated by educational or professional achievement standardized by White Supremacy Culture, People of Color may pervert their attempts to support BIPOC communities by employing tactics that are paternalistic and individualistic.

Identity Development

Various psychological models have been developed as a means to describe the stages or statuses pertaining to social identity progression relevant to a particular trait. Racial identity development models demystify intrapersonal conceptualizations of race and their resulting manifestations in interpersonal and societal relationships (Helms, 1995). Helms's (1995) white and people of color racial identity development models, in particular, offer a developmental framework for the ways in which the manifestations of saviorism demonstrated in the previous section are discernible and predictable.

Helms's White and People of Color Racial Identity Development Models

In her racial identity development models for White people and people of color, respectively, Helms (1995) outlined the continuous developmental statuses of individuals in relation to racial stimuli across the lifespan. The primary developmental task according to Helms (1995) is for individuals to dismantle their intrapersonal relationships to White Supremacy which are observed as efforts to protect entitlement for White people and variations of internalized inferiority for People of Color. The journey of maturation toward achieving this task, even if situational rather than sustained permanently, is marked by distinguishable but indiscrete statuses ranging from least to most sophisticated cognitive and affective socio-racial competence (Helms, 1995). Additionally, each status is associated with particular Information Processing Strategies (IPS) that offer insight into an individual's intrapsychic world based on the particular schemata used for responding to racialized events (Helms, 1995). Helms's (1995) White Racial Identity Development Model includes 6 ego statuses and the related IPS:

> a) Contact – denial, obliviousness, or avoidance of anxiety-evoking racial information; b) Disintegration – disorientation, confusion, and suppression of information; c) Reintegration – distortion of information in an

> own-group-enhancing manner; d) Pseudoindependence – reshaping racial stimuli to fit one's own "liberal" societal framework; e) Immersion-Emersion – reeducating and searching for internally defined racial standards; and f) Autonomy – flexible analyses and responses to racial material. (p. 188)

Helms's (1995) People of Color Racial Identity Development Model also includes 6 ego statuses and the correlated IPS:

> a) Conformity – denial, minimization, and selective perception; b) Dissonance – anxiety, ambivalence, or disorientation; c) Immersion – hypersensitivity and dichotomous thinking; d) Emersion – vigilance and energized collectivism; e) Internalization – intellectualization and abstraction; and f) Integrative Awareness – flexible analyses and responses to racial stimuli. (p. 190)

In addition to her Racial Identity Development Models, Helms (1995) proposed a Racial Identity Interaction Model in which the racial identity statuses not only communicate critical information about an individual's internal process, but may be used as prescient information for anticipating, interpreting, and intervening in interpersonal dynamics where race is a perceived factor. Helms (1995) outlined the premises of the Racial Identity Interaction Model as follows:

> a) racial identity statuses structure people's reactions to one another as well as to external events, b) people form harmonious or disharmonious alliances with one another based on the tenor of their expressed racial identity, c) racial reactions occur within the context of direct or vicarious interpersonal activities, and d) patterns of reactions within an interpersonal context can be classified according to quality. (p. 191)

Harmonious alliances include *Parallel* and *Progressive* relationships, while disharmonious alliances are categorized as *Regressive* and/or *Crossed* (Helms, 1995). Despite possible connotations, harmonious relationships do not necessarily imply interactions that are productive or without conflict. Parallel relationships indicate an interaction in which individuals share the same predominant racial identity development status or one analogous to the other if there is a White/BIPOC interracial dynamic (Helms, 1995). It is just as likely from this theoretical perspective for individuals with more sophisticated racial identity statuses to partner in endeavors of racial liberation as it is for individuals from less sophisticated racial identity statuses to collude in the perpetuation of racism, either knowingly or unknowingly. In Progressive, Regressive, and Crossed interactions, individuals inhabit disparate spaces on the respective continuum of racial identity status. Progressive interactions occur when an individual ordained with social power or authority in the context of a relationship (e.g. a teacher-student relationship), has a more sophisticated conceptualization of race than the person with less positional authority and can use their influence to advance the other person through the continuum of racial identity development statuses (Helms, 1995). Regressive relationships hold implications of social power beyond race inversely to Progressive relationships. In the case of a teacher-student relationship, a Regressive interaction would indicate that the teacher has less sophisticated cognitive and affective structures pertaining to race in comparison with the student. In these interactions, the person with less power but more knowledge experiences subjugation and repression of ideas by the authority figure, intensifying the experience of racial oppression if the person with less authority is also Black, Indigenous, or another Person of Color. Crossed interactions are a subset of Regressive interactions in which individuals are at polarized ends of their respective racial identity development continuums, though without the additional implications of social authority (e.g. student-student) (Helms, 1995). Because these relationships are likely to be contentious and there is no social hierarchy confining either individual to the connection, these interactions typically dissolve quickly and prevent the formation of a sustained relationship (Helms, 1995). In relationships characterized by a social power differential where the person with less authority maintains agency to discontinue the relationship at their discretion, such as in the relationship between a nonmandated client and their counselor, the relationship may be viewed as either Regressive or Crossed depending on the client's initiation of early termination of the therapeutic alliance.

Helms (1995) stated that the racial identity development and associated racial identity interaction models are intended to be used as diagnostic tools to create predictability around responses to racial stimuli. In consideration of the professional identities of helping professionals and their propensity to engage in saviorism, Pseudoindependence for White people and the combination of Conformity and Internalization for People of Color are arguably the most salient and predictable of the ego statuses. These statuses have implications for the professional themselves as well as the *interpersonal environment* they are poised to create with those to whom they provide services (Helms, 1995). Among these implications is the omnipresence of liberalism in the helping professional's identity.

Professional Identity and Liberalism

If we are to accept Helms's (1995) assertion that the primary socioracial developmental task is to relinquish internalizations of White superiority, and inversely the inferiority of People of Color, it is reasonable to infer that this developmental task is critical in the professional identity development of individuals in helping roles. More pointed than simply suggesting introspection of cultural values and the expressed commitment to avoid the imposition of those values onto others, this assertion renders helping professionals ineffectual if they have yet to develop relatively sophisticated skills to interpret and respond to racial stimuli without relying on the assumptions of Whiteness. One of these assumptions is a typology in which conventional liberalism endows helping professionals with an upright moral and political character that uniquely qualifies them for service-oriented roles to marginalized communities. Helms (1995) referenced this phenomenon generally in her statement that "typologies typically assign people to one or another of mutually exclusive personality categories (e.g. racist or nonracist), from which race related behavior (in this case) is inferred" (p. 182). For White people this assumption is most apparent during the Pseudo Independence status of racial identity development. Pseudo Independence is characterized by white people aligning themselves with People of Color through self-professed allyship while maintaining an "intellectualized commitment to one's own socioracial group" (Helms, 1995, p. 185). Maintenance of

Pseudo Independence as a dominant racial identity status at both the individual and societal levels is dangerous for White helping professionals and those they intend to serve given the insidiously racist rhetoric they are prone to perpetuate. DiAngelo (2018) referred to this typology as the *good/bad binary* in which the racism of White people is not easily challenged based on their attachment to their self-concept as "good (White) people" deserving of the benefit-of-the-doubt as opposed to the "bad (White) people" identified by their unequivocal support for racism. As we have discussed in previous sections, people of color also have the capacity to perpetuate pro-racist ideology in inter- and intra-racial relationships with one another, though this must not be conflated with the erroneous notion of "reverse racism". When Black, Indigenous, and other People of Color consciously espouse a commitment to improve the lives of communities of color through service (Internalization status) yet uphold standards of Whiteness (Conformity status), whether due to personal convictions, woeful professional obligation or some combination of the two, they may also rely on the recursive logic of liberalism and neoliberalism. Dismantling the integration of unchallenged liberal beliefs within the helping professions is paramount to mitigating saviorism.

Practical Implications

Throughout this chapter it has been my goal to expose saviorism in the context of benevolent or liberal racism and sensitize us to its otherwise subtle nature. Taking heed to Helms's (1995) encouragement to diagnose racial issues so as to provide more meaningful interventions, I have intended to unearth the innate reality of saviorism in the helping professions to mitigate its detrimental effects on marginalized communities. The most pertinent interventions educators and supervisors can implement to support the development of helping-professionals- in-training include deconstructing pathological myths, dismantling egocentrism, and utilizing racial identity assessment and power analysis in the training process.

Deconstructing Pathological Myths

I have already begun the work of deconstructing pathological cultural myths in this chapter. I have examined or alluded to false dichotomies relevant to perpetrators of White Supremacy versus non-perpetrators, the myth of meritocracy, the deceit of rugged individualism and exceptionalism, as well as the unreliable heuristics of typologies such as liberalism. Because the convergence of White Supremacy, Patriarchy, and Capitalism are enduring systems of oppression in the U.S. encompassing the totality of the public and private lives of its inhabitants, critical analysis of its manifestation in the helping professions must be as indefatigable. Ask probing questions about why someone has chosen to embark on a career in the helping professions while challenging them to go beyond the superficial. Personalize conversations by exploring the investments you and others may have in the myths uncovered. Problematize the intended kindnesses that wound the intended recipients.

Evolving Beyond Egocentrism

Egocentrism and saviorism are mutually inclusive concepts as helping professionals may implicitly embody the characteristics when they prioritize their own needs, desires, and goals to help rather than prioritizing the communities with whom they work. In the counseling profession, we refer to the work of differentiating our experiences, needs, desires, and goals from that of the client's as attending to issues of countertransference to avoid value imposition as well as other consequences of overidentification and figure representation. We intend to recognize that left unchecked, our own egocentrism can wreak havoc on the therapeutic relationship and engender a harmful, rather than helpful, environment. Cultural immersion offers one answer to the question of evolving beyond egocentrism. Rather than simply participating in the cultural events of the communities they intend to serve, however, helping professionals must do so in the role of learner while the cultural community offers expertise. This learning must not be mistaken as an opportunity for colonial appropriation, but as an opportunity to have a model for behavior that is functional and adaptive despite the potential difference in approach from the helper which may ordinarily create a deficit perspective. Relatedly, the expertise of an individual or community should be consulted and respected before any service is provided.

Utilizing Racial Identity Development and Interaction Models for Power Analysis

Evaluating the professional quality of individuals in the helping professions is a standard gate-keeping practice, though not without issues of its own. Critical evaluation of one's responses to racial stimuli, however, is an integral step to cultivating professions that will aid the progression of racial liberation. Self-assessments of racial identity development status and comparable assessments from authorities in the profession are predictive tools that can mitigate harm and promote wellness when used consistently. These assessments not only support leaders in advancing burgeoning professionals' developmental levels through Progressive relationships, but prevent Regressive, Crossed, and oppressive Parallel dynamics. Of course, this implies that one intervention is the exclusive promotion of individuals with sophisticated racial conceptualizations to positions of power and influence.

Conclusion

It is true that there are local and global humanitarian crises resulting from colonialism, cultural imperialism, and Capitalism that require urgent attention from helping professionals. The imperative to act in resolution of these violations is often what calls us to our professional roles. The same oppression responsible for the support needed, however, permeates the culture of the helping professions through saviorism, endemic to the helping professions in the context of White Supremacy, Patriarchy, and Capitalism. This is manifest in our behavior when we avoid critical investigation of our complicity in oppressive dynamics. This cultural phenomenon perpetuates pro-racist ideology, regardless of benevolent intentions, and is manifest in our behavior when we avoid critical investigation of our complicity in oppressive dynamics.

Antiracist helping professionals must not be derelict of their responsibility to subvert saviorism by intervening in its dominance across settings. In their respective fields, helping professionals can develop a formalized practice of discussing and assessing saviorism in their discipline's training process through both direct education and supervision. More conscientious and deliberate engagement with the communities we intend to serve beyond the desire or authority to 'help' and understanding how our helping behaviors are sometimes self-serving, allows helping professionals to better honor the agency of marginalized community members and realize antiracist practice.

Guiding Questions

1. What are some racial disparities that exist within your discipline and contribute to the oppression of BIPOC communities?
2. How might you discern the difference between a professional in your discipline who has deconstructed their internalized sense of saviorism and one who has not?
3. Discuss the implications of a helping professional of color participating in the 'saviorism industrial complex' compared to a white helping professional.

Quiz Questions

1. How is benevolent racism defined according to Esposito and Romano (2016)?
2. T/F: White Supremacy and racism require overt action and conscious hatred toward people of color.
3. Name three characteristics of White Supremacy Culture according to Okun (n.d.).
4. Regarding saviorism, internalized superiority is to white helping professionals as ——— and ——— are to BIPOC helping professionals.
5. Why should helping professionals in positions of authority be required to have a sophisticated understanding of race?

References

Bonilla-Silva, E. (2015). The structure of racism in color-blind, "post-racial" America. *American Behavioral Scientist, 59*(11), 1358–1376. https://doi.org/10.1177/0002764215586826

Cole, T. (2012, March 21). The white-savior industrial complex. *The Atlantic*. Retrieved from: https://www.theatlantic.com/international/archive/2012/03/the-white-savior-industrial-complex/254843/. Accessed 13 Feb 2021.

Comas-Díaz, L. (2000). An ethnopolitical approach to working with people of color. *American Psychologist, 55*(11), 1319–1325. https://doi.org/10.1037//0003-066x.55.11.1319

DiAngelo, R. (2011). White fragility. *International Journal of Critical Pedagogy, 3*(3), 54–70.

DiAngelo, R. (2018). *White fracility: Why it's so hard for white people to talk about racism*. Beacon Press.

Esposito, L., & Romano, V. (2016). Benevolent racism and the co-optation of the black lives matter movement. *The Western Journal of Black Studies, 40*(3), 161–173.

Helms, J. E. (1995). An update of Helm's white and people of color racial identity models. In J. G. Ponterotto, J. M. Casas, L. A. Suzuki, & C. M. Alexander (Eds.), *Handbook of multicultural counseling* (pp. 181–198). Sage Publications.

Okun, T. (n.d.). *White supremacy culture*. Dismantling Racism Works. Retrieved December 30, 2020, from https://www.dismantlingracism.org/uploads/4/3/5/7/43579015/okun_-_white_sup_culture.pdf

Sondel, B., Kretchmar, K., & Dunn, A. H. (2019). "Who do these people want teaching their children?" White saviorism, colorblind racism, and anti-blackness in "no excuses" charter schools. *Urban Education, 00*(0), 1–30. https://doi.org/10.1177/0042085919842618

Sue, D. W., Capodilupo, C. M., Torino, G. C., Bucceri, J. M., Holder, A. M. B., Nadal, K. L., & Esquilin, M. (2007). Racial microaggressions in everyday life. *American Psychologist, 62*(4), 271–286. https://doi.org/10.1037/0003-066X.62.4.271

Section II

Antiracist Pedagogy in Helping Professions

7

Antiracist Pedagogy for Helping Professionals

Shuntay Z. Tarver

U.S. social systems such as health care and education have continuously produced outcomes of health inequalities (Owens-Young & Bell, 2020), disproportionate access to resources (Paradies, 2006), and discrepancies in the quality of existing services (Williams & Mohammed, 2009). The visibility of such trends has been heightened by the COVID-19 pandemic, economic disparities, and grotesque displays of racial injustices, such as the murder of George Floyd (Tarver Robinson, & Brown 2022). Helping professionals across various disciplines have responded with disciplinary commitment to examining how professional practices contribute to systemic inequalities. Such response is evidenced by a resurgence of attention to integrating antiracist approaches for teaching discipline specific theories, skills, and practices within helping professions such as counseling (Mason et al., 2021), health professions (Garneau et al., 2017; Godley, et al., 2020), and social work (Phillippo & Crutchfield, 2021).

S. Z. Tarver (✉)
Department of Counseling and Human Services, Old Dominion University, Norfolk, VA, USA
e-mail: smccoy@odu.edu

© The Author(s), under exclusive license to Springer Nature Switzerland AG 2022
K. Johnson et al. (eds.), *Developing Anti-Racist Practices in the Helping Professions: Inclusive Theory, Pedagogy, and Application*,
https://doi.org/10.1007/978-3-030-95451-2_7

While such attention has resulted in a new call to antiracist action, beyond the field of education, less attention has been devoted to deconstructing how racism and structural inequalities are transmitted pedagogically through helping professionals' curricular language, classroom climates, and white supremacists' content across disciplines. Such oversight renders the most well-intentioned helping professionals vulnerable to overlooking how racism is transmitted into helping professions through teaching and learning practices, and thus ill-equipped to engage in antiracist pedagogy. However, employing antiracist practices through teaching methodologies and curricular content that effectively identify and disrupt racism embedded within helping professions requires an understanding of the pervasiveness of racism across disciplines. Such understanding constitutes a multifaceted and interprofessional approach to engaging in antiracist pedagogy (Johnson, et al., 2021).

This chapter introduces antiracist pedagogy as a framework for identifying and dismantling systemic inequities embedded within various helping professions. First, critical race theory (CRT) is used to deconstruct the perpetuation of systemic inequalities across U.S. social systems, and to reveal how racism is foundational to U. S. helping professions. Antiracist pedagogy is then defined as an essential framework for dismantling systemic racism. Next, an introduction to antiracist interprofessional collaboration is provided. Consideration of antiracist interprofessional collaboration emphasizes the relevance of discipline-specific chapters for the collective advancement of antiracist pedagogy across helping professions. Finally, this chapter concludes with an introduction to six chapters within this section that collectively offer illustrations for engaging in antiracist pedagogy.

A Critical Race Examination of the United States Helping Professions

Disparate outcomes reflecting systemic inequalities are translated through White supremacist theoretical content, teaching methodologies, and professional curriculums across the U.S. helping professions. Persistent inequitable outcomes of marginalized populations, across U.S. social systems, can best be deconstructed through the lens of Critical Race Theory (CRT). As noted in Chap. 2 by Vajda, Belcher, Borden, and Rivas, CRT was developed as a legal framework for deconstructing how the purported objective constitutional law consistently resulted in unjust outcomes for individuals who were not White (Delgado & Stefancic, 2017; Crenshaw et al., 1995). Thus, the utility of CRT with respect to unveiling the prevalence of racism, through the transmission of White supremacy into disciplinary training of helping professionals is ideal. While multiple tenets are beneficial for analyzing how white supremacy is maintained and transmitted, the CRT postulation of the endemic nature of racism is most apropos. I begin with a discussion of white supremacy, utilizing the CRT lens of the endemic nature of racism, to deconstruct the insidious transmission of White supremacy into helping professions within the United States.

White Supremacy

According to the Merriam-Webster dictionary, White supremacy is "the belief that the White race is inherently superior to other races and that White people should have control over people of other races" (Merriam-Webster, n.d.). It is also "the social, economic and political systems that collectively enable White people to maintain power over people of other races" (Merriam-Webster, n.d.). CRT scholars that study racism within U.S. social systems argue that White supremacy is far more than an individual overt activity that clearly communicates inferiority of all persons who are non-white (Bonilla-Silva, 1997). Rather, within the U.S., White supremacy is institutional and operates within social systems to produce racist outcomes despite societal shifts sanctioning overtly racist behavior (Crenshaw et al., 1995). White supremacy has been systematically embedded in all U.S. social systems and reflects changing manifestations that continue to produce racist outcomes. It ensures that aligning with whiteness affords individuals societal privileges and access to resources such as health care, quality education, mental health services, and other assets to enhance one's quality of life. Conversely, those who are not perceived to align with standards of whiteness are stratified into a racial hierarchy where accessing resources and privileges within society is more easily achieved by one's proximity to whiteness. The further one is perceived to be from the standard of whiteness, the more barriers and societal marginalization they are likely to experience. From the CRT perspective of the endemic nature of racism, it is apparent that societal marginalization is defined by race irrespective of economic classifications that may be more in line with Whiteness (Ladson-Billings & Tate, 1995). For example, research indicates that a wealthy Black woman, with optimal health care is likely to experience worse health outcomes than a poor White woman despite how economically similar she may be to her White male counterpart (Paradies, 2006).

Endemic Nature of Racism Within Helping Professions

The endemic nature of racism makes salient how simultaneously pervasive and inconspicuous White supremacy is within United States social systems, and by proxy within helping professions (Ross, 2016). It does not just happen one way, it is nuanced and manifests in insidious multi-dimensional ways. White supremacy is as characteristic to the United States as capitalism (Smith, 2016). In an explanation of White supremacist logic embedded within the foundational origins of the United States Smith describes this analogy by explaining,

> the capitalist system ultimately commodifies all workers—one's own person becomes a commodity that one must sell in the labor market while the profits of one's labor are taken by someone else. To keep this capitalist system in place—which ultimately commodifies most people—the logic of slavery applies a racial hierarchy to this system (Smith, 2016, p. 67).

Although virtually all U.S. citizens, including White people, participate in capitalism, the economic establishment of the United States primarily relied on the commodification of Black people through chattel slavery. Thus, the logic of White supremacy suggests that Black people are inferior. Consequently, their outcomes across all social systems such as health care and education remain the worst in comparison to other racial groups. Considering the established racial hierarchy embedded within social systems, an examination of the polar opposites of the hierarchy can be used to describe inequitable outcomes across various social systems. For example, it stands to reason that within education, the contributions of Black people to U.S. history are minimized and reduced to subservient passive roles of slavery and within health care (both physical and mental health) diagnoses are normed on White people and Black people are over and misdiagnosed. Collectively, "the black/white binary is central to racial and political thought and practice in the United States, and any understanding of white supremacy must take it into consideration. However, if we look at only this binary, we may misread the dynamics of white supremacy in different contexts" (Smith, 2016, p. 71). As a result, dismantling White supremacy across helping professions requires a critical examination of how White supremacy is embedded across all helping professions, and how it contributes to perpetuating inequities across the existing racial hierarchy beyond the polar opposites. Thus, while our issue is not just Black and White, history suggests we must include a deconstruction of the foundation of the racial hierarchy to effectively disrupt existing inequities across social systems (Smith, 2016).

Resistance to Dismantling White Supremacy

It is imperative that helping professionals understand that just as the manifestations of White supremacy have shifting institutional manifestations, so too does the resistance to its dismantling. Disrupting White supremacy across social systems is an arduous task that has been systemically resisted. Kendi's (2019) description of antiracism, framed systemically, offers an explanation of this resistance by postulating:

> Racist power produces racist policies out of self-interest and then produces racist ideas to justify those policies. But racist ideas also suppressed the resistance to policies that are detrimental to White [supremacy] by convincing average people that inequity is rooted in "personal failure" and is unrelated to policies. Racist power manipulates ordinary people into resisting equal-

> izing policies by drilling them on what they are losing with equalizing policies and how those equalizing policies are anti-White. White [supremacy] do[es] not want to define racial hierarchy or policies that yield racial inequities as racist. To do so would be to define their ideas and policies as racist instead they define policies not rigged for white people as racist. Ideas not centering White lives are racist (Kendi, 2019, pp 129- 130).

As a result, societal advancements to dismantling White supremacy consistently face opposition that threatens the regression of societal shifts toward equity. One example of systemic resistance is the political controversy surrounding CRT as a theoretical framework for deconstructing White supremacy. Strategies of systemic resistance have resulted in misrepresentation of the theoretical origins, scholarly meaning and reframed it as a racist theory that teaches hate within educational settings (Fortin, 2021). For example, a Texas Public Policy Foundation publicly disseminated a flyer that identified words that should be considered synonymous with CRT, and thus rallied against the impact it was having on children within K-12 educational settings (Ramsey, 2021). These identified words included terms such as "equity, diversity, inclusion, identity, social constructs, anti-racism, and white privilege/fragility/supremacy/ culture/ prejudice, and social justice or restorative justice" (Ramsey, 2021). The growing political controversy of CRT has resulted in federal, state, and local legislation successfully enacted to ban its utilization in various contexts from federal training to inclusion of experiences outside of those supporting White supremacy. In a recent interview Kimberlé Crenshaw, a founding CRT scholar, expressed her growing concern for the progress of institutional resistance to dismantling White supremacy through mischaracterization. She stated,

> The biggest risk is that this tried-and-true framing of antiracism, as racist against White people, is going to win again. It won at the end of the civil war, when civil rights were framed as reverse discrimination against White people. It won after Brown versus Board of Education when integration was framed as damaging White children, and it could win now if people don't wake up and have a sense of what's at stake. You're not going to hear, and you should, what is happening with these bans you're not going to hear that an essay by Ta'Nahashi Coates was the reason why a teacher was fired,

you're not going to hear about the affinity groups in colleges and universities and the educational programs that are being canceled" (Crenshaw, 2021).

The resistance to CRT that Crenshaw critiqued has often been rooted in the assumed dissonance between the historical origins of U.S. social systems and the current inequitable outcomes that they produce. However, current trends suggest that not only is there a connection between systemic racial hierarchies, and the disparate outcomes that they are producing; but maybe an implication that systems are doing what they were, by design created to do—maintain White supremacy through the perpetuation of systemic inequities. Thus, while a complete historical analysis of the social systems that helping professionals are situated in is beyond the scope of this chapter, it is important to note that across helping professions there is an urgent need that requires a multi-faceted intervention. Although the establishment of existing social systems that produce inequitable outcomes far outdates any readers of this chapter, the pervasiveness of White supremacy embedded in the foundations is undeniable. This is evidenced by the ways that White supremacy has continually resulted in outcomes of racial disparities across social institutions. Such trends emphasize the need for strategies that dismantle White supremacy through the adoption of antiracist educational practices. Helping professionals committed to antiracism are well positioned to engage in the identification and institutionalization of antiracist approaches within the educational practices of helping professions that work toward dismantling White supremacy.

Antiracist Pedagogy

Antiracist pedagogy is an action oriented approach for engaging teaching and training professionals in ways that dismantle White supremacy within the educational curriculum. Rooted in this approach is an acknowledgment that instructional methods, professional curriculum, and developing skills influence the systemic outcomes. As Kendi (2019) asserted, "movement from racist to antiracist is always ongoing—it requires understanding and snubbing racism based on biology, ethnicity, body, culture, behavior, color, space, and class. And beyond that, it means standing ready to fight against racism's intersections" (p. 10). Thus, antiracist pedagogy requires taking these actions to address White supremacy within the curriculum, classroom, and training contexts of helping professionals. Because helping professions have White supremacy steeped in their theoretical foundations, disciplinary practices, and curricular methods, antiracist pedagogy requires critical analyses of the disciplinary traditions and procedures that contribute to the maintenance and perpetuation of White supremacy, beyond the articulation of professional standards attempting to mitigate inequitable outcomes (Matais & Mackey, 2016). Antiracist pedagogy is also characterized by a nuanced understanding of the various manifestations of White supremacy over time. It requires critical self-reflection, acknowledgment of emotionality, and activism.

Critical Self-Reflection Antiracist pedagogy requires critical self-reflection both at the individual and systemic levels (Bonilla-Silva, 1997; Garneau et al., 2017; Tarver & Herring, 2019). Individually, helping professionals must recognize their "ability to influence, control, and access resources within their respective roles" (Tarver & Herring, 2019, p. 8). Interpretation of such influence must be understood and situated within the complexities of systemic racial hierarchy because of the influence it yields to the client-helper interaction. Thus, how helping professions were socialized to understand race and how they consider, or not, the impact it has on how they serve their clients directly contributes to the systemic outcomes their clients will experience. Systemic experiences are transmitted through interactions of individual helping professionals. Systemically, critical self-reflection requires an understanding of broader structural inequities. Garneau et al. (2017) suggest that systemically antiracist pedagogy requires "the need to understand issues of racism as extending well beyond individualistic explanations as imbricated with broader social trends" (p. 3). The interconnection between individual professional actions contributes to a broader systemic issue. Collectively, from an antiracist perspective, there is no neutral ground.

> One endorses either the idea of a racial hierarchy as a racist, or racial equality as an antiracist. One either believes problems are rooted in groups of people, as a racist or locates the roots of problems in power and politics as an antira-

> cist. One either allows racial inequities to persevere as a racist, or confront racial inequities as an antiracist. There is no in-between safe space of "non racist" the claim of "non racist" neutrality is a mask for racism (Kendi, 2019, p. 9).

Considering this notion, helping professionals must decide between passively conforming to White supremacist instructional content and practices embedded in the foundations of their profession, without critical self-reflection as to how they are racist as a racist; or critically self-reflect and commit to how they can and will engage in antiracist resistance to White supremacy through their professional practice, as antiracist.

Acknowledgment of Emotionality Antiracist pedagogy is emotional work that requires humanizing the experience of racism (Grosland, 2019; Matais & Mackey, 2016). Disrupting the transmission of White supremacy through educational practices and persisting amidst various manifestations of institutional resistance, is difficult work (Matais & Mackey, 2016). Matais and Mackey (2016) emphasized that "in order to *completely* teach diversity and antiracist theories in our course, we first committed ourselves to teaching the manifestations of whiteness that lie underneath the mere recognition that whites hold racial privilege" (p. 34). To address this issue, they utilized a teaching methodology that acknowledged the emotional work that deconstructing White privilege requires including "1) understanding social complexities: getting emotionally invested; 2) sharing the burden: expectations, strategies, and moving beyond basic; and 3) visions of humanity: demonstrations of a loving education" (Matais & Mackey, 2016, p. 37). Collectively, the engagement in antiracist pedagogy requires difficult emotional work strong enough to endure and persist amidst institutional resistance.

Activism Antiracist pedagogy requires action that advances the dismantling of White supremacy. As previously stated, Kendi (2019) critiques inaction as aligning with racist action that perpetuate systemic inequities. He asserts, "the only way to undo racism is to consistently identify and describe it and then dismantle it" (Kendi, 2019, p. 9). Thus, antiracist pedagogy requires helping professions to consider all aspects of their respective specialized curriculum, disciplinary content, instructional methods, and professional practices to interrogate where White supremacy is being transmitted. Then once identified, action(s) are essential to dismantling White supremacy in ways that will translate into equitable systemic outcomes. Collectively, the chapters in this section will offer various illustrations of and strategies for engaging in antiracist pedagogy. Collectively they offer ways in which the endemic nature of racism across helping professions can be disrupted in ways that advance equitable systemic outcomes.

The systemic nature of White supremacy substantiates the simultaneous need for action across social systems. In the same way that no one person could effectively dismantle White supremacy, no one helping profession can dismantle it alone. As a result, antiracist pedagogy requires helping professionals across social systems such as education, counseling, human services, social work and health care to work together. While this book attempts to encourage considerations for such collaboration, we remain fragmented in our disciplinary presentation; and thus, present discipline-specific examples of antiracist pedagogy. Nevertheless, our contribution lays the groundwork for envisioning ways in which helping professions can collaboratively engage in the unifying task of dismantling systemic White supremacy to advance societal equity. The following section introduces interprofessional collaboration as an antiracist tool for dismantling White supremacy.

Introduction of Antiracist Interprofessional Collaboration

Through interprofessional collaboration, various helping professionals have reduced the discipline-specific barriers to collaboratively meeting the societal needs for mental and physical health, education, and resource accessibility. Interprofessional collaboration, is defined as an educational strategy and best practice clinical approach, in which 'helping professionals' from two or more professions work collectively outside of professional silos to interact, learn, and practice together to enhance quality client/patient care. Within the professional training of helping professions such as medicine, pharmacy, nursing, counseling psychology (Boland et al., 2016), counseling (Johnson

& Mahan, 2020), human services (Johnson et al., 2017), and social work (Jones & Philipps, 2016) interprofessional collaboration has been integrated as a framework for collaborating across disciplines to provide optimal holistic care for clients. This growing field is also well positioned to establish partnerships that work towards dismantling White supremacy through utilizing interdisciplinary antiracist approaches to pedagogy. Interprofessional collaboration sets a precedence for understanding the unique professional language, filling existing gaps in service provision, and working to mitigate structural barriers for care. However, as it currently exists, the field of interprofessional collaboration has been limited in its ability to disrupt White supremacy inherent across helping professions (Cahn, 2020). Nevertheless, examining the strengths of the framework for interprofessional collaboration may provide a foundation upon which helping professionals may incorporate discipline-specific antiracist strategies that could strengthen existing interprofessional collaborations (Cahn, 2020). Although providing specific strategies for engaging an interprofessional collaboration is beyond the scope of this book, we offered a brief introduction to heighten the relevance of all chapters included, beyond the specific disciplines within which readers may be situated. Thus, from the perspective of interprofessional collaboration, all chapters utilize discipline-specific knowledge that advance the common goal of engaging in antiracist pedagogy.

Engaging in Antiracist Pedagogy Across Helping Professionals

In conclusion, this chapter introduces Section II of this book by defining antiracist pedagogy. Rarely do helping professionals deconstruct how White supremacy is transmitted through educational processes where they learn the skills of their respective professions. As a result, helping professions tasked with training emerging helping professionals inadvertently engage in White supremacist ideologies through institutional practices such as, "biased curricula, empirical misrepresentations, and oppressive ideological practices of exclusion" (McCoy, 2018, p. 327). Consequently, helping professionals develop professional behaviors that do little, or nothing, to disrupt systemic inequities, and by proxy will contribute to the perpetuation of racist professional practices that maintain White supremacy. As a result, antiracist examinations of pedagogical practices across helping professions are critical to identifying and disrupting the myriad of ways that professional practices contribute to the maintenance of existing inequities. Without a thorough understanding of how helping professionals are trained, little can be done to effectively disrupt the perpetuation of white supremacist behaviors that are transmitted through professional pedagogy. As a result, outcomes of professional intervention, prevention, and advocacy across helping professions have continued to be plagued by systemic inequalities that stem from misunderstood, unacknowledged, or completely ignored pedagogical practices across disciplines. To mitigate this issue this section provides strategies for engaging in antiracist pedagogical practices that have the potential to disrupt systemic inequalities. Although each chapter is situated within the context of a specific discipline, they each deconstruct white supremacist manifestations within their respective disciplines and respond to Kendi's (2019) call to action by offering strategies for actively engaging in antiracist pedagogy. By addressing antiracist pedagogy across counseling, social work and medicine we seek to unify helping professionals through common language, in ways that encourage antiracist engagement in interprofessional collaboration that will dismantle White supremacy and advance equitable outcomes across U.S. social systems.

References

Boland, D. H., Scott, M. A., Kim, H., White, T., & Adams, E. (2016). Interprofessional immersion: Use of interprofessional education collaborative competencies in side-by-side training of family medicine, pharmacy, nursing, and counselling psychology trainees. *Journal of Interprofessional Care, 30*(6), 739–748. https://doi.org/10.1080/13561820.2016.1227963

Bonilla-Silva, E. (1997). Rethinking racism: Toward a structural interpretation. *American Sociological Review, 62*(3), 465–480.

Cahn, P. S. (2020). How interprofessional collaborative practice can help dismantle systemic racism. *Journal of Interprofessional Care, 34*(4), 431–434. https://doi.org/10.1080/13561820.2020.1790224

Crenshaw, K. (2021). Creator of term 'critical race theory' Kimberle Crenshaw explains what it really is [Interview]. The ReidOut Joy Reid on MSNBC. https://www.youtube.com/watch?v=n4TAQF6ocLU

Crenshaw, K., Gotanda, N., Peller, G., & Thomas, K. (Eds.). (1995). *Critical race theory: The key writings that formed the movement*. New Press.

Delgado, R., & Stefancic, J. (2017). *Critical race theory: An introduction* (3rd ed.). New York University Press.

Fortin, J. (2021, July 27). Critical race theory: A brief history. *New York Times*. https://www.nytimes.com/article/what-is-critical-race-theory.html?searchResultPosition=2

Garneau, A. B., Browne, A. J., & Varcoe, C. (2017). Drawing on antiracist approaches toward a critical antidiscriminatory pedagogy for nursing. *Nursing Inquiry, 25*(1), 1–9. https://doi.org/10.1111/nin.12211

Godley, B. A., Dayal, D., Manekin, E., & Estroff, S. E. (2020). Toward an anti-racist curriculum: Incorporating art into medical education to improve empathy and structural competency. *Journal of Medical Education and Curricular Development, 7*, 1–6. https://doi.org/10.1177/2382120520965246

Grosland, T. J. (2019). Through laughter and through tears: Emotional narratives to antiracist pedagogy. *Race Ethnicity and Education, 22*(3), 301–318. https://doi.org/10.1080/13613324.2018.1468750

Johnson, K. F., Blake, J., & Ramsey, H. E. (2021). Professional counselors' experiences on interprofessional teams in hospital settings. *Journal of Counseling & Development, 99*, 406–417. https://doi.org/10.1002/jcad.12393

Johnson, K. F., & Mahan, L. B. (2020). Interprofessional collaboration and telehealth: Useful strategies for family counselors in rural and underserved areas. *The Family Journal: Counseling and Therapy for Couples and Families, 28*(3), 215–224. https://doi.org/10.1177/1066480720934378

Johnson, K. F., Sparkman-Key, N., & Kalkbrenner, M. T. (2017). Human service students' and professionals' knowledge and experiences of interprofessionalism: Implications for education. *Journal of Human Services, 37*(1), 5–13.

Jones, B., & Philipps, F. (2016). Social work and interprofessional education in health care: A call for continued leadership. *Journal of Social Work Education, 52*(1), 18–29. https://doi.org/10.1080/10437797.2016.1112629

Kendi, I. X. (2019). *How to be an antiracist*. Random House.

Ladson-Billings, G., & Tate, W. F. (1995). Toward a critical race theory of education. *Teachers College Record, 97*(1), 47–68.

Mason, E., Robertson, A., Gay, J., Clarke, N., & Holcomb-McCoy, C. (2021, July). Antiracist school counselor preparation: Expanding on the five tenets of the transforming school counseling initiative. *Teaching and Supervision in Counseling, 3*(2), 4–14.

Matais, C. E., & Mackey, J. (2016). Breakin' down whiteness in antiracist teaching: Introducing critical whiteness pedagogy. *The Urban Review, 48*(1), 1–9. https://doi.org/10.1007/s11256-015-0344-7

McCoy, S. Z. (2018). The intellectual war zone: An autoethnography of intellectual identity development despite oppressive institutional socialization. *Journal of Diversity in Higher Education, 11*(3), 325–346. https://doi.org/10.1037/dhe0000062

Merriam-Webster dictionary. (n.d.). *Merriam-Webster.com dictionary*. Retrieved October 29, 2021, from https://www.merriam-webster.com/dictionary/white%20supremacy

Owens-Young, J., & Bell, C. N. (2020). Structural racial inequities in socioeconomic status, urban-rural classification, and infant mortality in US counties. *Ethnicity & Disease, 30*(3), 389–398. https://doi.org/10.18865/ed.30.3.389

Paradies, Y. (2006). A systematic review of empirical research on self-reported racism and health. *International Journal of Epidemiology, 35*(4), 888–901. https://doi.org/10.1093/ije/dyl056

Phillippo, K. L., & Crutchfield, J. (2021). Racial injustice in schools: Underscoring social work's obligation to promote antiracist practice. *Social Work, 66*(3), 226–235. https://doi.org/10.1093/sw/swab020

Ramsey, R. (2021, July 1). Analysis: A critical culture war over how to teach history. *Texas Tribune*. https://www.texastribune.org/2021/07/01/critical-race-theory-texas/

Ross, L. J. (2016). The color of choice: White supremacy and reproductive justice. In INCITE! Women of Color Against Violence (Ed.), *Color of violence: The INCITE! anthology* (pp. 53–65). Duke University Press.

Smith, A. (2016). Heteropatriarchy and the three pillars of White supremacy: Rethinking women of color organizing. In INCITE! Women of Color Against Violence (Ed.), *Color of violence: The INCITE! anthology* (pp. 66–73). Duke University Press.

Tarver, S. Z., & Herring, M. (2019). Training culturally competent practitioners: Student reflections on the process. *Journal of Human Services, 39*(1), 7–18.

Tarver, S. Z., Robinson, D., & Brown, D. (2022). Triple pandemic: How COVID-19, racial injustices, and economic inequalities worsen ACEs for black families. [Manuscript submitted for publication].

Williams, D. R., & Mohammed, S. A. (2009). Discrimination and racial disparities in health: Evidence and needed research. *Journal of Behavioral Medicine, 32*(1), 20–47. https://doi.org/10.1007/s10865-008-9185-0

8

The Linguistic Gospel Truth: Implementing Inclusive Language Practices for Navigating the Educational Space

Sarah Earlene Burford and Bridget L. Anderson

Introduction

Linguistics, the scientific study of language, is a field that reveals truths for the ways in which the world, its people, and their cultures all come together through language to navigate the spaces in which we live. It is a discipline that holds a depth and breadth of information about how language works, both technically and socially. Linguistics often falls prey to the ultimate sin with regards to knowledge—relegated to platforms unable to disseminate these truths to the world so that teachers and other helping professionals, politicians, journalists, and everyday people can

S. E. Burford
Virginia Beach Public Schools, Old Dominion University, Norfolk, VA, USA
e-mail: sarah.burford@vbschools.com

B. L. Anderson (✉)
Old Dominion University, Norfolk, VA, USA
e-mail: blanders@odu.edu

© The Author(s), under exclusive license to Springer Nature Switzerland AG 2022
K. Johnson et al. (eds.), *Developing Anti-Racist Practices in the Helping Professions: Inclusive Theory, Pedagogy, and Application*,
https://doi.org/10.1007/978-3-030-95451-2_8

have the opportunity to benefit from a raised awareness of how language works and why and how it matters in social struggle. The concepts linguists study and discuss are terminology-heavy and jargon-dense, with complex subfields which require formal training in methods and theories—such as phonology (the study of sound systems), phonetics (the study of production and perception of speech sounds), syntax (the study of grammatical systems), sociolinguistics (the study of language in society), etc.—the list goes on. In this paper, we aim to make linguistics more accessible by sharing a message of linguistic "gospel truths" using a framework that can be put to use by educators across all levels and disciplines and by other helping professionals as well. Language matters to us all.

The first truth which must be addressed when taking up a position as an educator in the classroom is this: language is the foundation of education. It is the base from which we build. It is at the heart of our methods and our results. Though discussions of language use in education often center around English classrooms and English pedagogy, language is ubiquitous—it permeates all subjects and genres and must be utilized to convey all aspects of the educational experience. This basic educational act of sharing and receiving knowledge through language must be carried out in a manner that is anchored in an inclusive and explicitly antiracist linguistic approach. This paper demonstrates that language is not just transactional; it is also social. The linguistic hierarchy reflects the cultural hierarchy and is justified through misinformation about language, which is enshrined in institutions. Therefore, antiracist language practices are vital and urgent and should be implemented cross-disciplinarily. They must not be singularly limited to the English classroom.

The inclusion of antiracist speech in education is paramount, as language is both a linguistic system and a cultural resource. Language *is* culture, and how we use, evaluate, and educate through this medium is reflective of our own cultural blind spots and also, crucially, institutional blind spots. As Milroy and Milroy (1985) point out, there is an appalling (they use the word "depressing") amount of ignorance in the educational system about both the technical aspects of language as well as its social functions. Students listen and absorb the words we share—especially the words that seemingly extend beyond the confines of the assigned curriculum, and, as teachers, it is our duty to take the utmost care when projecting our voices into the educational space. It signifies the ways in which we value the cultures of our students while simultaneously revealing the ways in which we impress our ideas of culture upon those students.

The time is now to utilize language as a cultural resource to empower classroom learners, celebrate the ways in which non-white users of language display the command and expertise of their dialects, and be a vocal protestor of policies that aim to enforce hegemonic practices by way of factually misinformed standard language ideologies. As a society and as a people, Americans have reached a defining moment in our centuries-long antiracist social justice journey. Taking up a position of neutrality is no longer viewed as a symbol of peace, but is in fact an act of weakness, indecision, and at times, betrayal. The notion that ideas can be categorized as *non-racist* has been challenged. For example, Kendi (2019) argues that individuals fall only within the binary categories of *racist,* "one who is supporting a racist policy through their actions or inaction or expressing a racist idea" or *antiracist,* "one who is supporting an antiracist policy through their actions or expressing an antiracist idea." Our analysis of and commentary on the current Mainstream English Only models of language education in the American educational sector utilizes Kendi's definitions of these terms to establish the principles of antiracist language use needed in classrooms that aim to exercise the tenets of linguistic justice (Baker-Bell, 2020a). Educators must vocally and deliberately pick up the baton of action and intentionally act in favor of antiracist policies to establish an antiracist culture within the classroom. Silence as an alternative for action in the face of discriminatory practices is the equivalent of complacency (Kendi, 2019).

Ideology used for purposes of language discrimination is defined by Lippi-Green (2012) as "the promotion of the needs and interests of a dominant group or class at the expense of marginalized groups, by means of disinformation and misrepresentation of those non-dominant groups" (67). Language is the mechanism by which we express these ideologies, and as such, speech must also be established within the racist/antiracist binary, and cannot exist in a neutral purgatory. Family is the foundational source of ideology, but education has the power to either break those chains or reinforce them. In order to free oneself from the confines of such harmful language ideologies, an understanding of the systematic exposure students experience in the educational setting will be outlined as the Mainstream Model of Language Education in America.

Language is a powerful cultural resource that can either impact and improve the social and ideological climate in education or continue the cycle of reinforcing the status quo. The status quo for language at present is the cultural and educational oppression of members of non-mainstream cultural groups. Just as positions of racism cannot exist in a state of neutrality, cultural resources are never power-neutral and do not exist in a power vacuum. The dominant language reflects the dominant cultural group, and enforcement of "prestige" language plays a key role in elevating elite groups and their language in our institutions, including in education. The reality that whiteness is the current stakeholder of power in our classrooms is a core tenet of the power dynamic at play in the current mainstream model of education and is the result of a long history of racism in education. It is past time to challenge a culturally and materially oppressive status quo of linguistic hegemony (domination) of marginalized cultural groups by the dominant power-holders, through misinformation about language so factually incorrect that it amounts to propaganda, in our educational system. This chapter proposes an antiracist linguistic model for education based on basic and well-established linguistic facts that all helping professionals, and certainly all educators, should come to know.

Linguistic Facts and How Language Actually Works

Educators, regardless of discipline, must be in command of linguistic truths and understand how language impacts the larger system of reinforcing toxic norms when language is wielded as a tool to spread misinformation by those we trust as the arbiters of knowledge within the learning environment. Despite the exigencies of language-use consciousness in the classroom, unfortunately, many pre-service programs for aspiring educators do not include the requirement to enroll in a course that would aid in developing an understanding of how people think about language and how language works (Baker-Bell, 2020b; Lippi-Green,

2012). As a result, a dissonance exists between what linguists *know* to be true, and what non-linguists *believe* to be true. The first step in developing linguistic understanding is to come to terms with concepts Lippi-Green coins the "Linguistic Facts of Life," the undeniable truths of language (2012). Once an educator is made aware of these facts, it is essential that these truths be shared—explicitly amongst colleagues in the workplace. Then utilize these linguistic facts as foundational when developing norms for how language works in your classroom pedagogy.

As mentioned in the introduction, the broader field of linguistic study has many schools of thought when discussing the syntactic, phonological, sociolinguistic, and semantic systems of languages, how language is represented in the brain, and other matters of theory and practice. Linguistics is a science and is thus technical. However, the facts of life are where we, as a unified discipline, come together in agreement (Lippi-Green, 2012):

1. All spoken language changes over time and through history.
2. All dialects (both stigmatized and mainstream/standard) are "equal in linguistic terms." This means that stigmatized dialects are fully formed language systems and are just as functional as mainstream/standard varieties of a language.
3. Written language and spoken language are "historically, structurally, and functionally fundamentally different."
4. Spoken language shows variation at all levels, and this is normal and natural. Spoken language is inherently variable. (*adapted from Lippi-Green,* 2012)

Non-linguists are largely familiar with the reality that there are a variety of dialects within the larger scope of the English language (i.e. African American English, Chicano English, Appalachian English, Southern English, etc.) which are often stigmatized and viewed as being less respectable than other mainstream varieties of English. While there has always been a wide *acknowledgment* of language variation by non-linguists, in other words, the understanding that a variety of dialects exist and are used by a large percentage of the American population, public opinion largely renders these dialects "unprofessional, inappropriate for respectable speech communities, and grammatically incorrect." These perspectives hold fast to the (mis)belief that there is exclusively a single variety of English, often referred to as "Standard American English," which is viewed as "correct" and "appropriate" for professional and educational settings (Milroy, 1999, as cited in Hill, 2008, p. 35). We will refer to this "standardized" variety of English as "Mainstream English" (ME). This (mis)belief is in fact a myth. Ideologies of standardization, which will be further elaborated below, simply create a supposition of perceived dialect inferiority and inappropriateness, which results in unequal treatment of non-mainstream dialects. This misinformation is widely reinforced in classroom policies and is upheld as truth in education, adding further to the legacy of misinformed, harmful, and non-inclusive language ideologies. The time has come for education to relinquish a stronghold on dialect discrimination and begin operating in the truth that *all* dialects are rule-governed languages in their own right that have the ability to convey meaning and adapt as necessary (Lippi-Green, 2012). The English language, like all languages, is not a monolith. There are many varieties, and all are valid communicative systems worthy of dignity and respect.

This standard of Mainstream English, which our institutions hold dear as a status quo, thrives as a result of misinformation about "grammatical correctness." In other words, its superiority is upheld under the belief that it is the spoken equivalent of written language, or more specifically, the written form of academic English. However, grammaticality is an issue independent of communicative effectiveness. Chomsky (1957, as cited in Lippi-Green, 2012, p. 13) famously illustrates the difference between what is likely recognizable as "grammatically correct" and whether or not a string of words conveys meaning.

1. Colorless green ideas sleep furiously.

adj adj N V adv

English speakers will immediately recognize that while this sentence is *grammatically* correct, it lacks *semantic* meaning. In other words, the lexical word classes (or parts of speech) are in the correct slots, but together they have no meaning. Dialects and languages rely on far more than "grammatical correctness" to be communicatively effective and add value to a conversation. And these elements of meaning-making will adapt across time and circumstance.

On the level of the individual speaker, all spoken languages are inherently and inevitably variable and will adapt both structurally and socially to the speaker's environment. Likewise, just as time has caused young generations of speakers of the English language to change the way they express enjoyment and excitement over the last 60 decades from *swell*, to *groovy*, to *rad*, to *lit*, dialects as a shared mode of communication which are to be acquired by future generations of humans will continue to change over time. Understanding and internalizing the linguistic "facts of life" serve as necessary prerequisites to facing the current mainstream (and nothing else) language approach in education. In order to grapple with the realities of the teaching profession, one must see the situation in its true form: an oppressive ideology that impersonates truth, impressed upon us by repressive forces and enforced through language. Fairclough (2015) urges "raising people's consciousness of how language contributes to the domination of some people by others, as a step towards social emancipation" (p. 3). We agree, and elaborate on this theme below.

The Mainstream Model of Language Education in America

It is undeniable that language is power—an act that holds the capacity to harm, remedy, indoctrinate, educate, and interpolate ideology, or "the promotion of the needs and interests of a dominant group or class at the expense of marginalized groups, by means of disinformation and misrepresentation of those non-dominant groups" (Lippi-Green, 2012, p. 67). As an institutional entity, the education system has threads of white supremacy woven throughout its policies, traditions, ideologies, and pedagogy which have been continuously sewn from its inception, and is reinforced and perpetuated through the status quo of mainstream language hegemony.

America's history is responsible for the creation of a white supremacist language system in our schools. A widespread belief that non-white cultures are subservient and should remain segregated from the mainstream was established as the status quo and bolstered by language and educational practices which began the tradition of schooling in our country—first intended only for white males. As time passes, an additional constant has remained tried and true: the consistent and large presence of whiteness as the predominant participant (students) and facilitator (teachers) of learning. The dominant group has inherently developed and sustained the prestige of white language, so much so that it has become the governing language "standard" of our education system that encapsulates the inherent power dichotomy which characterizes it as a hegemonic practice to maintain the dominance of mainstream (privileged) language in education.

Hegemonic, culturally dominating ideology advances the needs and interests of a dominant group or class and works to spread misinformation to continue to suppress marginalized and non-dominant groups (Lippi-Green, 2012). By definition, in America, the land of colonization and intentional disenfranchisement of people of color, by way of traditions which were built upon slavery, segregation, and the gate-keeping of information, whiteness prevails as a dominant cultural force in our society. Indeed, it is, at this historical moment, being vigorously defended through a dedicated movement to literally erase (ban) non-white histories and literatures in our schools.

While people of color have spent centuries going through the process of *disenfranchisement*, we argue that society has implemented a promotional system that functions to create and maintain the *superenfranchisment* of whiteness. These ideologized processes characterize the fabric of our ideological landscape, which consequently permeates into our schools at both classroom and administrative levels. The presence of racist ideology does not just manifest in actions; it is perpetuated through our speech, and the classroom is the foundation of standardization. Schools will often implement policies that encourage and promote assimilation of marginalized groups to deny them of their languages and suppress their cultures in order to achieve and succeed in schools (Paris & Alim, 2017). This is nothing new in American education. Native Americans were historically prohibited from speaking their native languages in boarding schools (yet another example of "banning" non-white history, culture, and literature in a white supremacist educational model), as is well documented by the BIA (Bureau of Indian Affairs), and as a result, many Native languages are now lost forever or endangered.

The classroom is a space almost all American children experience over an extended period of time throughout their formative years. While students learn and develop, cultural norms begin to take shape, ideologies are adopted, and identities are formed which will determine how they make sense of the world around them. As generations of students have entered the classroom over time, a cultural imbalance has been a constant reality facing students and teachers (D.O.E, 2016; NCES, 2019a, 2019b)—a memento of the country's racist heritage passed down through the generations. With each passing decade, many Americans look back and relish in the small steps we have taken from darker, racially motivated events from days long gone. In fact, the twenty-first century has been inaccurately described as a "post-racial" society as the memories of segregation and enslavement seem to be faded and relegated to the past. As mentioned earlier, in some places in America these memories and histories are actively being "banned" from being included in school curriculum. Whitewashing of education seems to be, unfortunately, having a moment. The patterns of racial inequality that have left their mark in our classrooms have remained. In 2016, the US Department of Education (D.O.E.) released its most recent report which detailed the state of diversity in the educator workforce between 1987 and 2012. This study found that while the United States education system has become increasingly diverse over time, it still exhibits an overwhelming disparity of racial homogeneity evidenced by the large percentage of white teachers and students who continue to vastly outnumber the other ethnicities represented in America's school systems. While the D.O.E. has not released a version of the diversity report in the last 4–5 years, the National Center for Education Statistics has continued to collect demographic data, and the findings continue to align (Fig. 8.1) with those that determined a racial disparity in the 2016 study which utilized data from 2012.

Despite diversity being an overarching goal in education, a buzzword ever-growing in popularity as a designated goal for schools seeking to

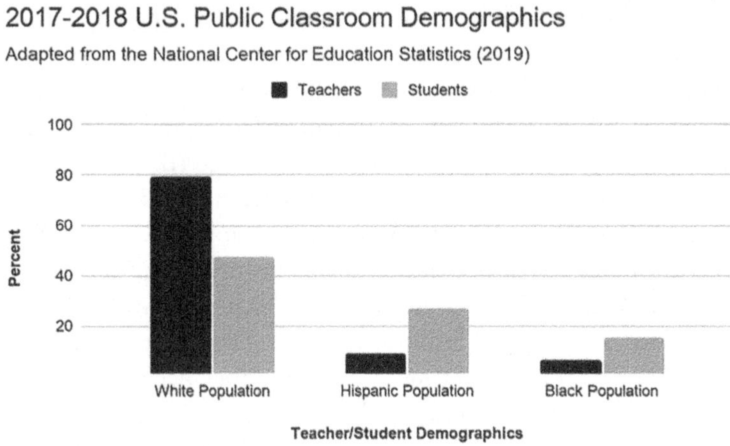

Fig. 8.1 2017–2018 U.S. Public classroom demographics (NCES, 2019a, 2019b)

diversify both faculty and student body, the majority of the demographic marketplace is comprised of white teachers (79.3%) and students (47.6%). While the Black and Hispanic populations disproportionately represent far lower percentages of both teachers and students present in the American public school system, the white demographic continues to be the predominant presence in classrooms across the country. Simultaneously, the representation of Black (6.7%) and Hispanic (9.3) teachers are critically low as white teacher voices outnumber the voices of teachers of color. Per these percentages, white voices receive more representation than any other in education, making it crucial to take up positions of inclusive and antiracist language practices and to exercise linguistic justice not only for students but in the workplace, to advocate and serve as examples for colleagues as well. With such an incongruity, it is important that we as educators are intentional with our language choices and make actionable linguistic strides to take up a position of antiracism.

While the language of education—learning spaces and the language which govern them—overwhelmingly amplifies white ideals, the implementation of an antiracist model of education is urgent for creating a pluralistic and inclusive classroom. Educators must be intentional and explicit in the inclusion of anti-racist language use in the education setting and commit these strategies to daily consciousness and practice if we ever wish to expel the systemic presence of language as a tool for promoting racism in the larger context of our society. The inclusion of black and brown language varieties in our classrooms is crucial as it serves as a tool to explain, implement, and reproduce the realities of these students as they express their perspectives of the world (Smitherman, 1998a).

Our educational system assists in the reinforcement of the larger societal status quo which places whiteness at the top of the metaphorical "cultural food chain." Dominant groups are powerful and can exercise influence over what is allowable and appropriate in society, and take great steps to afford prestige to societal norms and attitudes about appropriateness—including language. The mainstream model of language has a foundational "ideology of tradition" which serves as the basis of all other language ideologies. This ideology is a practice in which individuals seek to preserve, often blindly and without logic or reason, long-standing archaic policies, actions, beliefs, and norms that are viewed as iconic to their dominant group. Those who subscribe to an ideology of tradition may be unaware that their beliefs and subsequent practices are oppressive, and may therefore have greater difficulty recognizing their participation in a model that reinforces a frankly and rankly oppressive status quo. Like all ideologies, the ideology of tradition is most effective when it is rendered invisible through unquestioning acceptance. Such unquestioning acceptance is the root of hegemony (cultural domination) in general and the Mainstream Model of Language Education in particular. As Fairclough (2015) cautions, anything to do with language that is deemed "common sense" is a red flag of ideology used in the service of the domination of some groups by others.

Instead of shifting language perspectives and policies toward what linguists *know* to be true as described with respect to the linguistic "facts of life" above, many of society's views on language are based on what speakers *believe* to be true, likely based on the tradition of these ideals being passed down to subsequent generations. The ideology of tradition's existence within America perpetually "justifies" the continuance of mainstream language ideologies and racially hierarchical policies within education. These policies are measures that cultivate and produce racial inequity and disparity between racial groups (Kendi, 2019) and work to maintain a non-diverse and non-inclusive model of language education in America. Kendi also argues that "race creates new forms of power: the power to categorize and judge, elevate and downgrade, include and exclude" (38). Language is the way in which we commit these acts. We argue that the weaponization of Mainstream English creates forms of power in the classroom: to include/exclude, elevate/downgrade, and validate/invalidate which function to implement and sustain the oppressive model of language education we see in our schools. Any incorporation of these forms of power in a classroom indicates a model of language in the classroom which elevates the language of privilege, thus negating any claims that the classroom is an antiracist one. The inclusion of traditional non-inclusive policies in the classroom materializes in six forms of power implemented in two phases. The first phase will contain purposeful and calculated attacks on Black & Brown varieties of English in an attempt to maintain mainstream language supremacy in the classroom (Table 8.1):

Table 8.1 The mainstream model of language education in America

Phase 1: Overt and purposeful acts to maintain mainstream language ideologies
1. *Exclude speakers of Black and Brown varieties of English*
Peripheralizing speakers who do not conform to mainstream English (ME).
Subtle, yet repeated verbal mention of a student's non-ME features. This establishes a pattern of 'othering' a student drawing continued attention toward linguistic differences
The promotion of exclusively mainstream language conventions in the classroom.
Only speakers who utilize ME are celebrated and lauded for their ability to be "well-spoken" and "articulate."
2. *Downgrade speakers of Black and Brown varieties of English*
Establish a relationship of teacher authority/student dependency.
Students are no longer viewed or treated as experts of language. The teachers establish themselves as the expert who can bridge the gap between the subordinate mother tongue and the prestige of ME.
3. *Invalidate speakers of Black and Brown varieties of English*
Implement standard language ideology, promote forced code-switching.
Upholds a policy that students should abandon their non-ME features when entering the learning arena. Teaches that there are appropriate and inappropriate dialects for specific spaces.

To exclude and downgrade speakers of Black and Brown varieties of English (BBVE) is an isolationist technique to encourage the assimilation of BBVE speakers into ME. When their dialects are marked as salient while speakers of ME are receiving praise, it is a subtle way to stigmatize these non-standard varieties. The implication that a student is no longer an expert of language with respect to their mother tongue is an example of what has been referred to as "linguistic violence" (Martinez, 2017; Skutnabb-Kangas, 1995) which are acts to encourage individual "linguicide" in the classroom which label students with a deficit perspective. These acts seek to promote the domination of the preferred language variety at the expense and erasure of another. In fact, the educational governing bodies have had a history of upholding a "separate but equal" policy towards dialect variation (NCTE, 1996, as cited in Lippi-Green, 2012), and education scholarship frequently advocates codeswitching in the classroom (Elbow, 1999). Separate but equal is not equal, and it never has been and never will be. We strongly reject "separate but (un)equal" approaches to language.

In the Mainstream Model of language, ideologies of language prestige and subsequent language discrimination exist and are reinforced in the classroom. Both educators and linguists have determined that effects (both structurally and symbolically) have contributed to "the longstanding and persistent racial, class-based, and regional achievement/opportunity gaps among U.S. youth, (Mallinson et al., 2011, p. 444). This acknowledgment that the repercussions of using such a model has lasting and detrimental side effects further supports the notion that this is not simply a standard language ideology at play, but an outright attack on speakers of BBVE to uphold a mainstream, non-diverse, and non-inclusive model of language not only in education but in society's vast linguistic marketplace. Language is not only culture, but identity, and to deliberately exercise power to enact corruption of marginalized individual's language system they use to make meaning in the world, understand the value of their identity, and experience/share unique expressions of the self (Eckert, 1989), is in fact an act of BBVE linguicide to sustain the institutional norm of elitist language prestige. An individual's language is an individual's identity. It is personhood. It is group and cultural affiliation. Being deprived of language as self-determined identity and a symbolic system of group and cultural identity is oppressive.

And victims of linguistic discrimination are well-aware that criticism and contempt for their language is a rejection of their authentic selves. It is also a criticism of everybody in their social network who speaks their dialect. As we have said before, ideology is most effective when it is presented and absorbed as "common sense," and thus language discriminators are often well-intentioned and ignorant of the harm they cause. We nevertheless consider rejection of non-mainstream voices and vernaculars to be state-sponsored abuse when it occurs in public institutions such as schools.

The second phase in the mainstream model (Table 8.2) features more covert modes of promoting self-censorship and assimilation in the classroom. These three acts of power operate under the guise of positive reinforcement while rewarding the adoption of language myths and the acceptance of linguistic misinformation.

The bastardization of BBVE features begins when teachers responsible for the establishment of traditional ideologies of language in the classroom begin to incorporate elements of BBVE themselves as a means of rapport building. This act simultaneously condemns nonstandard varieties while also utilizing varieties such as Black English, Mock Spanish, and other marginalized varieties. The hypocrisy of this act is another corrupt

Table 8.2 The mainstream model of Language education in America

Phase 2: Covert, misleading acts to maintain mainstream language ideologies
1. *Include speakers of Black and Brown varieties of English*
Acts of linguistic bastardization take place.
The teacher begins to appropriate and incorporate those non-ME features she/he regards as inferior as a rapport-building technique. This is an act of rank linguistic hypocrisy.
2. *Elevate speakers of Black and Brown varieties of English*
The conflation of spoken and written language conventions.
Ideology of language prestige is reinforced and rewarded by teaching students that they should aim to speak how they write, and model writing after speakers of ME
3. *Validate speakers of Black and Brown varieties of English*
Surrender to/justify mainstream standards of language use in the classroom.
Because of classroom norms, students accept they must achieve mastery by way of native language abandonment. Mastery is believed to be a result of the adoption of ME conventions.

use of linguistic violence which not only oppresses BBVE users but also pillages the culture of students as they relinquish control to the teacher in an act that mirrors the long-standing tradition of suppression and seizure of marginalized identities and cultures to elevate and maintain the superiority of whiteness. Hill (2008) describes "mock-Spanish" as an act of covert racism, and we argue that the appropriation of other forms of BBVE such as Black English is a form of mock-Black English and an additional form of covert racism. For example, many Black English words and phrases have been appropriated by the white community to serve as a source of comedic relief (i.e. *on fleek, I love your outfit—it's the shoes for me, it be like that,* etc.). This suggests that Black English is inferior in intellectual spaces, but its slang and turn of phrase is made freely available for play and consumption for the purposes of white speakers to viewed as street-smart, funny, cool, etc. by white speakers while also abusing the language and pilfering the members of the donor group (Baker-Bell, 2020a; Hill, 2008). Black terms and phrases which have been misappropriated by white language users are rendered uncool once stolen and implemented into ME use (Simtherman, 1998b). The term goes through a transformation that would classify this appropriated form as "mock-Black English." Black English is the most important dialect in creating new, hip, young, street-wise language for ME users to source for their own use, all while being viewed as unvalued and deficient by those same users who loot their language. As Geneva Smitherman states, "Whites pay no dues, but reap the psychological, social, and economic benefits of a language and culture born out of struggle and hard times" (Smitherman, 1998b, p. 218).

The ideology of language prestige views ME as a variety of status and is falsely perceived as being the spoken equivalent of written English. Teachers not only reinforce this harmful ideology which completely goes against the linguistic "facts of life", but have also had this ideology interpolated via curricular policy. Governing curricular entities have advocated that a key to success in education is the standardization of both written and spoken English (Lippi-Green, 2012; NCTE, 1996). Once teachers have justified this practice establishing the supremacy of mainstream English standards as well as displaying a positive bias toward students who assimilate, the ideology will often be accepted and adopted by the student (Charity-Hudley & Mallinson, 2011). The elevation of ME as the standard language imbues it with connotations of respect and prestige, which then carry social and economic benefits (Hill, 2008), and the cycle of tradition will continue on the basis of misinformation and normalized privilege. By teaching under the Mainstream Model, these ideals and biases continue to be interpolated and injected into future generations in a recursive cycle of linguistic oppression. This justification of the continued permittance of this discriminatory and culturally oppressive model must stop. Teachers must break free of the standardization trap camouflaged in tradition which leads them to believe that these practices are necessary for the future success of students. Their futures depend on this model because we continue letting this serve as the foundation for the ways in which we teach and view language. It is time to walk away from these covertly racist traditions; otherwise, the promised land of anti-racist language equality can never be reached (Inoue, 2019).

The Linguistic Gospel Truth

Walking away from a system drenched in tradition is never easy. There is a reason why so many students, teachers, and adults out in the world have chosen to assimilate, code-switch, and encourage the standardization of language in the classroom and in the workplace. These linguistic gospels will provide an action-oriented approach for teachers and other helping professionals trying to navigate the murky waters of systemic racism to the promised land of linguistic equality. If we are to ever truly achieve language equality in education and carry a new model and mindset into other social spaces, teachers must understand these gospels and commit them to action. All of these gospels are able to be implemented when the power is taken from the mainstream model and traditional ideologies and applied to new practices on the basis of one overarching revelation: language is power.

Gospel 1: *Linguistic mother tongues provide formative identity work.* Identity is formulated as individuals make meaning in the world. The mother tongue a speaker is born into situates them in relation to others—those who share the same dialect and those whose dialects differ. This helps to shape a person's perspective on the world, and the interactions they experience help to shape his or her understanding of self-worth (Eckert, 1989). Teachers must be intentional in the choices made with regards to a student's mother tongue. We must be mindful of how we characterize the tool our students will use to socialize themselves into this world and how they will see themselves through their own lens of the world (Baker-Bell, 2020a). It would be a miscarriage of linguistic justice to mishandle and abuse such an integral piece of self-identity for another human being. Committing acts of cultural and linguistic erasure crosses the line and falls outside of our role as educators.

Gospel 2: *It is essential to foster positive language attitudes in the classroom.* In order to break the cycle of racially and culturally discriminatory language practices in education, educators must adopt attitudes opposite of the mainstream model. It is considered a basic and fundamental fact in linguistics, the language science, that all dialects of a language are valid and worthy language systems. It is somewhat depressing that incorporating language science into the classroom will be considered radical. The dominant cultural group is what determines the dominant ("mainstream") language, and this power is likely not going to be relinquished in a spirit of humility and atonement. But educators are often at the forefront of change. The shift in attitudes on behalf of teachers will result in positive outcomes in students, such as linguistic pride and elevated senses of self-worth. Likewise, the shift away from the white supremacist language ideology that might makes right & that the dominant group can force its language on everyone else towards a culture of respect and celebration of non-mainstream varieties will also benefit speakers of Mainstream English. Everyone benefits from being linguistically informed and from an inclusive and caring classroom environment. Privilege, linguistic or otherwise, does no favors when it comes to accurately being able to understand the world in which we live and to truly hear the voices of fellow humans who are different than ourselves. It is time to take off the cultural blinders that cause harm to us all. A classroom culture of language equity is one in which all dialect groups can stand on equal footing and have equal access to mastery and to education (Kendi, 2019).

Gospel 3: *Standardized English is the language of privilege because **what** is not allowed is reflective of **who** is not allowed.* This gospel is based on Lippi-Green's discussion of appropriacy arguments (2012). Educators will too often determine what is appropriate and inappropriate for language use based on a rationalization that it is better to linguistically conform, given that language discrimination exists. This rationalization both acknowledges and rejects speakers of stigmatized dialects (pp. 85–88). It is an acknowledgment of their language, but an attempt to coerce conformity to the dominant language. It is an acquiescence to prejudice.

One of the take-home messages of this paper is that all dialects are valid language systems with full expressive and communicative functions. The "big lie" about ME is that it is inherently better than other varieties of language. The language scientists (linguists) can assure you that if you study the technical aspects of language (the sound system, grammatical system, vocabulary, meaning system, etc.) of different language varieties for a living (as we do), it is a scientific fact that all language varieties are fully formed, sophisticated, and nuanced language systems. Every little piece and every little variation in a language matters and has meaning.

Linguists have a long academic tradition of studying the different pieces that make up complex and varied language systems. So elevating some dialects over others is not based on the superiority of the language itself but is based on cultural dominance and power. We are not supposed to notice that varieties of human language that are deemed "stigmatized" happen (not coincidentally) to be spoken by culturally stigmatized and marginalized groups of our fellow human beings whose voices would be heard with dignity and respect if we lived in a more just society. It is time to get on the road to language equality. Conforming to prejudice and misinformation is never the correct path for positive and transformative social change. Policing language use in the classroom has been a cornerstone of educational practices for quite some time. It is an inherently problematic position to filter the language use of stigmatized student populations to such an inequitable degree. The dominant language of Mainstream English is dominant not because of some inherent linguistic superiority. It is dominant because our public institutions say it is. Public institutions continue to privilege the dominant language, and in this way language discrimination is state-sponsored oppression.

Gospel 4: *Diversity is more than having a variety of student identities in your classroom, it must also include the acceptance of diverse language varieties.* As has been established in Gospel 1, language is identity. Institutional reform demands linguistic equality. Diversity is a mainstay in discussions surrounding education in recent years. Schools have put plans in place to diversify the gender and ethnic identities in the workplace, English classrooms have adapted reading lists to diversify authorship and genre, and an overall push is being made for educational spaces to become more inclusive. It is essential that diversity of language varieties and appreciation of linguistic differences take place. Non-performativity of anti-racism in institutions is dangerous (Ahmed, 2006), in that it can cheapen the mission to diversify education, and warp students' understanding of the value their differences bring to the classroom community. Meaningful language contribution in the classroom is more than just hanging a colorful poster celebrating differences. Making room for BBVE and other non-mainstream varieties and celebrating those features through your own language adds the necessary layer of action behind the words we say and the posters on our walls.

In adopting and applying these linguistic gospels, teachers will have the necessary understanding to move forward into an education model of linguistic equality. Let the by definition non-inclusive mainstream model serve as a cautionary tale and motivate you to leave behind the mindset of needing to be a linguistic savior for students who speak marginalized languages, and instead take action to empower students of color to liberate themselves.

Linguistic Equality: An Antiracist Model of Language Education

Many educators who implement the mainstream model of language education have unconscious biases and allegiances which may disguise nefarious practices as helpful techniques aiming to better a student's understanding of language use. Well-intentioned teachers can still perpetuate discriminatory and non-inclusive language ideologies simply by being an authority figure who exercises a Mainstream English Only approach and is present in the classroom (Inoue, 2019). Therefore, one must take a temperature-check of their ideologies and address those difficult beliefs, and be ready to leave some personal and engrained traditions behind. To anchor this model in principles, the following definitions will be used (Kendi, 2019):

1. Antiracist: "One who is supporting an antiracist policy through their actions or expressing an antiracist idea" (p. 13)
2. Antiracist ideas: "any idea that suggests the racial groups are equals in all their apparent differences" (p. 20)
3. Antiracist policies: "any measure (written and unwritten laws, rules, procedures, processes, regulations, and guidelines that govern people) that produces or sustains racial equity between racial groups" (p. 18)

Schools have a long, sordid history as being institutions that promote white-supremacist policies intent on eradicating and erasing the languages, cultures, and histories of students of color (Paris & Alim, 2017). For example, government-run boarding schools for Native Americans were explicit about aggressively attempting to eradicate indigenous language, religion, and cultural traditions. Assimilationist rhetoric was vile then, and we contend assimilationist rhetoric in the current historical moment is also inappropriate. The linguistic gospels, when welcomed as an inclusive element to help teachers interact with students and navigate language in their daily lives, equip teachers with the knowledge and tools to value marginalized languages as part of a truly pluralistic democracy. All students benefit from linguistic diversity; for our society is linguistically diverse. April Baker-Bell's Antiracist Linguistic Black Language

Table 8.3 Linguistic equality: An anti-racist model of Language education (adapted from Baker-Bell, 2020b)

Explicit and actionable norms to dismantle white-supremacist language hegemony
1. *Center the disenfranchised (speakers of BBVE)*
Elevate the linguistic consciousness of Black and Brown students.
Reinvigorate the languages, histories, literacies, and cultures that have been silenced and subject to erasure in white-supremacist classroom models, and place the needs of students of color at the center of language education
2. *Confront the language of mainstream cultural hegemony*
Explicitly names tactics used to normalize BBVE language suppression.
Provide students with the language needed to confront the language and ideologies of white supremacist language hegemony, and dispel language myths
3. *Contest anti-blackness*
Dismantle the normalization of linguistic racism in the classroom.
Empower Black and Brown students to engage in Black/Spanish linguistic freedom by including and celebrating their language in classroom discourse by providing opportunities to learn about and play with their own language
4. *Implement classroom antiracist language policy*
Collaboratively and explicitly establish inclusive language norms in the classroom.
Engage students in establishing an antiracist language policy. Teach these policies as normative and foundational practices and encourage students to uphold these policies and establish these norms in all linguistic arenas

Pedagogy (2020b) hones in on three essential components. An Antiracist Language Pedagogy must (1) center Blackness, (2) confront white linguistic and cultural hegemony, and (3) contest anti-Blackness (p. 8). In other words, this model requires that teachers not simply take up the task of inclusivity, but place a specialized focus on those target ethnic groups which have been marginalized, and the educator must utilize their own language to confront and contest dominant language ideologies. In keeping with Baker-Bell's model, we advocate for and cosign these three components, and suggest the addition of a fourth standard (Table 8.3).

Elevating the linguistic consciousness of students who speak dialects with ties to their ethnic identities is essential to linguistic justice. Teachers using this model are honest with students about the ills of dialect discrimination and work with colleagues to dispel these language myths. As educators, we must not only understand but verbalize that students are linguistically rich, not linguistically deficit. While some may be hesitant to center the disenfranchised, it is essential that educators replenish those students who have been forced to assimilate and abandon language competencies and identity markers throughout years of exposure to mainstream language hegemony. As these students are regaining their linguistic consciousness and navigating linguistic equity, white speakers of ME are also experiencing new language norms to reintroduce out in the world. There is power in students learning that when using features of their language *all* speakers have the agency to make authentic language choices. There is power in understanding the new paradigm that their dialectal speech acts are language choices, not language mistakes. The empowerment that frees one student has the capacity to free all students. Part of being a free person is being able to present an authentic linguistic self to the world without being oppressed as part of gaining an "education."

In addition to Baker-Bell's components, we add to the model the importance of implementing an antiracist language policy within your classroom culture for all students—of all cultures and creeds. It is imperative that educators instill and establish critical competencies, so all students are armed with the language necessary to seek out and identify, investigate, and help to dismantle linguistic hegemony (Baker-Bell, 2020b). The ultimate goal of this model is to empower students' voices and equip them with tools that help to serve linguistic justice out in the world. However, educators must first establish and model policy and social norms and set a precedent for the classroom communication style. In this model, teachers first establish that acts and ideology consistent with the mainstream model have no place within the classroom discourse community. As part of the social norms, educators must seek to explicitly teach students the hallmarks of dominant language warfare and provide strategies detailing how to effectively identify and combat oppressive tactics such as dialect and language policing, language suppression, and the bastardization of non-mainstream dialects. By implementing the antiracist language classroom policies, we can empower all students to develop positive language attitudes.

In an inclusive model which practices antiracist language policies and encourages antiracist ideas by students, teachers must adjust and revise their standardized tests, and advocate for these changes at the district and state level. For some, it may be a no-brainer to implement these seemingly radical policies in the privacy of one's own classroom, but some will also experience hesitation when advocating for antiracist ideas and change at the school, division, or state level. Educators must break free of these hesitations. It is not enough to implement an antiracist language model at the classroom level; while that is a necessary and valued starting point, education is an institution, and the classroom is only a piece of the puzzle in dismantling institutionalized racism (Inoue, 2019). While we can make meaningful changes in our classrooms, institutional change often comes from the top-down. Passage-based assessments must include culturally relevant information by utilizing examples relevant to a variety of cultures. Processing of these passages and determining a response are processes heavily reliant on cultural beliefs and moral values—which are shaped and experienced by the language used to navigate and make sense of the world. For instance, a commonly used 6th grade standardized test featured a passage and question set about yoga. While yoga is a widespread activity, there are certain student populations who have a higher likelihood of being familiar with or having family members who practice yoga. Those students would be equipped with specialized vocabulary words, but students who do not have this cultural background may have to take longer to respond (Charity-Hudley & Mallinson, 2011). This is simply one of many examples that highlight the inequity of standardized testing resulting in Black and Brown students being limited by their cultural backgrounds and experiences. Teachers must speak up against these traditional forms of "language and experience" standardization and further emphasize the need for equitable language experience test items for our students.

Looking Ahead: The Promised Land of Language Equality

Being an advocate for change in a systemic and institutionalized arena can be a frightening role. It means being in the minority, and being one of few change agents working to turn the tide of centuries-long racism, tradition, and an established status quo. Basic linguistic facts will be treated as radical, especially at first, but you have the knowledge to push back and to help normalize linguistic equality. Though it is not easy to be a catalyst for institutional reform and cultural acceptance, it will put you on the right side of history. These gospel truths must be implemented in order for the mainstream language tradition to be rejected and disrupted, and for antiracist models to be implemented. A teacher who empowers is one who does not settle into a role of talking *at* students but must stand up and talk *with* them—in the classroom and in traditionalized educational arenas to advocate for systemic change (Shor, 1992). Only by implementing this model of antiracist language use and explicitly teaching/incorporating language equality can we have any hope of reaching the promised land of language equality in our society.

Insisting on Mainstream English Only in our public institutions was never meant to invite people in; it is meant to keep non-dominant cultural groups out. It is past time for linguistic pluralism as social justice. Helping professionals could lead the way. The linguistic gospel truth asks that the power behind language be redistributed from just the voices of the dominant to the voices of the many. We hope you will join linguists in promoting and disseminating the truth about language. Only the truth will set us **all** free.

Guiding Questions

1. How do you perceive Black and Brown Varieties of English (BBVE) in your everyday life? Based on your observations, how do your colleagues perceive BBVE in everyday life? Use the following framework:
   a. *What was said?*
   b. *Which features of BBVE were used?*
   c. *In what setting did the conversation take place?*
   d. *Who was present during the conversation?*
   e. *What stance was taken* (e.g. *Did you view these language features as inappropriate for the setting? Was your instinct that this was a display of incorrect language use??)*
2. Reflect on the aforementioned discussion, and establish which model of your language ideology you practice.

3. Whose language would you be comfortable correcting in the professional space? Consider not only their rank with respect to your position in the workplace but also their status as a marginalized speaker in a traditional, marginalized setting. What qualifies them for correction?
4. How are we able to take mainstream views of language as well as prescriptive language use in the classroom and shift the language culture *in our own classrooms*?
5. How are we able to take dominant views of language as well as prescriptive language use in the classroom and transform the language culture in *institutionalized educational spaces*?

Quiz Questions

1. When considering both the Mainstream Model of Language Education and the Antiracist Model of Language Education in America, organize the following educational practices into each ideological framework:

Mainstream Model Framework	Antiracist Framework
•	•
•	•
•	•

1. *The use of marginalized language features by white teachers as a means of rapport-building and humor*
2. *The inclusion of multicultural works in the classroom (books, interviews, artists, etc.) and the subsequent discussion and celebration of language differences*
3. *Discussing language as a tool for enslavement during relevant history lessons*
4. *Mentor texts exclusively written by speakers of mainstream English*
5. *Elimination of forced code-switching in the classroom*
6. *Celebrate native language norms in relaxed settings (e.g. classroom discussion), advocate for temporary language abandonment for achievement of mastery*

2. In the space below, identify the four "linguistic facts of life" as developed by Lippi-Green (2012):
    a.
    b.
    c.
    d.

3. In the space below, identify the four "linguistic gospel truths" outlined in this chapter:
   a.
   b.
   c.
   d.
4. In considering the Anti-Racist Model of Language Education (Table 8.3), which of the following practices would be an example of the way a teacher could *confront the language of mainstream cultural hegemony?*
   a. Celebrating the language of BBVE speakers by allowing them to explore their language norms through written classroom assignments
   b. Working collaboratively with students to establish classroom norms with respect to language inclusivity
   c. Stress that language abandonment need only be practiced during summative assessment
   d. Explicitly naming common language myths and dispelling them using student-friendly language
5. In considering the Mainstream Model of Language Education, which of the following practices would be an example of an *overt* practice utilized by educators to maintain hegemonic practices of language in the classroom?

   a. The teacher positions oneself as an arbiter of language use—to be used as a tool to bridge the gap between inferior dialects and prestigious white mainstream varieties of English.
   b. Rewards speakers who speak how they write
   c. Celebrates the adoption of ME conventions
   d. Uses linguistic appropriation to bond/relate to students of color

References

Ahmed, S. (2006). The nonperformativity of antiracism. *Meridians, 7*(1), 104–126.

Baker-Bell, A. (2020a). *Linguistic justice: Black language, literacy, identity, and pedagogy*. Routledge.

Baker-Bell, A. (2020b). We been knowin: Toward an antiracist language & literacy education. *Journal of Language & Literacy Education, 16*(1), 1–12.

Charity-Hudley, A., & Mallinson, C. (2011). In J. Banks (Ed.), *Understanding English language variation in US schools*. Teachers College Press.

Eckert, P. (1989). *Jocks and burnouts: Social identity in the high school*. Teachers College Press.

Elbow, P. (1999). Inviting the mother tongue: Beyond 'mistakes', 'bad English', and 'wrong language'. *Journal of Advanced Composition, 19*(2), 359–388.

Fairclough, N. (2015). *Language and power* (3rd ed.). Routledge.

Hill, J. H. (2008). *The everyday language of white racism*. Wiley-Blackwell.

Inoue, A. (2019). 2019 CCCC's address: How do we language so people stop killing each other, or what do we do about white language supremacy? *College Composition and Communication, 71*(2), 352–369.

International Reading Association & The National Council of Teachers of English. (1996). Standards for the english language arts. International Reading Association and the National Council of Teachers of English.

Kendi, I. X. (2019). *How to be an antiracist*. Random House.

Lippi-Green, R. (2012). *English with an accent: Language, ideology, and discrimination in the United States* (2nd ed.). Routledge.

Mallinson, C., Charity-Hudley, A., Rutter Strickling, L., & Figa, M. (2011). A conceptual framework for promoting linguistic and educational change. *Lang & Ling Compass, 5*(7), 441–453.

Martinez, D. C. (2017). Imagining a language of solidarity for Black and Latinx youth in English language arts classrooms. *English Education, 49*(2), 197–196.

Milroy, J., & Milroy, L. (1985). *Authority in language: Investigating language prescription and standardization* (2nd ed.). Routledge.

National Center for Education Statistics. (2019a). *Table 203.50. Enrollment and percentage distribution of enrollment in public elementary and secondary schools, by race/ethnicity and region: Selected years, fall 1995 through fall 2029*. [Data set]. Digest of Education Statistics. https://nces.ed.gov/programs/digest/d20/tables/dt20_203.50.asp?current=yes

National Center for Education Statistics. (2019b). *Table 209.10. Number and percentage distribution of teachers in public and private elementary and secondary schools, by selected teacher characteristics: Selected years, 1987–88 through 2017–18*. [Data set]. Digest of Education Statistics. https://nces.ed.gov/programs/digest/d19/tables/dt19_209.10.asp?current=yes

Paris, D., & Alim, H. S. (Eds.). (2017). *Culturally sustaining pedagogies: Teaching and learning for justice in a changing world*. Teachers College Press.

Shor, I. (1992). *Empowering education: Critical teaching for social change*. University of Chicago Press.

Skutnabb-Kangas, T. (1995). Multilingualism and the education of minority children. In O. Garcia & C. Baker (Eds.), Policy and practice in bilingual education: Extending the foundations (pp. 40–62). Multilingual Matters.

Smitherman, G. (1998a). Ebonics, King, and Oakland: Some folk don't believe fat meat is greasy. *Journal of English Linguistics, 26*(2), 97–107.

Smitherman, G. (1998b). Word from the hood: The lexicon of African-American Vernacular English. In S. S. Mufwene, J. R. Rickford, G. Bailey, & J. Baugh (Eds.), *African-American English: Structure, history, and use* (pp. 203–225). Routledge.

U.S. Department of Education, Office of Planning, Evaluation and Policy Development, Policy and Program Studies Service. (2016). *The state of racial diversity in the educator workforce*. [dataset]. U.S. Department of Education. https://www2.ed.gov/rschstat/eval/highered/racial-diversity/state-racial-diversity-workforce.pdf

9

Decentering Whiteness in Teaching Psychopathology: Challenges and Opportunities

Stephanie Z. Chen

Introduction

Psychopathology is a foundational course for graduate-level studies often taught in the first year of a clinical psychology, counseling psychology or social work program. One of the key reasons for the early timing is that this class is a formative course, which teaches students the professional terminology of diagnosis and diagnostic criteria. Such knowledge is useful and necessary in the process of destigmatizing mental illness and disorders, the art and science of diagnosis, communicating with other professionals, and for future acquisition of clinical knowledge. This is especially true for programs whose graduates pursue licenses of the helping professions[1] where they will be actively working with clients, and

[1] Such as Marriage Family Therapist (MFTs), Professional Clinical Counselor (LPCCs), Clinical Social Worker (LCSW) and Clinical and Counseling Psychologists.

S. Z. Chen (✉)
The Wright Institute, Berkeley, CA, USA

© The Author(s), under exclusive license to Springer Nature Switzerland AG 2022

K. Johnson et al. (eds.), *Developing Anti-Racist Practices in the Helping Professions: Inclusive Theory, Pedagogy, and Application*,
https://doi.org/10.1007/978-3-030-95451-2_9

assessing, diagnosing, and providing treatment. Using an antiracist framework when teaching this course would then be even more an imperative and an ethical obligation to our students and all the helping professions.

An antiracist framework is fundamental, and is a calling for many in the helping professions. The murders of George Floyd, Breonna Taylor, Ahmaud Arbery, and countless others in 2020 created a nation-wide examination on race relations and topics related to diversity, equity, inclusion and social justice. Many professions and academia were also affected, and propelled active examination of culpability and accountability to address systemic, historical and current injustices within their own organizations and institutes (Jones, 2020).

This chapter is a needed reckoning of the course and teaching of psychopathology and other similar courses. I will discuss how key principles of psychopathology replicate and perpetuate White supremacy, and how to capitalize on opportunities to revise, adapt and to change this course towards an antiracist frame. I will also propose several recommendations and practical tips that I have learned, and have utilized in teaching this course for almost 10 years.

Challenges: How Course Itself Reflects White Supremacy

There are many ways a psychopathology course perpetuates a White-supremacist framework. For example, the historical and current use of diagnosis is embedded in a medical model that focuses on identifying pathology. The medical model itself is reductionist and solely locates the problem (e.g. disorder) in the individual, with little to no attention paid to systemic impacts, or non-medical or pharmaceutical interventions and healing. The characterization of abnormal psychology or subpar functioning is predicated on what is considered "normal" and normal functioning (Fernando, 2017; Kurtis & Adams, 2015). And common among all fields of study, what is normal are based on being White, male, and college-educated. Henrich, Heine, & Norenzayan (2010) introduced the acronym of WEIRD (Western, Educated, Industrialized, Rich,

Democratic), which has been commonly used in the literature of multicultural, decolonization and liberation psychology as a way to highlight the highly subjective and narrow generalizability of existing scientific data and knowledge. In addition, Fernando postulated that the roots of Western science specific to psychiatry and psychology drew heavily from the age of Enlightenment which espoused values and beliefs in White superiority (2017, p. 22).

In other words, norms are not neutral. Baselines are not neutral. In her seminal article about the field of psychopathology, Cosgrove reminded us "diagnostic categories are constitutive; they construct, rather than represent, reality. That is, psychiatric labels create certain realities and marginalize others and in the process, may inadvertently sustain unjust social relations" (2005, p. 284). The construction of what constitutes normal has perpetuated the definition and characteristics of what is then abnormal, which have been commonly used to diagnose and label the "other" (meaning nonwhite) as defective and abnormal. Words such as primitive, hysterical, and perverted, have been used to categorize and to stereotype BIPOC (Black, Indigenous, and People of Color), women and LGBTQ+ (Lesbian, Gay, Bisexual, Transgender, Queer and all other members within this community) folks, respectively. Indeed, diagnoses such as drapetomania and homosexuality are such key examples. For example, drapetomania, as conceptualized by Dr. Samuel Cartwright in 1851, was "the disease causing slaves to run away" (Tripathi et al., 2019, p. 702). This medical diagnosis pathologized enslaved people who desired and sought freedom, and provided scientific legitimacy to the institution of slavery (Tripathi et al., 2019).

It is even more problematic when we consider the trend of misdiagnosis within psychiatry, and psychology (American Psychiatric Association, 2021a, b; Fernando, 2017). Misdiagnosis (including under- and over-diagnosis) is a common occurrence, especially of individuals and communities who are, or identify as BIPOC (Delphin-Rittmon et al., 2015; Hays et al., 2010; Liang et al., 2016). Researchers have indicated that African American clients were more likely to be diagnosed with schizophrenia, and drug-related disorders when demographic variables were controlled (Delphine et al., 2015). Similar data is reflected in clinical adolescent populations. African American youths were more likely to be diagnosed with psychotic disorders, disruptive behavior disorders and conduct related problems (Liang et al., 2016; Nguyen et al., 2007). Lastly, Hays et al. demonstrated that women were disproportionately diagnosed with personality disorders (2010).

DSM-5 Considerations

Another challenge to teaching the psychopathology course to future professionals is the importance of having some competence in utilizing the *Diagnostic and Statistical Manual of Mental Disorders* (5th ed.; DSM–5; American Psychiatric Association, 2013). Diagnosis is a requirement for third-party reimbursement and for mental health treatment, and the DSM-5 is often used to help students learn the diagnostic criteria of mental disorders. The DSM-5 is purposefully "atheoretical" (American Psychiatric Association, 2013) and yet, the medical model has perpetually promulgated the belief that pathology resides solely in the individual, and then treatment and healing occur only within that individual.

There is also an assumption that DSM categories are constructed from scientific evidence, and therefore bias-free and neutral. In Fernando's critique of the psychiatry and psychology fields, he remarked "the 'psy' disciplines only mimicked objectivity whereas many of the methods they used for understanding individuals were clearly subjective" (2017, p. 22). Even revisions of the DSM to its current fifth edition still categorize normal and abnormal standards and functioning via a WEIRD lens. Therefore, DSM categories are not neutral but are constructs that reflect implicit values, beliefs, interests and ideologies, and of a particular culture in time (Cosgrove, 2005, p. 290).

Remnants and perpetuation of Whiteness and White supremacy have real-life impacts and consequences. Jones reminds us "racist research kills people. It ends lives and destroys communities" (2020). Her statement summons to the forefront the various horrific research and experimentation on Black bodies in the name of scientific progress. From surgeries performed without anesthesia on enslaved women, the Tuskegee Syphilis Study to Hoffman et al.'s study of white medical students (2016), black bodies were degraded, dispensable, and continue to be provided with substandard care. Specific to psychological treatments, several governmental reports have indicated that equitable care is not consistently available to BIPOC clients (Delphine et al., 2015). The American Psychiatric Association also recently issued an apology to the BIPOC community for its silence and use of "abusive treatment, experimentation, victimization in the name of "scientific evidence"" (2021a).

In sum, the roots of White supremacy are deep in the field of psychology, and the impacts continue to reverberate in research, quality of clinical care, and in education. Training institutions play a significant role in how information is taught to their students, and it is a vital investment to not perpetuate implicit bias and beliefs among future professionals and within the field.

Opportunities: Building an Antiracist Approach

> "Racist" is not—as Richard Spencer argues—a pejorative. It is not the worst word in the English language; it is not the equivalent of a slur. It is descriptive, and the only way to undo racism is to consistently identify and describe it—and then dismantle it. The attempt to turn this usefully descriptive term into an almost unusable slur is, of course, designed to do the opposite: to freeze us into inaction. (Kendi, 2019, p. 9)

This passage from Kendi's book (2019) is an important reminder to start this section about opportunities. After summarizing all the ways how psychopathology teaches and perpetuates White supremacist beliefs and prejudices, it can be debilitating to confront the enormity of the profoundly problematic and deep-rooted perspective and pedagogy of psychology towards an antiracist one. Kendi proposes that real change and conscious movement away from racism (and other isms) require active practice (2019). We must move past stages and feelings of shame, embarrassment, or overwhelm in order to address and start dismantling racism and other White supremacist practices.

The first opportunity in engaging with an antiracist framework to teaching psychopathology is to make explicit certain facts: the primary being the assumption that psychology and psychiatry (and their practitioners) are neutral. As instructors, we have to challenge the idea of the "colorblind mentality in mental health" (Gottlieb et al., 2021). Kurtis & Adams (2015) encouraged instructors to *"de-normalize* or *denaturalize* [their italics] patterns of experience that mainstream research tends to treat as standard" (p. 395). In other words, WEIRD is not a reflection of universal human nature but a very select slice, and yet is still used disproportionately to inform psychological sciences and thinking (Kurtis & Adams, 2015, p. 395).

One way to do this is to provide a more comprehensive and critical history of psychology and psychiatry, which also includes an acknowledgment and confrontation with the racist foundations of the science of psychology. We must teach our students how to deconstruct the implicit beliefs espoused by the medical model and various diagnoses; we can help students assess and critique long-held standards of what constitutes as abnormal vs. normal; who have/had the power to create such labels; and who are continually impacted and why.

The recent press release published by the American Psychiatric Association (APA) could be one starting point. The APA issued a formal apology to BIPOC communities (2021a, b). As "the oldest national physician association in the country," the APA accounts the various ways they contributed to and perpetuated racism onto BIPOC bodies and communities. They close their apology with a commitment to social and human equity and practices from direct care, research and their teaching institutions (APA, 2021a). This press release provides many overtures for critical thinking and discussions.

Another opportunity to move towards an antiracist frame is to insert and to integrate our client's individual contexts throughout the processes of assessment, diagnosis and treatment planning. Prilleltensky et al. warned that without context, students and therapists miss "intrapsychic forces, injustice, and power dynamics potentially oppressing clients from the inside and outside" (2007, pp. 37–38). Cosgrove reminded mental health counseling programs of their "ethical responsibility to teach students to think about the sociopolitical context in which behaviors become understood as symptoms of mental disorders" (2005, p. 283).

Mann & Himelein (2008) also cautioned that "labeling at the exclusion of personal information" sharpened students' diagnostic skills but at the expense of having no knowledge of how to use them (p. 549). Labels created more reliance on categorization, very little understanding of the individuals with the mental health diagnosis, and increased students' own stigma of mental illness (Mann & Himelein, 2008).

In addition to contexts, instructors should normalize patterns of experience, especially of marginalized folks, whose behaviors and lived experiences have been historically judged and treated as suboptimal or deviant (Kurtis & Adams, 2015, p. 395). One of the results of civil rights protests of 2020 was the burgeoning of numerous trainings and writings by BIPOC professionals and experts who focused on this theme (Academics4Black Lives, 2020; Bryant-Davis, 2020; Coates, 2020; Gottlieb et al., 2021; Holman, 2020; ISPRC, 2020; Jones, 2020; Moore-Lobban & Green, 2020; Murray-Browne, 2020; Smith et al., 2020; Spann et al., 2020). Several of these presentations featured the historical and current impacts of racial trauma and minority stress on the daily functioning of BIPOC communities (Academics4Black Lives, 2020; Holman, 2020; ISPRC, 2020; Moore-Lobban & Green, 2020; Murray-Browne, 2020; Smith et al., 2020; Spann et al., 2020). The associated symptoms and lived experiences (and across generations) are bestowed new and more fitting definitions and meaning: a much-needed transformation from attributions based on pathology and individual weakness to emphasis of enduring resiliency of individual and communal spirit to live despite systemic inequities.

There is also an expansion of not only who and how normal functioning is defined, but also more options for treatment and healing. We are just starting to include and to spotlight indigenous and ancestral healing practices as just as worthy as lab-tested and empirically supported treatments (Charlton et al., 2020; Zapata, 2020).

Another opportunity to create an antiracist framework is to engage students in examining their own implicit biases. The field's own reliance on having (multi)cultural competence skills and guidelines are important foundations and beginnings, and are also inadequate. As a BIPOC panelist remarked, cultural competence [training and courses] do not mean antiracist (Gottlieb et al., 2021).

This quote is even more poignant when we consider existing studies and findings. Hoffman et al.'s study on racial bias in pain assessment and treatment indicated White medical students and residents who endorsed false beliefs that white and Black patients (based on a vignette) had different biological bodies also provided different recommendations on levels of pain medication to their patients (2016). Specifically, White medical students and residents believed the Black patient would feel less pain and were then recommended less dosage of pain medication when compared to the White patient (Hoffman et al., 2016). Hoffman et al. also concluded that the study's results are "consistent with research on intergroup bias demonstrating that discrimination often occurs due to ingroup favoritism rather than outgroup hostility (p. 4300). They postulated that White medical students and residents' identification with "white fragility (of the white patient) may shape racial bias in pain perception as much, if not more, than perceptions of blacks' strength" (Hoffman et al., 2016, p. 4300). Hays et al. showed a similar finding in their mixed methodological analysis of the role of culture in the clinical decision-making process (2010). The results indicated that there were disproportionately diagnoses of particular cultural groups; specifically, participants diagnosed more severe diagnoses on vignettes with patients of oppressed statuses, and underdiagnosed those vignettes "who were not oppressed" (Hays et al., 2010, p. 115). Participants also reported that culture did not influence presenting problems or diagnoses even though findings indicated that culture did matter (Hays et al., 2010, p. 119). Hays et al. highlighted the need to address "cultural blindness" in the clinical decision-making process (2010, p. 119).

If we center the comprehensive history of psychology, importance of context(s) of clients, patterns of experience/lived experience of marginalized folks, and examine our own implicit bias including cultural evasiveness,[2] then we can truly move into the active work of dismantling racism and racist structures.

[2] Color-evasiveness is the more current and inclusive language that has replaced the former and ableist term of 'color-blindness'. For further analysis, read through Annamma et al.'s work (2017).

Practical Tips & Recommendations

In this final section, I share recommendations and approaches that I have utilized to demonstrate the key tenets of what I believe are opportunities to build an antiracist approach to teaching a psychopathology course.

- Research, implement and cite nonWEIRD authors, experts and professionals.

I am grateful for the generosity and the flourishing of publications, webinars and trainings in 2020, and some of which are listed in my references. Use these references in the construction and preparation of this course as well as insert them (e.g., writings, videos, etc.…) into your lectures and assignments. I would also like to note that before 2020, there is quite a selection of nonWEIRD works available, while not as prolific. Many of the concepts I've discussed are not new or ground-breaking but rather a re-examination and drawing attention back to them.

It is important to be thoughtful and inclusive of what you choose to use including graphics and visuals to PowerPoint slides and other multimedia clips (i.e., videos, podcasts, etc.…). It might seem like a small action, and the impact is resounding especially to my BIPOC and other marginalized students. Representation matters especially in a field of academic instruction and practice where WEIRD is still the norm.

- Pair conventional references and texts with critiques

With the use of references such as the DSM-5 (APA, 2013), I recommend using other sources that critique the actual system of diagnostic criteria. Being able to take in and analyze another and multiple perspectives are instrumental in teaching our students to be critical thinkers. Ishibashi's collection of essays (2015) could be an excellent start. The authors of that collection were moved to provide a counter-narrative and critique of existing DSM-5 diagnostic categories and overall diagnoses.

I do not eliminate the DSM-5 from my course because my students will need to know diagnostic criteria, and still work in our current system of managed health care where a diagnosis is required for most mental health treatment. I also have used these opposing texts/sources as a way to introduce a class exercise. I have students engage their critical thinking skills by first weighing the pros and cons of diagnosis and the use of the DSM, and then presenting their findings to each other. In such activities students can practice with dialectical thinking, particularly that multiple and conflicting truths can exist (Wong, 2006), and to help students and move beyond a dichotomous method of "either-or" thinking.

In a similar vein, we must acknowledge other venues and opportunities for healing. CBT and pharmaceuticals are not the only efficacious treatments. How could this be when most random-controlled research and studies have been based on WEIRD participants? Comparable to diagnosis and diagnostic categories, I explicitly ask students their opinions on touted treatment recommendations as well as how these recommendations make sense, or have applicability in their own lives. I also query why certain treatments are highlighted whereas others are not.

While controversial, I have used the use of recreational drugs (i.e. cannabis) and emerging data on psychedelics to prompt curiosity and debate. The possibility of psychedelic in treating several mental diagnoses is a beginning to many rich discussions. Psychedelics have been used as traditional healing practices in several cultures and communities for centuries, were disparaged and pathologized because of it, and only in the past 10 years, psychedelics have been reframed and legitimized as real treatment options in both scientific studies and mainstream discussions. There is a similar trend with the practice of mindfulness and yoga, too. There are valid critiques of these practices as "white washed" due to appropriation-like actions of disconnection or lack of acknowledgment from its origins of Hindu, Buddhist and other spiritual practices (Gottlieb et al., 2021; ISPRC, 2020).

Lastly, because I teach and practice in Northern California, there are more readily resources available (e.g. The Sage Institute, n.d.) which other colleagues in different parts of the country and the world do not. Nonetheless, incorporating these alternative treatments do seem to capitalize and capture student interests and offer a level of relatability that pharmaceuticals and random-controlled studies do not. And, of course instructors would need to be mindful of the messaging behind the use of non-prescribed drugs, especially if they teach in institutions with certain restrictions and guidelines.

- Insert real life narratives with the teaching of diagnosis and diagnostic criteria.

There is a plethora of resources of first person's narrative of their experience with mental diagnoses. When possible, invite mental health consumers to share their lived experiences with your class. Depending on your geographical location, there are city/county or private organizations that support and create speaking opportunities for people with mental health diagnoses to talk about their experiences with others. The mission of these speaking groups is to help destigmatize mental illness and people with mental health diagnoses across various communities (LEVS, 2020). A consistent highlight for my students is listening and interacting with such panelists as it bridges the gap between intellectual learning (i.e. diagnostic criteria) to affective/emotional relating. Students start to learn that their knowledge and skills will be utilized and applied to real people with complexities and rich details and nuances that do not fit neatly into diagnostic criteria or text-book descriptions.

If this is not possible, there are existing literature, from personal essays (Wang, 2019) to searing critiques (Green & Ubozoh, 2019), that center the individual experience with mental disorders. In addition, add a writing or discussion component with questions prompting reflections on what students have learned from other texts and sources, and how that might compare or contradict what they just read or heard (e.g., what was surprising, what did you learn, etc.…). I know that there are other mediums such as documentaries, movies, music and artwork that can prompt similar learning, and my students have shared their resources with me as a way to further enhance my course. For example, this past term I was invited by a student to be a part of and to add to a list of graphic novels that focused on mental health and disorders. My student believed the medium of graphic novels was more inclusive of younger age audiences, of other learning abilities, and would provide an age-appropriate version of bibliotherapy to latency, adolescent, and adult clients. I couldn't agree more.

- It's never too early to introduce practice on addressing implicit bias and color-evasiveness

Some colleagues have argued with me that a psychopathology course is not a place to work on students' bias. Antiracist work in academia cannot be accomplished without a self-assessment of how much of what I am promoting is actually being implemented in every course I teach including psychopathology. And, I believe that the whole course on psychopathology presents prime opportunities for instructors and students to start and engage with this essential work. Singh's handbook includes concrete worksheets and activities (2019). Greenwald et al.'s Implicit Associations Test (IAT) could also be another starting point (1998). Project Implicit has made variations of the IAT available and free (2001). Regardless of actual worksheet or activity, what is more important is the instructor's role in making connections of implicit bias to actual life applications and implications. It is important to normalize that everyone (including instructors) has implicit bias, and that addressing and working on implicit bias is an on-going and liberating endeavor.

To combat color-evasiveness, I insert a query on multicultural consideration in every assignment (i.e., vignettes and papers), any use of other media, and when facilitating large to small group discussions. I encourage students to think about how social identities and the intersectionality of those identities impact (e.g., exacerbating and protective factors) people's experiences with mental disorders, the reception to treatment and overall prognosis. I actively require students to practice with this analytic muscle so it becomes part of the rhythm and overall process of rapport building, assessment, diagnosis and provision of treatment of every clinical encounter. This is an example of one of my pedagogical tenets: the teaching of psychopathology and psychology cannot be done without consideration and integration of sociocultural and political contexts and realities. If we are in the science of researching, treating and teaching about the human experience, we cannot ethically or comprehensively do so without such considerations.

Final Words

In the writing of this chapter, I continue to struggle with the question and dilemma of what does antiracist really mean and look like. One resounding question: is it even possible for psychopathology to be antiracist if diagnostic criteria still exist, and the DSM-5 is still used? Tuck & Yang presented a very convincing argument that true liberation is not possible if we continue to hold on to the colonial legacy such as categorizing mental disorders (2012). Nonetheless, I hold on to this ideal with the hopes that my approach in an antiracist frame in teaching psychopathology is one step closer towards liberation including the creation of a new system of talking, creating and using diagnosis embedded in antiracist, decolonized and liberation principles.

Lastly, I am honored to be part of this collection of writing. How revolutionary to be compiling works that promote helping professions as an antiracist one! And similar to the sentiments expressed in the various panels of BIPOC academics and professionals, there is worry that the tidal wave of 2020 will ebb (Academics4Black Lives, 2020; Bryant-Davis, 2020; Coates, 2020; Gottlieb et al., 2021; ISPRC, 2020; Jones, 2020; Moore-Lobban & Green, 2020; Murray-Browne, 2020; Smith et al., 2020; Spann et al., 2020). That the current national and individual receptiveness to diversity, the spotlight on BIPOC experiences and active work towards decolonizing and liberation of academic curricula etc.... are only a trend. I hold on to that fear and to the hope that like me, readers of this collection are connected in a long-term commitment to action and sustaining antiracist work. This connection is what sustains and revitalizes my love of teaching and to be in community with you all.

Guiding Questions

1. As you review your current curriculum, identify areas (e.g., topics, activities, readings, etc....) that perpetuate Whiteness.
2. Identify 2–3 areas of your syllabus where you can insert suggestions made in the Practical Tips & Recommendations of this chapter.
3. Examine what is your own relationship to Whiteness or White supremacy in your role as instructor/professor.

Quiz Questions

1. True or False: The field of psychiatry and psychology is neutral and addresses the experiences of all people.
2. What does WEIRD stand for?
3. True or False: It is important to decenter Whiteness in a psychopathology class.
4. Which is the more updated and inclusive term: color-blindness or color-evasiveness?
5. True or False: Being culturally competent means that one is not racist.

References

Academics4Black Lives. (2020, August 1–21). *Academics for Black wellness and survival: The rewind and remix* [Virtual training].

American Psychiatric Association. (2021a, January 18). *APA's apology to Black, Indigenous and People of Color for its support of structural racism in psychiatry* [Press Release]. https://www.psychiatry.org/newsroom/apa-apology-for-its-support-of-structural-racism-in-psychiatry

American Psychiatric Association. (2021b, January 18). *Historical addendum to APA's apology to Black, Indigenous and People of Color for its support of structural racism in psychiatry* [Website]. https://www.psychiatry.org/newsroom/historical-addendum-to-apa-apology

American Psychological Association. (2013). *Diagnostic and statistical manual of mental disorders* (5th ed.). https://doi.org/10.1176/appi.books.9780890425596

American Psychological Association. (2017). *Multicultural guidelines: An ecological approach to context, identity, and intersectionality.* Retrieved from https://www.apa.org/about/policy/multicultural-guidelines.pdf

Annamma, S. A., Jackson, D. D., & Morrison, D. (2017). Conceptualizing color-evasiveness: Using dis/ability critical race theory to expand a color-blind racial ideology in education and society. *Race Ethnicity and Education, 20*(2), 147–162.

Bryant-Davis, T. (2020, July 24). *Antiracism therapy: Moving beyond cultural competence* [Webinar]. Redwood Psychological Association.

Charlton, J. E., Michell, J. E., & Acoose, S. L. (Eds.). (2020). Decolonizing mental health: Embracing indigenous multi-dimensional practice. Journal of Charlton Publishing.

Coates, R. (2020, July 30). *A 12-step program for decolonizing the university: A conversation with Dr. Rodney Coates* [Web conversation]. Sage Publications.

Cosgrove, L. (2005). When labels mask oppression: Implications for teaching psychiatric taxonomy to mental health counselors. *Journal of Mental Health Counseling, 27*(4), 283–296.

Curtis, D. A., & Kelley, L. J. (2019). Myth-checking: Evaluating teaching activities in abnormal psychology. *North American Journal of Psychology, 21*(2), 245–252.

Delphin-Rittmon, M. E., Flanagan, E. H., Andres-Hyman, R., Ortiz, J., & Amer, M. M. (2015). Racial ethnic differences in access, diagnosis and outcomes in public sector inpatient mental health treatment. *Psychological Services, 12*(2), 158–166.

Fernando, S. (2017). *Institutional racism in psychiatry and clinical psychology: Race matters in mental health*. Palgrave Macmillan.

Gottlieb, R., Cabral, C., Despradel, R., & Touisaint, S. (2021, January 18). *Beyond cultural competence: Decolonizing clinical constructs* [Zoom Webinar].

Green, L. D., & Ubozoh, K. (Eds.). (2019). *We've been too patient: Voices from radical mental health*. North Atlantic Books.

Greenwald, A. G., McGhee, D. E., & Schwartz, J. L. K. (1998). Measuring individual differences in implicit cognition: The implicit association test. *Journal of Personality and Social Psychology, 74*(6), 1464–1480.

Hays, D. G., Prosek, E. A., & McLeod, A. L. (2010). A mixed methodological analysis of the role of culture in the clinical decision-making process. *Journal of Counseling and Development, 88*(1), 114–121.

Henrich, J., Heine, S. J., & Norenzayan, A. (2010). The weirdest people in the world? *The Behavioral and Brain Sciences, 33*(61–83), 111–135. https://doi.org/10.1017/S0140525X0999152X

Hoffman, K. M., Trawalter, S., Axt, J. R., & Oliver, M. N. (2016, April 19). Racial bias in pain assessment and treatment recommendations, and false beliefs about biological differences between blacks and whites. *Proceedings of the National Academy of Sciences of the United States of America, 113*(16), 4296–4301.

Holman, A. (2020, December 9). *Antiracist psychological assessment: Acknowledging the harmful history and working towards honesty, humility and healing* [Webinar]. The Collaborative Assessment Association of the Bay Area.

Institute for the Study and Promotion of Race and Culture (ISPRC). (2020, October 23–24). *Diversity challenge: Goodbye "isms," hello future*. Boston College Lynch School of Education.

Ishibashi, N. L. (Ed.). (2015). *Critical perspectives of the DSM-5*. lulu.com

Jones, C. (2020, June 15). Not just the syllabus, throw the whole discipline in the trash. *Medium*. Retrieved from https://medium.com/the-faculty/not-just-the-syllabus-throw-the-whole-discipline-in-the-trash-777d19201cb5

Keith, K. D. (2018). *Culture across the curriculum: A psychology teacher's handbook*. Cambridge University Press.

Kendi, I. X. (2019). *How to be an antiracist*. One World.

Kurtis, T., & Adams, G. (2015). Decolonizing liberation: Toward a transnational feminist psychology. *Journal of Social and Political Psychology, 3*(1), 388–413.

Liang, J., Matheson, B. E., & Douglas, J. M. (2016). Mental health diagnostic considerations in racial/ethnic minority youth. *Journal of Child and Family Studies, 25*, 1926–1940.

Lift Every Voice and Speak (LEVS). (2020, October 29). *Peers envisioning and engaging in recovery services* [Speaker's Bureau]. Retrieved from https://peer-snet.org/programs/levs/

Mann, C. E., & Himelein, M. J. (2008). Putting the person back into psychopathology: An intervention to reduce mental health stigma in the classroom. *Social Psychiatry and Psychiatric Epidemiology, 43*, 545–551.

Moore-Lobban, S., & Green, C. (2020, September 11). *Race, racism & racial trauma: Speaking to the unspeakable in professional psychology* [Webinar]. Washington DC Psychological Association.

Murray-Browne, S. (2020, June 28). *6 crucial steps to decolonize your therapy practice* [Webinar]. Self-business.

Nguyen, L., Huang, L. N., Arganza, G. F., & Liao, Q. (2007). The influence of race and ethnicity on psychiatric diagnoses and clinical characteristics of children and adolescents in children's services. *Cultural Diversity and Ethnic Minority Psychology, 13*, 18–25.

Prilleltensky, I., Dokecki, P., Frieden, G., & Wang, V. O. (2007). Counseling for wellness and justice: Foundations and ethical dilemmas. In E. Aldarondo (Ed.), *Advancing social justice through clinical practice* (pp. 19–42). Lawrence Erlbaum Associates Publishers.

Project Implicit. (2001). *Implicit Association Test (IAT)*. Harvard University. Retrieved from https://implicit.harvard.edu/implicit/index.jsp

Singh, A. A. (2019). *The racial healing handbook: Practical activities to help you challenge privilege, confront racism, and engage in collective healing*. New Harbinger Publications.

Smith, C., ORourke, S., & Richards, D. (2020, July 20). *Multicultural counseling & allyship* [Panel]. American Counseling Association.

Spann, R. T., Davis, H., & Akinyela, M. (2020). *Mental health and Black men* [webinar]. American Counseling Association.

The Sage Institute. (n.d.). Retrieved from https://sageinst.org

Tripathi, S., Messias, E., Spollen, J., & Salomon, R. M. (2019). Modern-day relics of psychiatry. *The Journal of Nervous and Mental Disease, 207*(9), 701–704.

Tuck, E., & Yang, K. W. (2012). Decolonization is not a metaphor. *Decolonization: Indigeneity, Education, & Society, 1*(1), 1–40.

Wang, E. W. (2019). *The collected Schizophenias: Essays*. Graywolf Press.

Wong, W. C. (2006). Understanding dialectical thinking from a cultural-historical perspective. *Philosophical Psychology, 19*(2), 239–260.

Zapata, K. (2020, February 27). Decolonizing mental health: The importance of an oppression-focused mental health system. *The Calgary Journal*. Retrieved from: https://calgaryjournal.ca/more/calgaryvoices/4982-decolonizing-mental-health-the-importance-of-an-oppression-focused-mental-health-system.html

10

An Antiracist Approach to Social Work Education at HBCUs

Melissa E. Buckley, Malcolm Drewery, and Gary Jones

History of Whiteness

Eurocentrism seeks to impose a European perspective into the consciousness of other people across the world (Asante, 2012). The Eurocentric ideology makes its way into every aspect of other people's lives, assimilating them into and erasing the diverse history of those who are considered other. This process started with the European conquest of the Americas and has unfortunately continued to this day. Eurocentric education affects all people but in very different ways. It influences their worldviews, their culture, their self-esteem, and their physical, mental, and spiritual well-being by reproducing the racist status quo and reinforcing racist beliefs that people of color have less rights to agency and self-determination.

M. E. Buckley (✉) • M. Drewery • G. Jones
Coppin State University, Baltimore, MD, USA
e-mail: mbuckley@coppin.edu; mdrewery@coppin.edu; gajones@coppin.edu

© The Author(s), under exclusive license to Springer Nature Switzerland AG 2022

K. Johnson et al. (eds.), *Developing Anti-Racist Practices in the Helping Professions: Inclusive Theory, Pedagogy, and Application*,
https://doi.org/10.1007/978-3-030-95451-2_10

The major theories of the helping professions taught in higher education emerged from eurocentric theoretical and conceptual frameworks. Erik Erikson's psychosocial development, Sigmund Freud's psychoanalysis, David Kolb's experiential learning styles, Lawrence Kohlberg's moral development theories, and Carl Jung's analytical psychology are considered by many to be the pillars of helping professions. In an open letter to the editor of the Journal of Analytical Psychology (2019), a group of researchers called for the journal to confront the issue of Jung's racist ideologies and to apologize for the continued use of Jung's colonial and racist ideologies, particularly in clinical and academic circles. The researchers asserted that Jung's explicit and implicit racist ideologies have contributed to internalized and interpersonal conflicts for those represented by his racist thought (Journal of Analytical Psychology, 2019). Jung's ideologies are not the only ones to have inflicted psychological harm on non-white people. In 2021, the American Psychiatric Association (APA) issued a statement acknowledging the history of explicit and implicit racism within psychiatry and committed to working towards social equity and fairness for all (American Psychiatric Association, 2021).

Historically, the notion of "whiteness" has largely influenced non-white people. Radd and Grossland (2019) suggest that in order to address racism, one must also address whiteness. Lindsay (2007) defines whiteness as what is considered to be the normal or correct state of being and that it is deeply embedded in political systems that it goes unnoticed or simply regarded as the normal way of being.

Whiteness has negatively influenced academic settings, thus creating a potentially hostile learning environment for non-whites and whites because the absence of an antiracist pedagogy creates a toxic learning environment (Lindsay, 2007). It is for this reason that abolitionists, anti-racists and religious leaders aligned to establish Historically Black Colleges and Universities (HBCUs) (Crewe, 2017; Mobley, 2017).

HBCUs created spaces for former slaves to obtain skills and networks to transition towards some type of independence after years of enslavement, trauma, and exploitation (Bowles et al., 2016; Crewe, 2017; Williams, 2005). The establishment of these institutions was antiracist in nature, yet they still maintained eurocentric influences. Though the institutions were established for Black scholars, it is important to note the model they replicated draws from or perpetuates Eurocentric power or privilege and exclusion is at their very foundation (Arroyo & Gasman, 2014). To that end, HBCUs and other institutions of higher education need to adopt antiracist pedagogy, such as Critical Race Theory (CRT), to undo the damage caused by whiteness. Whiteness is described as historical, institutional, structural, and emotional and CRT will illuminate the ways whiteness and racism have been normalized and harmful to non-whites (Radd & Grosland, 2019).

Using Critical Race Theory (CRT)

Traditional theoretical frameworks and ideologies steeped in whiteness tend to pathologize Black and Brown communities and ignore the cultural strengths, assets, and influences of these communities. These theoretical approaches are harmful to the pedagogical process because it establishes a deficit perspective in the learner (Arroyo & Gasman, 2014). Viewing the experiences of others from a Eurocentric perspective may lead to exclusion, marginalization, and discrimination when individuals do not possess and display traits valued within European American culture. Eurocentrism can occur at individual, cultural, and institutional levels and can be manifested in overt and covert ways (Cunningham et al., 2004). Hamilton-Mason and Schnieder's (2018) study on antiracist social work pedagogy suggests that in order to engage in antiracist pedagogy, whiteness and white privilege must be addressed. To achieve this, pedagogy must be equitable and inclusive (Trifonas, 2002).

CRT is the singular movement within higher education that unapologetically calls for the study of race to be the primary focus. Yet, this theory is one that students may never be taught or exposed to which places students at risk of continued exposure to racist pedagogy (Crenshaw et al., 1995). This is of particular concern in disciplines of the various helping professions. Social work pedagogy must follow the example of social justice set forth by the APA and boldly confront issues of race and racism. The Council on Social Work Education (CSWE) announced in September 2020 that a task force will examine social work pedagogy and make recommendations for diversity and inclusion for the 2022 Educational

Policy and Accreditation Standards (EPAS) (Hymans et al., 2020). These recommendations must be inclusive of antiracist language and strategies for how to activate antiracist social work pedagogy.

Social Work Education: A Call for Antiracist Pedagogy

In his seminal work, "The Miseducation of the Negro", Carter G. Woodson (1990) asserts that education is intended to inspire people to want to learn more and to desire to enhance life. He further suggests this has not been the reality for Blacks in higher education who have in fact been "miseducated" and have perpetuated the cycle of miseducating countless others. Beasley, Chapman-Hilliard, & McClain (2016) explain that for many Black students attending Predominantly White Institutions (PWIs), both their academic and social outcomes can be negatively impacted as they matriculate at these institutions due to the absence of pedagogy that acknowledges their historical foundation, identity, and existence. These students earn an education that is shaped by the influences of the white society and are rarely given the opportunity to explore their lived experiences within those pedagogical frameworks. While HBCUs have their challenges and are not inherently antiracist, many Black students elect to attend HBCUs for their cultural relevance and to further their own racial development (Holland, 2020). Thus, it is imperative to the social and academic evolution of Black students, particularly at HBCUs that they have the benefit of a well structured and developed antiracist education, not an education bolstered by whiteness and patriarchy that reinforces the erasure of their lived experiences.

Social work, as a profession and pedagogy, is in a state of evolution which has been brought on by the cries for change, justice, and equality. At the time of this writing, the United States has been grappling with the unjust murders of Black men and women, healthcare disparities, evictions, non-liveable income, unemployment, and the disproportionate impact of the COVID-19 pandemic on Black communities. During the first 8 months of 2020, 164 Black people were unjustly killed by police

(Cohen, 2020). That means that each week, Black men and women, either through mainstream news reporting or through local news, learned that another Black person was killed by the police. The rapid public dissemination of these traumatic events reinforced the reality of racial injustice, and Black communities were yet again left to find a way forward (Wagaman et al., 2019).

At the time of this writing, the White House was attacked by predominantly white protestors who believed their rights, power, and status in this country were at risk. The sitting President did not initially condemn these acts, which further incited bigotry and racism. Of note is the fact that the event was caught on live television and images of the men and women who stormed the Capitol went viral. Their guilt was evident, yet their actions were met with sympathy by the President of the United States as well as certain mainstream news outlets. In some instances, the rioters were even gently escorted out of the restricted areas they unlawfully entered.

The death of George Floyd in May of 2020 prompted hundreds of protests nationwide over the summer. In many cities, including the nation's capital, police met protesters with tear gas, violence, and arrests. National Guard troops were deployed to the Lincoln Memorial on June 2, 2020, during protests held in Washington, DC, over the death of George Floyd. However, the insurrection by white protesters was very different.

The response by the police was one more example of the hypocrisy in our country's law enforcement response to protest. There was no call for the National Guard, there was no tear gas, there was no pepper spray, and no one was beaten by the police or shot with rubber bullets. During the summer of 2020, a number of legislatures pushed for punitive policies against protesters challenging police brutality, inequities in our society, and white supremacy. The intent behind the policies that emerged during this tenure was to deter multigenerational and multiethnic groups uniting to address systemic issues. Florida Governor Ron DeSantis's passage of what is called House Bill 1 was the catalyst for over 92 anti-protest bills across the nation since the death of Mr. George Floyd (Craig, 2021; Solomon, 2021). Rather than addressing the concerns of the protesters, politicians have taken actions to deter individuals from practicing their freedom to peacefully assemble.

Members of the DC National Guard, armed and wearing camouflage uniforms, stood on the steps of the Lincoln Memorial in June of 2020, as crowds of demonstrators held a peaceful protest following several days of demonstrations. During the January 6 insurrection, rioters had already made it inside the building before the DC National Guard was activated. There was a livestream video of the January 6 insurrection showing a Capitol Hill police officer taking a selfie with a rioter inside the building. There is video footage of Missouri Senator Josh Hawley walking from the Capitol encouraging rioters to keep fighting.

According to CNN News analyst, Nicole Chavez, in an article she wrote comparing the Black Lives Matter (BLM) movement protest and the Capitol insurrection, last June, protesters in Washington, DC, repeatedly faced tear gas. Many were detained. One protest, on one day, led to 88 arrests. By comparison, the Metropolitan Police Department Chief said that on January 6, police had made 52 arrests, only 26 of which were made on U.S. Capitol grounds. The George Floyd protests were largely peaceful and law abiding while the Capitol insurrectionists blatantly broke laws, yet there was an obvious difference in how police handled both incidents (Chavez, 2021).

These incessant reminders that Black lives do not matter has a significant impact on the mental and emotional health of those who recognize that their protests would not have been received with sympathy and the likelihood of loss of life would have been imminent. The fear of becoming the next hashtag can be crippling. These high rates of loss of life at the hands of police should have a profound impact on emerging social workers and those who are currently in practice and it should inspire a call to action.

Antiracist Social Work Pedagogy

Traditional social work pedagogy tends to assess challenges faced by Black people through a pathological lens. This is the approach that emerging social workers take into the field of practice and unless given the opportunity to deconstruct, most will continue with this Eurocentric approach that lacks cultural insights. Two of the three contributors to this article, Drs. Buckley and Jones are social workers trained at accredited social work programs. They both matriculated at three institutions respectively, two of which are HBCUs and are current faculty members at an HBCU. They have been confronted with the need to deconstruct much of the teachings learned during their matriculation due to pathological influences. They now have an understanding of the need to elevate the values and strengths of the Black community and to employ non-oppressive methods and interventions. Martin and Martin noted (1985) social workers who adapt middle class values to "fix" Black families, rather than viewing their values and strengths, are pathologizing and traumatizing the Black community. The narrow focus on pathology without the integration of holistic, asset-based, and historical analysis in the classroom will prevent the elimination of disparities and dismantling of oppressive systems. It is for this reason that HBCU social work programs were established to increase the likelihood of social workers being better equipped to understand the diverse needs of their Black clients (Crewe, 2017). Research suggests that practitioners' conceptions of cultural responsiveness, cultural relevance, or other widely used terms like "diversity" and "multiculturalism" may center more on honoring difference, celebrating diversity, and ensuring representation, with less attention to racism, injustice, or the systems and structures that create disparate outcomes for students of color and other minoritized groups (Galloway et al., 2019). It is imperative that inequities, racism, and structural oppression measures are explicitly integrated into the curricula that prepare nurses, social workers, educators, and other helping professionals so they can serve and educate individuals, families, and communities effectively and efficiently, with an understanding of existing oppressive structures. When these measures are not taken, practitioners can cause additional trauma and harm to clientele.

Social work programs cannot afford to miss opportunities to bolster their pedagogy with content that generates dialogue around social justice and race issues. Faculty must create spaces for students to confront the impact of racism on individuals and communities to counteract the conflicting information about the status and impact of race relations of this era. On one hand, they are told they are seeing the manifestation of a post-racial society; however, the daily account of the value of Black lives tells another tale (Mueller, 2012). The images of successful people of color, the emphasis on Black empowerment, and the influence of "Black culture" on mainstream society give the impression that Black people are better now than they have ever been. This perception may reduce the urgency of the cries for racial justice among Black people and diminish the need for antiracist pedagogy (Mueller, 2012). Ultimately, emerging social workers should be prepared for activism as that is an ethical principle according to the National Association of Social Workers (NASW) Code of Ethics.

Racism has been the cornerstone of American society since its inception and is evidenced in its structures and institutions. Mueller (2012) says white people are benefactors of racism while people of color experience unjust and racist treatment. This definition of racism is subtle; yet, the depths of the influences of racism are profound in this definition. This definition is the very reason social work pedagogy must have a strongly stated antiracist approach. Social work instruction at the undergraduate, graduate and doctoral levels must demonstrate an awareness of the barriers to justice, equality, and cultural humility. Unfortunately, social work historically has done a poor job of addressing racism on a macro level and has instead left the burden of responsibility on micro interventions to confront this social ill (Corley & Young, 2018).

Studies have reported 72.6% of masters prepared social workers are white, compared to 19.1% who are Black or African American and 67.4% of bachelors prepared social workers are white, compared to 25.7% who are Black or African American (Salsberg et al., 2017). These numbers are unequal and while these social workers have learned the competencies and the knowledge, values and skills set forth by the CWSE, the lack of an antiracist education will make it challenging for them to recognize and respond to the deeply entrenched racism that oppresses and binds their non-White clients (Corley & Young, 2018).

Smith et al. (2017) suggest that white professors have limited or no guidance in their attempts at antiracist pedagogy development which contributes to their selection of eurocentric and pedagogical approaches. If social workers are mandated by the NASW Code of Ethics to address social problems and challenge social injustice, social work pedagogy must be more intentional in integrating these ethical principles. Social work pedagogy must fully embrace an antiracist approach that espouses anti-Black racism and cultural humility.

Higher education programs have done very little to change their programs from a Eurocentric based curriculum. While most higher education programs have had new policies and frameworks that speak about equality, equity, transformation, and change, institutional cultures, and epistemological traditions have not considerably changed. Policies might be there but the willingness to implement them is lacking. This is why it is of paramount importance to bring about fundamental epistemological change at institutions of higher learning. Antiracist pedagogies and theories challenge structures and systems that have historically upheld European ideas, identity, culture, and values (Gourdine & Brown, 2016; Trinidad, 2014). Steps must be taken by institutions to include students' lived experiences in the campus culture in a non- oppressive manner. In addition, the hiring of professors with expertise and interest in antiracism and dismantling of white supremacy is a necessary step (Gourdine & Brown, 2016).

All CSWE accredited programs are required to uphold the Education Policy and Accreditation Standards (EPAS) in order to remain in good standing and to be able to award accredited social work degrees. With respect to antiracism, the program should demonstrate this mandate by reinforcing three competencies in particular: engaging diversity and difference in practice, advancing human rights and engaging in policy practice (Council on Social Work Education, 2015). It should seem peculiar that a values-based profession that speaks to its commitment to address social justice would then be accused of being tone deaf at best and racist at worst. Social work researchers for over 25 years have conducted research and have asserted that social work as a profession and social work education are racist based on the way in which the profession operates and provides classroom instruction (Corley & Young, 2018; McMahon & Allen-Meares, 1992; Woo et al., 2018). A study by McMahon & Allen-Meares (1992) found that only 6% of the 4 major social work journals in the 1980s addressed race and ethnicity. Barretti's (2015) study as reported by Woo et al. (2018) found that there was an underrepresentation of

Black women in social work literature. The failure of the profession to address issues of race and inequalities has a negative impact on the men and women of color who are social workers and on aspiring social workers. If their experiences of injustice are not even validated by their profession, how can they truly engage in the work and fight for social justice? The responsibility to establish the rubric for combating racial injustice should not rest solely on the backs of those affected by this endemic. It is the responsibility of the social work profession and the CSWE to strengthen their interventions and approaches to antiracism.

Why Critical Race Theory (CRT) Essential to HBCU Curriculum

People of color in the United States have been made to understand the world through a Eurocentric curriculum. Eurocentric curriculum is defined as a curricular narrative that utilizes the social history and understandings of the dominant white race to communicate and sustain white construction of society (Carruthers, 1994; Scheurich & Young, 1997; Shujaa, 1998). From this perspective, the focus of the Eurocentric curriculum is on the complex and contextual comprehension of ideology, race/ethnicity, the school, society, and curricula. The Eurocentric curriculum explores how these ideologies and institutions intersect to create and foster intellectual disadvantages and the lack of self-knowledge among students of color, families, and communities. Historically, the miseducation of Blacks in the United States has been used to preserve white supremacist ideology through curriculum standards that communicate the dominant societies norms, values, and expectations (Carruthers, 1994; Shujaa, 1998; Watkins, 2001).

Black people have been forced into a system of learning that has caused them to struggle with their identities because history is taught from a Eurocentric perspective. The Eurocentric curriculum sustains multiple forms of racism—cultural, individual, interpersonal, institutional, structural, and systemic (Bell, 2019). Carter G. Woodson (1990), found that the Eurocentric curriculum of the U.S. education system was propaganda to instill conformity and inferiority into Black students which he considered a form of mental slavery. The fact that most Black people do not know the complete history of African people demonstrates that Eurocentric education has pervaded the education system. Blacks have been forced to take on a frame of reference that is not natural or familiar to them, which is a manifestation of oppression. This mindset has led to the oppressive structural and functional issues that exist in the United States (Grier & Cobbs, 1992). In general, Blacks are devalued in the educational system of the United States, and the lack of interest in this system can stem from their inability to see the benefit from learning from a Eurocentric perspective. This perspective tells Blacks they only can be valued and rewarded in society if they assimilate into the culture and ways of the white mainstream, which essentially means giving up their blackness.

Learning from an Afrocentric perspective fosters a psychological liberation characterized by a conceptual shift from a narrative rooted only in oppression to a narrative that acknowledges the strengths, accomplishments, and creativity of Black people throughout their history (Baldwin, 1989; Myers & Speight, 2010). CRT's main thesis is that racism is much more endemic than an isolated incident. It asserts that racism is rooted in American institutions, culture, and concepts of self-identity and group identity (Vargas, 2003). CRT posits that time and good faith alone are not sufficient to cope with the race problem that exists in the United States. Therefore, it is essential for Blacks to reclaim their historical narrative of reference starting from the transatlantic slave trade to the current crisis of mass incarceration and police brutality. Without these references, Black people will continue to operate from a Eurocentric perspective. CRT shifts the center of focus from notions of whiteness to the cultures of people of color.

What Is CRT?

In general, the aim of CRT is to analyze, deconstruct, and transform power by using race as its point of engagement. CRT is rooted in social constructionism and critical theory and converges with feminist thought, critical legal studies, and the Civil Rights Movement (Vargas, 2003). Specifically, for CRT, race is not just an additional variable; instead, it is at the center of the research perspective. CRT is composed of four perspectives. First, it posits that "race" is largely a social experience, and racial groups experience and understand race in different ways. Second, it theorizes that the racial experiences of racial minority groups are subordinate relative to a white racial experience. Third, much of the work of CRT applies insights to how race functions to critique rules, norms, standards, and assumptions that appear "neutral," but it systemically disadvantages or "subordinates" racial minorities. Finally, CRT describes and theorizes about the causes that maintain racial minorities' relative subordination in a post-Civil Rights Movement American culture that has come to embrace the equality norm (Crenshaw et al., 1995; Delgado & Stefancic, 2001).

CRT origins are in legal studies that examine the continued impact of race and racism on society particularly after the Civil Rights Movement (Harris, 2012). Legal scholars Derrick Bell, a former Harvard Law professor, and Alan Freeman were foundational in the start of CRT studies (Delgado, 2005; Delgado & Stefancic, 2001). Criticism of CRT often centers on Bell's assertions that race is a central discussion in the United States from law to politics and social concerns (Delgado, 2005). Ensuing research by numerous scholars have focused a lens on racism and its impact through laws and the court where racism can sometimes be perpetuated by the legal process in which justice is arguably supposed to be blind. For example, Critical race theorists and others claimed that under New York's stop and frisk policy the police were unconstitutionally relying on people's race in making judgments about who seems suspicious and dangerous. Critical race theorists attempt to show how contemporary law—including contemporary antidiscrimination law—Intentionally or unintentionally encourages discriminatory thoughts and actions in the legal system (Harris, 2012). This is a recurring theme in CRT research. Harris's (2012) work on CRT points to themes and issues that legal studies sought to elucidate whether implicit bias, unconscious or unintentional racism, or structural racism which structures are in place through laws, policies, and programs continue to limit improvements for Blacks and others in different aspects of society.

Although CRT's roots are in the law, CRT scholarship draws on data from various disciplines – sociology, history, feminist and postcolonial studies, ethnic and cultural studies, economics, and political science. This information helps researchers understand how relations of power based on racial hierarchies can be deconstructed and challenged by calling into question fundamental assumptions about social structures in American society and the nature of any injustices perpetrated (Harris, 2012; Baciu, 2020).

Critical Race Theory Usage and Implications in Social Work

According to Hiraldo (2010), CRT's framework originally consisted of five major tenets: the permanence of racism; counter-storytelling; whiteness as property; interest conversion; and the critique of liberalism. CRT scholars have added to the list three tenets including intersectionality, commitment to social justice (McCoy & Rodricks, 2015), and race as a mechanism for organizing society (Delgado & Stefancic, 2001; Ladson-Billings, 2016a, b; Ladson-Billings & Tate, 1995; Ledesma & Calderón, 2015; Lynn, 2005; Smedley & Smedley, 2012; Solórzano & Yosso, 2016; Taylor, 2016; Yosso et al., 2009; Zamudio et al., 2011). These tenets of CRT can be used to uncover the ingrained societal disparities that support a system of privilege and oppression reinforced through the institution of higher education. Although CRT varies in theory and usage, there are three major tenets of CRT that are of significance for the profession of social work and should be included in social work curricula:

- Inherent racism (permanence of racism)
- Race as a social construct (race is a mechanism for organizing society)
- Differential racialization (counter-storytelling)

Inherent Racism

Inherent racism stipulates that racism and race-based judgements, evaluations, and practices are rooted at every level of the society and are embedded in the everyday life of individuals. The prescriptions and stereotypes about race and inter-racial or intra-racial relations are absorbed by the individual through culturalization and socialization processes. These prescriptions and stereotypes are put into practice in their daily activities and feed the loop indefinitely by the repeated thoughts, words, and actions (Abrams & Moio, 2009). These prescriptions and stereotypes are applied by individuals when fulfilling their various social and professional roles which permeate institutional arrangements and practices. These beliefs lead to structural racial oppression of ethnic and racial minorities and socio-economic inequality between people from different ethnic and racial backgrounds (Campbell, 2014). Simultaneously, the fact that race-based judgments and practices have become such an integral part of ordinary social arrangements and structures makes racism invisible, and thus, it is prone to spread.

Inherent racism teaches us that, when laying the foundations of the helping relationship with Black clients, social workers have to pay extra attention to the risk of allowing their own stereotypes to permeate their professional decisions about the ways and means involved in assisting their clients (Baciu, 2020). Campbell (2014) urges social workers to deepen their knowledge of the growing impact systemic racism has on the community and national level; for members of racial and ethnic minority groups and communities in order to improve the effects of their intervention with these clients.

The social workers who are aware of this CRT tenet will re-examine their own beliefs and values constantly and will reflect critically about the potential bias of these beliefs and values on their professional judgments. They also will scrutinize institutional practices and arrangements that potentially could foster discriminatory climates and advocate for their improvement.

Race as a Mechanism for Organizing Society

Race as a social construct has real life implications. The associations and meanings of race inevitably are shaped by political, social, and economic processes and historically have served to justify exploitation, inequality, and oppression of ethnic and racial minority groups (Campbell, 2014). Race as a mechanism for organizing society teaches us how labels arbitrarily associated with Blacks strengthen over the course of time. Once produced, these labels become inextricably linked, in the collective imagination, to a certain race and start defining each and all members of a racial or ethnic group (Campbell, 2014). The social workers who absorb and internalize these labels inevitably will come to enact them in their professional activities and will subsequently alter the principle of individualization of their intervention. They will produce parameters for the collective, regardless of race, rather than adapted interventions with actual people in need of support, that is based on geographic location (Baciu, 2020).

The social workers who are aware of this CRT tenet will sort out what is real and what is imagined about their clients' characteristics and will design intervention plans that respond to the actual needs of the beneficiaries. No matter where they are, they will not condone racial discrimination or race-based judgments and evaluations.

Differential Racialization

Differential racialization holds that the various racial minority groups in the United States have been racialized in different ways in response to the different needs of the majority group (Abrams & Moio, 2009). These attributes may refer to various dimensions from expectations, to roles, behaviors, language, norms, or meanings and are labels that operate differently in the case of the various groups (Baciu, 2020). The groups feature different histories and struggles. They had to contend with different sets of discriminatory laws and practices put forth by the dominant group. For example, English-only laws for Latinos, alien land laws for Asians, and Jim Crow laws for Blacks. Thus, such attributes become inextricably linked, in the collective imaginary to a certain race and start defining each and all members of a racial or ethnic group. However, the racialization of a certain group of people can differ historically depending on the concrete needs and agenda (social, economic, political) of the dominant group (Campbell, 2014).

This tenet of CRT shows how the narratives of the dominant group changed accordingly over time to facilitate society's obtaining what it wanted from the group in question (Baciu, 2020; Delgado & Stefancic, 2001). For example, during slavery, when southern whites had total control of their slaves, the dominant narratives, songs, and stories about Blacks were heartening: Blacks were happy with their lives and pleased to serve whites. After the Emancipation Proclamation, when Blacks received their freedom and were perceived as a threat, social images of them changed. The research data used to exemplify how this tenet works in real life situations demonstrated that two opposing images about the minority group can coexist, in the collective imaginary of the majority, without being questioned. Such unquestioned wavering projections impede the members of the dominant group to take any type of stance in support of the minority group, when confronted with overt institutional abuse.

The social workers who are aware of this CRT principle will not tolerate discourses or narratives that are meant to justify racially oppressive behavior and to impede ethnic minorities in achieving their lawful rights. They will actively get involved in deconstructing such discourses and revealing their harmful nature and the negative effects they generate in the lives of their clients. Whenever possible, they will break down the labels and stereotypes and show their audience that beyond these labels are actual human beings with real vulnerabilities, needs, and feelings who are pursuing the same happiness as everyone else.

The commitment to equality and antiracism makes social work and CRT highly compatible in pursuing activities that lead to transformative social justice (Ortiz & Jani, 2010); while social work is dedicated to promoting human well-being and individualized approaches in improving the social functioning of people from various disadvantaged backgrounds, CRT seeks to understand and tackle the actual mechanisms and structures that create or maintain the social disadvantage by making the dominant group aware of inequities and how individuals are treated according to their race (Baciu, 2020). The use of the CRT framework is essential for social workers not only in teaching awareness of cultural humility and anti-racism, but also in representing the interests of the marginalized and stigmatized people.

Conclusion

In this chapter, we outlined the historical context of racist theoretical frameworks and perspectives used in social work education. We demonstrated the presence of these same pedagogical influences in social work programs at HBCUs and explained that though HBCUs were established to meet the educational needs and aspirations of Black scholars, those institutions were founded on oppressive and patriarchal structures. The persuasive culture of whiteness in higher education and in social work education has persisted and in some instances has even gone unchallenged. As a helping profession, social work education cannot be silent on issues of race and inequities. For social work programs to authentically adopt an antiracist pedagogy, they must do so by employing CRT as its guiding antiracist theoretical framework.

The three major tenets of CRT, inherent racism, race as a mechanism for organizing society, and differential racialization, not only provide insight into the systemic harm caused by racism, these tenets also provide social workers with a guide for how to become antiracist. An antiracist social work pedagogy must be integrated at the micro, mezzo, and macro levels of instruction to fully equip emerging social workers with the critical tools needed to identify, confront and respond to racism and anti-Black racism. The CSWE task force must include specific antiracist language in its 2022 recommendations for the new iteration of its EPAS. Failure to do so could result in a lack of trust from social work educators, professionals, and emerging social workers. Social work education and its pedagogy should follow the example of the APA in condemning whiteness and reinforcing its pillars with fairness and equity for all as its strategic framework for an antiracist pedagogy.

All helping professions must see the importance and value in adopting an antiracist approach in practice, not just social work. With the climate of racial tensions in the United States related to police brutality and health disparities, an increase in awareness regarding race and racism is critical for helping professions (Anabel, 2018). Color-blind [racial ideology] and universalist attitudes must be dismantled and helping professionals must consider how critical race theory and other similar theoretical frameworks emphasize racial justice and enhance the work of helping professions (Spainerman & Smith, 2017). Only then will individuals, groups, and communities that have been historically disenfranchised and pathologized be able to begin their journey to equality.

Guiding Questions

1. Is it possible for social workers to not recognize when they are being racist towards their clients and are operating within their best interest?
2. Is it possible for Black institutions or Black social workers to be racist? How is engaging in antiracist work different for white people than it is for people of color?
3. What steps do professors need to take to ensure that scholars are competent and confident in their understanding and application of CRT.
4. Should social work programs and other helping professions continue to use Eurocentric frameworks while integrating CRT or should they abandon use of Eurocentric frameworks altogether?
5. What steps can professors take to help non-Black and White students to understand Antiracism and its essentiality in social work as a profession?

Quiz Questions

1. What is the difference between a non-racist and an anti-racist social work program?
2. Can you share at least two reasons why a helping professional should have an understanding of various social inequities experienced by populations they will serve?
3. How have HBCUs failed to educate students of color from an anti-racist perspective?
4. Using the CRT tenets, describe an antiracist social work pedagogy.

5. What roles does eurocentrism play in our society?
6. What roles does eurocentrism play in our society?
7. Identify the impact of social workers and human service professionals who are not committed to taking steps to assess if policies and procedures utilized are non-oppressive and anti-exploitative.
8. What political, social, and economic factors contributed to the emergence of Historically Black Colleges and Universities?
9. Identify the impact of the promotion and indoctrination of racist and pathological frameworks in social work and human service curriculums.
10. What social work values align with critical race theory?

References

Abrams, L. S., & Moio, J. A. (2009). Critical race theory and the cultural competence dilemma in social work education. *Journal of Social Work Education, 45*(2), 245.

American Psychiatric Association. (2021, January 18). *APA's apology to black, indigenous and people of color for its support of structural Racism in psychiatry* [Press release]. Retrieved from https://www.psychiatry.org/newsroom/apa-apology-for-its-support-of-structural-racism-in-psychiatry.

Anable, R. by E. (2018). Racism in the United States: Implications for the helping professions, 2nd Edition. Smith College Studies in Social Work (Taylor & Francis Ltd), 88(2), 174–177.

Arroyo, A. T., & Gasman, M. (2014). An HBCU-based educational approach for black college student success: Toward a framework with implications for all institutions. *American Journal of Education, 121*(1), 57–85.

Asante, M. K. (2012). Reconstituting curricula in African universities: In search of an Afrocentric design. In C. Alvares & S. S. Faruqi (Eds.), *Decolonizing the university: The emerging quest for non-Eurocentric paradigms*. Penerbit University of Malaysia.

Baciu, L. (2020). Reading beyond the Label Implications of the Critical Race Theory for the Social Work Practice with Roma Persons. *Revista de Asistență Socială, 3*, 79–98.

Baldwin, J. A. (1989). The role of Black Psychologists in black liberation. *Journal of Black Psychology, 16*(1), 67–76. https://doi.org/10.1177/009579848901600106

Barretti, M. A. (2015). In search of women of color in the social work journal literature (1998–2007). *Affilia: Journal of Women & Social Work, 30*(4), 427–446.

Beasley, S. T., Chapman-Hilliard, C., & McClain, S. (2016). Linking the emancipatory pedagogy of Africana/black studies with academic identity outcomes among black students attending PWIs. *Journal of Pan African Studies, 9*(8), 9.

Bell, K. (2019). Transforming social work for environmental justice: Theory, practice, and education, *Australian Social Work, 72*(2), 242–244. https://doi.org/10.1080/0312407X.2019.1569080.

Bowles, D. D., Hopps, J. G., & Clayton, O. (2016). The impact and influence of HBCUs on the social work profession. *Journal of Social Work Education, 52*(1), 118–132.

Campbell, E. (2014). "using critical race theory to measure "racial competency" among Social Workers.". Journal of Sociology and Social Work, 2(2). https://doi.org/10.15640/jssw.v2n2a5

Chavez, N. (2021). *This was the police response when it was Black protesters on DC streets last year.* https://www.cnn.com/2021/01/07/us/police-response-black-lives-matter-protest-us-capitol/index.html

Cohen, L. (2020, September 10). Police in the U.S. killed 164 black people in the first 8 months of 2020. these are their names. (part I: January-April). CBS News. https://www.cbsnews.com/pictures/black-people-killed-by-police-in-the-u-s-in-2020/.

Corley, N. A., & Young, S. M. (2018, Oct 1). Is Social Work Still Racist? A Content Analysis of Recent Literature. *Soc Work, 63*(4), 317–326.

Council on Social Work Education. (2015). Educational policy and accreditation standards

Craig, T. (2021, April 9). *He was arrested at a black lives matter protest. Now, he's warning others about Florida's anti-riot proposal.* Washington Post. https://www.washingtonpost.com/national/florida-protest-bill-silences-activists/2021/04/09/5b5b252c-93c2-11eb-a74e-1f4cf89fd948_story.html

Crenshaw, K., Gotanda, N., Peller, G., & Thomas, K. (1995). *Critical race theory. The key writings that formed the movement.* New Press.

Crewe, S. (2017). Education with intent – The HBCU experience. *Journal of Human Behavior in the Social Environment, 27*(5), 360–366.

Cunningham, W. A., Nezlek, J. B., & Bananji, M. (2004). Implicit and explicit ethnocentrism: Revisiting the ideologies of prejudice. *Personality and Social Psychology Bulletin, 30*(10), 1332–1346.

Delgado, R. (2005). Critical race theory. *New dictionary of the history of ideas international encyclopedia*. Retrieved from http://www.encyclopedia.com/topic/Critical_Rce_Theory.aspx

Delgado, R., & Stefancic, J. (2001). *Critical race theory: An introduction*. New York: New York University Press.

Galloway, M. K., Callin, P., James, S., Vimegnon, H., & McCall, L. (2019). Culturally responsive, antiracist, or anti-oppressive? how language matters for school change efforts. Equity & Excellence in Education, 52(4), 485–501. https://doi.org/10.1080/10665684.2019.1691959

Gourdine, R. M., & Brown, A. W. (2016). *Social Action, advocacy and agents of change: Howard University School of Social Work in the 1970s*. Inprint Editions.

Grier, W., & Cobbs, P. (1992). *Black Rage: Two Black Psychiatrists Reveal the Full Dimensions of the Inner Conflicts and the Desperation of Black Life in the United States*. Westview Press.

Hamilton-Mason, J., & Schneider, S. (2018). *Journal of Social Work Education, 54*(2), 337–348.

Harris, A. P. (2012). *Critical race theory. From the selected work of Angela P Harris*. http://works.bepress.com/angela_harris/17/

Hiraldo, P. (2010). The Role of Critical Race Theory in Higher Education. *The Vermont Connection, 31*, 53–59

Holland, M. M. (2020). Black Students' College Preferences: The Role of the White Racial Frame in Perpetuating Integration. *Sociological Perspectives, 63*(4), 552–570.

Hymans, D., Spence Coffey, D., & McLean, A. (2020, September 25). *We "Have a Way To Go" to achieve racial equity in social work*. http://www.socialworkblog.org/advocacy/2020/09/we-have-a-way-to-go-to-achieve-racial-equity-in-social-work/

Ladson-Billings, G. & Tate IV, W.F. (1995). Toward a critical race theory of education. *Teachers College Record, 91*(1), 47–68.

Ladson-Billings, G. (2016a). Just what is critical race theory and what's it doing in a nice field like education? In E. Taylor, D. Gillborn, & G. Ladson-Billings (Eds.), *Foundations of critical race theory in education* (2nd ed., pp. 15–30). Routledge.

Ladson-Billings, G. (2016b). Critical race theory – What it is not! In E. Taylor, D. Gillborn, & G. Ladson-Billings (Eds.), *Foundations of critical race theory in education* (2nd ed., pp. 345–356). Routledge.

Ledesma, M.C. & Calderón, D. (2015). Critical race theory in education: Review of past literature and a look to the future. *Qualitative Inquiry, 21*(3), 206–222.

Lindsay, J. (2007). Talking whiteness: Representations of social justice in one school. *Urban Review, 39*(4), 425–453.

Lynn, M. (2005). Critical race theory, Afrocentricity, and their relationship to critical pedagogy. In Leonardo, Z. (Ed.) *Critical pedagogy and race* (127–139). Malden, MA: Blackwell Publishing.

Martin, E., & Martin, J. (1985). *Social work and the black experience.* NASW Press.

McCoy, D. L., & Rodricks, D. J. (2015). Critical race theory in higher education: 20 years of theoretical and research innovations. *ASHE Higher Education Report, 41*(3), 1–117.

McMahon, A., & Allen-Meares, P. (1992). Is social work racist? A content analysis of recent literature. *Social Work, 37*(6), 533.

Mobley, S. (2017). Seeking sanctuary: (re)claiming the power of historically black colleges and universities as places of black refuge. *International Journal of Qualitative Studies in Education, 30*(10), 1036–1041.

Mueller, J. (2012). Tracing family, teaching race. *Teaching Sociology, 41*(2), 172–187.

Myers, L. J., & Speight, S. L. (2010). Reframing mental health and psychological well-being among persons of African descent: Africana/Black Psychology meeting the challenges of fractured social and cultural realities. *Journal of Pan African Studies, 3*(8), 66.

Open Letter from a group of Jungians on the question of Jung's writings on and theories about "Africans". (2019). *Journal of Analytical Psychology, 64*(3), 361–366.

Ortiz, L., & Jani, J. (2010). Critical race theory: A transformational model for teaching diversity. *Journal of Social Work Education, 46*(2), 175–193.

Radd, S. I., & Grosland, T. J. (2019). Desirablizing whiteness: A discursive practice in social justice leadership that entrenches white supremacy. *Urban Education, 54*(5), 656–676.

Salsberg, E., Quigley, L., Mehfoud, N., Acquaviva, K. D., Wyche, K., & Silwa, S. (2017). *Profile of the Social Work Workforce.*

Scheurich, J. J., & Young, M. D. (1997). Coloring Epistemologies: Are Our Research Epistemologies Racially Biased? *Educational Researcher, 26*(4), 4–16.

Shujaa, M. J. (1998). *Too much schooling, too little education: A paradox of black life in White Societies.* Africa World Press.

Smedley, A. & Smedley, B. (2012). *Race in North America: Origin and evolution of a worldview*. Boulder, CO: Westview Press.

Smith, L., Kashubeck-West, S., Payton, G., & Adams, E. (2017). White Professors Teaching About Racism: Challenges and Rewards. *The Counseling Psychologist, 45*(5), 651.

Solomon, M. (2021, March 27). Controversial 'anti riot' bill approved by Florida House. *Politics*. https://www.local10.com/news/politics/2021/03/26/controversial-anti-riot-bill-approved-by-florida-house/

Solórzano, D. G. & Yosso, T. J. (2016). Critical race methodology: Counter-storytelling as an analytical framework for educational research. In E. Taylor, D. Gillborn, & G. Ladson- Billings (Eds.), *Foundations of critical race theory in education 2nd Edition* (pp.127–142). New York, NY: Routledge.

Spanierman, L. B., & Smith, L. (2017). Confronting white hegemony: A moral imperative for the helping professions. *The Counseling Psychologist, 45*(5), 727–736.

Taylor, E. (2016). The foundations of critical race theory in education: An introduction. In E. Taylor, D. Gillborn, & G. Ladson-Billings (Eds.), Foundations of critical race theory in education 2nd Edition (pp. 1–11). New York, NY: Routledge.

Trinidad, A. M. (2014). Critical indigenous pedagogy of place: How centering Hawaiian epistemology and values in practice affects people on ecosystemic levels. *Journal of Ethnic and Cultural Diversity in Social Work, 23*(2), 110–128.

Trifonas, P. P. (Ed.). (2002). *Pedagogies of Difference: Rethinking Education for Social Justice* (1st ed.).

Vargas, S. (2003). Critical Race Theory in Education: Theory, Praxis, and Recommendations. In Lopez, Gerardo & Ed, Parker, (Eds). *Interrogating Racism in Qualitative Research Methodology*. New York, NY: Peter Lang Inc., International Academic Publishers.

Wagaman, M. A., Odera, S. G., & Fraser, D. V. (2019). A Pedagogical Model for Teaching Racial Justice in Social Work Education. *Journal of Social Work Education, 55*(2), 351–362.

Watkins, C. (2001). *Learning about learning enhances performance*.

Williams, H. (2005). Self-taught : african american education in slavery and freedom. Chapel Hill: University of North Carolina Press

Woo, B., Figuereo, V., Rosales, R., Wang, K., & Sabur, K. (2018). Where Is Race and Ethnicity in Social Work? A Content Analysis. *Social Work Research, 42*(3), 180–186.

Woodson, Carter Godwin, 1875–1950. (1990). *The mis-education of the Negro. Trenton*. N.J.: Africa World Press.
Yosso, T., Smith, W. A., Ceja, M., & Solorzano, D. (2009). Critical race theory, racial micro-aggressions, and campus racial climate for Latina/oundergraduates. *Harvard Educational Review, 79*(4), 659–690.
Zamudio, M., Russell, C., Rios, F. A., & Bridgeman, J. L. (2011). *Critical race theory matters: Education and ideology*. New York, NY: Routledge.

11

Program Practices for Cultivating Antiracist Counselors

Eva M. Gibson and Jessica A. Fripp

Program Practices for Cultivating Antiracist Counselors

Racist policies have been in place throughout U.S. history and impact every institution. In fact, Ibram Kendi noted that, "Racism itself is institutional, structural, and systemic (2019, p. 18). America has a lengthy record of oppressive practices evidenced by the intentional institution of systemic barriers based on race (Sandifer et al., 2021). More recently, racially motivated policing and killing of Black men and women, along with racist educational and housing policies, demonstrate how prominent systems have unapologetically harmed the bodies and souls of Black people. Furthermore, these practices have consistently undermined and dehumanized Black communities, leaving limited to no opportunities for

E. M. Gibson (✉) • J. A. Fripp
Austin Peay State University, Clarksville, TN, USA
e-mail: gibsone@apsu.edu; frippj@apsu.edu

© The Author(s), under exclusive license to Springer Nature Switzerland AG 2022

K. Johnson et al. (eds.), *Developing Anti-Racist Practices in the Helping Professions: Inclusive Theory, Pedagogy, and Application*,
https://doi.org/10.1007/978-3-030-95451-2_11

advancement (Swain, 2018). This is also true for helping professions; historically, the helping professions have operated from a color-evasive approach, viewing the world from a Eurocentric lens and dismissing the value and identities of others (Chung & Bemak, 2012). Kendi (2019) also argued that good intentions and kindness are insufficient; rather an intentional antiracist approach is required to facilitate meaningful change and disrupt oppressive systems and practices. An antiracist approach supports policies and practices that reduce racial inequity. For those in the helping professions, it is not just about choosing to be non-racist; to be antiracist requires deep exploration of personal biases, an openness to the client's worldview, and an understanding of culturally appropriate interventions (Ratts et al., 2016). In an ever-diversifying world, it is critically important that an emphasis is placed on multicultural competence in professional counseling practice.

As the field of counseling first began in the 1950s, it is a relatively new area within the helping profession yet it has made significant developments in response to societal changes (Gibson & Sandifer, 2020). In fact, ethical guidelines for the counseling field directly address practice standards as it relates to diverse clientele (American Counseling Association [ACA], 2014). Practitioner work should also be informed by the Multicultural and Social Justice Counseling Competencies (MSJCC). These competencies provide a comprehensive framework for working with clients that include attention to privilege, oppression, and intersecting identities (Ratts et al., 2016). The MSJCC also calls for culturally responsive direct intervention at the individual and systems levels. With these directives in mind, counselor education programs should provide meaningful opportunities for students to develop antiracist attitudes/beliefs, knowledge, skills, and actions. Although significant advances have been made in the area of multicultural competence, more work is still needed in this space.

Historically, most counselor training programs attempt to address cultural responsiveness by requiring one multicultural course. However, students often report feeling unprepared to work with people of color, and course instructors may feel discouraged or retaliated against when met with resistance regarding the course content (Littleford et al., 2010). While this is a starting point, one course on this issue is not enough. Consistently communicating about and confronting racism can lay the groundwork toward social change (Tatum, 1997). Thus an enhanced focus should be placed on culturally responsive practice within preparation programs as well as the field to disrupt the cycle of oppressive policies and practices. As counseling programs work to build strong counselors, they must do so by dismantling racist beliefs, practices, and policies. This entails an intentional approach designed to confront white supremacist ideology and antiBlackness.

Counselor preparation programs must challenge students to examine their ingrained racist beliefs, introduce antiracist practices, provide remediation as needed, and connect students to community resources in an effort to support trainee development. Accordingly, this chapter will address the following topics: incorporating antiracist strategies into graduate programming, refining advocacy efforts for professional practice, and developing and sustaining community connections through a multipronged approach. The proposed multifaceted process integrates considerations for the development of antiracist attitudes/beliefs, knowledge, and skills. Specific recommendations for action are intertwined throughout the narrative.

Antiracist Strategies in Graduate Programming

Graduate programs should maintain a transformative approach to dismantling racism, as our society is ever-evolving. Furthermore, counselor educators need to provide deliberate programming that is culturally responsive and integrates social justice in an effort to create antiracist counselors. Programs committed to this goal move beyond simple introductory awareness activities and invest in consistent programming designed to instill antiracist attitudes/beliefs, knowledge, and skills for future practitioners. The recommendations below incorporate actionable items in each component to operationalize these aspirational competencies.

Attitudes and Beliefs

Counselor education programs are designed to assess student competence and potential success in the profession. Just as faculty members observe and address student dispositions, it is mutually beneficial for counselors-in-training (CITs) to engage in self-awareness as a means to collaborate with program faculty on areas of growth and continued development. Students are responsible for their active participation in the learning process and assessed on their progression. It is imperative that throughout this process, CITs explore their perspectives on a deeper level; additionally, counseling faculty support students towards their own identity and skill development. Attitudes and beliefs, particularly related to cultural competence, is one area that requires critique. As Chung and Bemak (2012) noted, it is important that students demonstrate the dispositions that reflect the program's mission and overall objectives of the profession. These dispositions are not reflections of strong textbook knowledge or choosing answers based on social desirability; rather faculty members must observe those traits in and outside of the classroom. A formal assessment and review of dispositions serve to provide feedback to CITs on traits not measured in classroom assignments.

For example, counselor educators can create a rating form that consists of desired dispositions reflecting counseling values from an antiracist lens. Likert responses may be used to determine a standard measure for competence. Students can utilize this form each semester as a routine self-assessment to rate their ability to exhibit professional dispositions. Faculty members may complete the same evaluation for each individual student then contrast and compare the faculty/student rating responses. Program faculty should explicitly include questions related to perceived demonstration of cultural competency and self-work related to cultural competence as a means to increase cultural competence and reflection. For students who demonstrate low scores in these areas, faculty members should explore strategies to address this on both the individual and program levels. Considerations for the program level are addressed below while considerations for the individual level are addressed in a later section.

At the program level, faculty members should provide brave spaces to acknowledge, address and grapple with the experiences of Black people when their communities are negatively impacted. The term "brave space" is intentionally used instead of "safe space" as resulting conversations may be uncomfortable, but required. As unarmed killings of Black citizens through state-sanctioned violence or supremacist vigilantes are continuously publicized, program faculty members should consider ways to provide support and hold weight to process these experiences. Utilizing class time appropriately can be one way to address emotions and responses as well as create learning opportunities for non-marginalized CITs to listen to those narratives from their Black peers. Chew et al. (2020) encouraged faculty to set student guidelines for antiracist discussions within the classroom. In an effort to facilitate productive discussions, these scholars recommended that faculty teach students to name the discomfort, understand the importance of impact rather than intent, maintain a leader's mindset, utilize sound academic arguments, use professional language, and make sure all voices are heard. These communication standards help create a space for critical inquiry into social justice issues. Faculty members can support Black students by allowing them to create connections through affinity groups that build community and foster the development of positive identities. More formal approaches to support Black students include coordinating a town hall meeting to connect meaningfully to their experiences. Faculty can also encourage the use of student-led brown bag sessions in which all students can engage in conversations, collaboratively process the weight of racial encounters, and co-conspire to promote change through research opportunities and scholarship.

Knowledge

Effective preparation programs integrate antiracist training throughout the graduate experience. This includes infusion within the required coursework, selection of culturally diverse texts and readings, discussion and application of the MSJCC along with other critical theoretical approaches (e.g., Critical Race Theory, Black feminist thought), and approaches to andragogy that elevate the Black experience (Arredondo et al., 2020; Ratts et al., 2016; Washington & Henfield, 2019). A commitment to antiracist pedagogy should be clearly reflected in the syllabus as it sets the tone for each class (Fuentes et al., 2021). The authors also noted that "classrooms often operate as a microcosm of greater society, and therefore, systems of oppression may be played out in classroom dynamics"'(p. 71). With this in mind, the development of syllabi and subsequent course content and activities should be intentional and focus on equity. Faculty may consider including the following components: a course-specific diversity statement, a supplemental course description if the bulletin version does not include references to diversity, communication expectations with specific notations that micro and macro aggressions will be used as teaching moments, antiracist learning objectives, and a statement that addresses the intentionality of readings from Black scholars. Faculty may also consider opportunities for a collectivist approach to knowledge acquisition, methods to reframe office hours as student hours, and development of a policy that allows for some flexibility in assignments in an effort to further promote student growth during course development. Faculty should also consider integrating resources within the syllabi that would reduce barriers to success (e.g. food pantries, mental health supports, career services, specialized student support centers, etc.). Additionally, program faculty can solicit feedback from current students about these efforts to ensure inclusive pedagogical practices. These strategies may help foster an optimal learning environment as CITs undertake topics that may cause some unpleasant, but necessary, discomfort. Moreover, it may also be beneficial for program faculty to share and review syllabi to ensure that courses reflect an antiracist pedagogy.

While students benefit from a coursework model that integrates antiracist pedagogy, they also learn from direct observations. Bandura's Social Learning Theory (1971) provided considerations for training programs. According to this theory, modeling is a significant influence on the learning process. Competent models who demonstrate how the expected activities should be performed allow students to examine standards in practice. As such, counselor educators should demonstrate a commitment to antiracist work and openly share these efforts with CITs.

Faculty activities can be highlighted through a variety of methods. Research supports the use of social media to engage students in higher education (Bal et al., 2015; Janoske et al., 2019; Roblyer et al., 2010). Accordingly, programs may consider creating social media pages (e.g., Facebook, Twitter, Instagram, etc.) as a means to connect with students and specifically share faculty contributions to antiracist work. Scholars maintain that social media is the most used method of communication for students so leveraging it for educational purposes would serve to enhance student engagement (Bal et al., 2015). Some programs utilize routine electronic newsletters to disseminate information to students. While this approach may be used to broadcast faculty work and antiracist resources, it may be especially advantageous for highlighting upcoming antiracist programming, events, and professional development opportunities. Traditional avenues such as program websites, bulletin boards, and postings in course shells may also be utilized to publicize relevant material.

Skills

Critical responsiveness is a key element in educational antiracist strategies. However, it requires introspection and the acquisition of new knowledge that might prove uncomfortable for its recipients. As programs transform their curriculum to reflect social justice and critical approaches to teaching, student responses to these modifications may result in resistance to the materials and the facilitator. Zinga and Styres (2019) described these shifts to decolonize curriculum as rejections of mainstream teaching practices. The author also noted that this entails a discussion of how those mainstream messages maintain the status quo and perpetuate false narratives about marginalized populations. Although this approach encourages students to resist the messaging embedded in mainstream education, inevitably some students adopt a counter-resistant stance. This counter-resistance reflects a reluctance to pedagogy that directly addresses oppression and racism. While it is useful to call out a student's resistance to material, it is equally beneficial to engage with "calling in". This concept allows for deeper reflection and interpretation of the student's perspective, utilizing opportunities to create meaning around their reactions to course content (Verduzco-Baker, 2018). Though it is common for CITs to experience discomfort when faced with new information, one might argue that to reject these cultural paradigm shifts is to reject continued multicultural competence. A refusal to engage with and accommodate this information would require immediate action on the part of the faculty as professional codes of ethics outlined clinician responsibilities to respect the diversity of clients.

While counselor education programs prepare individuals who uphold the counseling dispositions described previously, faculty must also address problematic behavior or racist ideology. Foster and McAdams (2009) identified this process as gatekeeping, whereby professional counselors and colleagues work to prevent the individual from causing harm to the future populations they serve. This is affirmed in the ACA Code of Ethics (2014) which not only encouraged counselors to assist colleagues in recognizing unacceptable behavior, intervening where necessary to prevent harm to others; but, it also encouraged CITs to recognize their own opportunities of growth and notify appropriate faculty about their problems. Thus, if performance proves too harmful, students limit, suspend, or terminate their professional responsibilities until proven capable of returning to work. According to Brown-Rice and Furr (2015), the process of gatekeeping includes determining which students are prepared for professional counseling based upon acquired skills, knowledge, and ability; furthermore, for those students who lack adequate preparation, a rehabilitation component is put into place to address attitudes, perspectives and harmful behavior that could disrupt their 'fitness' for the field. Though gatekeeping might look different across graduate programs, its goal remains the same: to prevent a person from causing harm to the communities they encounter.

Gatekeeping and remediation are nuanced, contextual procedures; therefore, recommendations should be executed from a culturally-informed approach. Furthermore, faculty members must consider how each student's cultural background, intersecting identities, experiences, and observable behaviors shape their potential as a future counselor. This gatekeeping process begins before the first class. Programs should consider the inclusion of questions on the application as well as during the interview to assess a candidate's stance on diversity-related issues. If responses are flagged for concern during this period then these candidates should be screened out at this point. However, if concerns do not emerge until later, programs must be prepared to respond accordingly at the individual level. As noted by Henderson and Dufrene (2011), counselor educators are often given resources for dismissing students from programs, but are not equipped with strategies for prevention or remediation. Therefore, some guiding concepts on remediation used by the authors in their training program are provided. Faculty members should utilize various methods to evaluate performance, including but not limited to coursework, measured dispositions (intrapersonal behavior), and connections to peers and colleagues (interpersonal behavior). If assessments and/or interactions raise concerns regarding the student's potential as a counselor, then faculty members discuss the student's behavior formally to identify consistent themes or patterns. Once a concern is identified, counselor educators should consider how to nurture and develop CITs and understand the source of behavior, negotiating what is being observed. Counselor educators may want to reflect on the following questions:

- Is this behavior passionate or disruptive?
- Is this student being resistant to change or are they misinformed and in need of further exposure?
- How might the student's cultural background impact their decisions and behavior?
- Is the observed behavior a matter of clinical skill set or personal/life issues?

As educators review their responses to those questions, appropriate interventions are developed. Additionally, these courses of action are determined in collaboration with the CIT. This collaborative process may be officially initiated through a remediation meeting designed to develop a targeted plan for growth. While the term "remediation" may trigger negative feelings, the purpose is to support student development and skills. Furthermore, programs must have procedures and processes for student grievances to ensure the use of fair and equitable practices.

Faculty members may utilize remediation meetings to review their concerns and observations with the student as an opportunity for shared meaning and understanding, as well as a guide for determining culturally-informed solutions. The faculty member should provide evidence for areas of concern during the evaluation period (e.g., papers, examinations, videos, evaluations from instructors or supervisors, classroom behavior) to review with the student; additionally, they should highlight disparities between desired outcomes with the student's current performance. It is imperative to connect the student's performance to measurable criteria to ensure the student understands how their performance did not meet expectations. Once areas of concern are addressed, the plan should connect the identified concerns with the following components: ethics, professional responsibility and accountability, cultural identity and competence, and future performance expectations. Some suggested activities include: repeating the course, increased supervision, workshops on antiracist strategies, personal therapy (if appropriate), and increased exposure to multi-ethnic communities through community programming and organizations. Students should explicitly detail their goals for increased cultural competence and submit it for faculty review and approval. As with a treatment plan, remediation plans should be time-sensitive, measurable, and relevant. The remediation procedure should be well-documented and reviewed as applicable throughout the duration of the remediation. Faculty members should reconvene to discuss the student's fitness to continue progressing toward the degree once the student completes the remediation terms. If progress is satisfactory, the terms of remediation are complete; however, the remediation plan is considered part of the student's academic record and kept on file for documentation purposes. Students who do not make necessary progress are subject to dismissal from the program. As gatekeepers, counselor educators are responsible for preparing counselors fit for the field. Being intentional with curriculum and program development, while incorporating a cultural competence framework, promotes the development of antiracist counseling practitioners. Although these strategies facilitate the process for individuals, the inclusion of a collectivist approach is critical for systemic change.

Sustaining Community Connections

While the primary focus of counselor training programs is intended to prepare professionals for the field, some scholars contend that these programs may also serve to provide educational opportunities to the public and contribute to the local community (Gibson & Sandifer, 2020). Intentionally engaging with the surrounding systems has the potential to foster a deeper community investment. These targeted interactions should be focused on meeting the unique needs of the area residents. Counseling programs can sustain community connections by contributing to the development of antiracist attitudes/beliefs, knowledge, and skills through a variety of methods and a multi-pronged approach. The recommendations below also incorporate actionable items for operational purposes.

Attitudes and Beliefs

The ACA Advocacy Competencies (Toporek & Daniels, 2018) provided an applicable framework to utilize as programs engage in community outreach efforts. More specifically, the Community Collaboration domain addressed strategies to implement that allow for shared contributions and joint efforts in response to social injustices. Such a response needs to be informed by the voices of those most impacted. The MSJCC called for counselors to take steps to become aware of the clients' worldviews, beliefs, and lived experiences with power, privilege, and oppression (Ratts et al., 2016). Competent counselors possess a curiosity for learning about these beliefs and look for ways to gain insight into the lived experiences of marginalized groups. The following case example illustrates program efforts of the authors and provides a model for consideration as others engage the community in this work.

In light of the recent prominent murders of Black citizens (e.g., Ahmaud Arbery, George Floyd, Breonna Taylor, etc.), program faculty partnered with community organizations, school system leaders, and school counselors to offer an open forum for middle school and high school students to create meaningful dialogues, identify the needs of marginalized students, and provide a brave place for processing the impact of recent racial events of social injustice. This forum was offered via Zoom (due to COVID-19), organized by the counselor educator, and co-facilitated by the counselor educator and school counselors. Community organizations and school system leaders co-partnered and assisted in marketing the free event. As students identified needs and concerns, these were passed along to respective bodies to better inform their work. Facilitators were also able to provide resources and connections for ongoing student support. Collaborations such as this one may serve to enhance communication, understanding, and services.

Knowledge

Counselor educators are tasked with the responsibility of providing learning opportunities beyond the university doors (Gibson & Sandifer, 2020). As such, they should remain actively engaged within the field through the production of antiracist publications, presentations, and professional development trainings (Gibson et al., 2021). Notably, faculty members largely influence and contribute to the professional literature. Therefore, authors should be intentional about referencing Black scholars and incorporating the contributions and perspectives of this underutilized group. Furthermore, intentionally establishing a diverse working group of collaborators adds to the richness of thought and may enhance the antiracist lens directed towards scholarly production. Counselor educators should provide opportunities for Black students and early professionals to engage in professional development, facilitating mentorship to underrepresented professionals. A similar approach may be applied toward the production of presentations as well. These engagements provide unique training opportunities for counselor educators to equip current and future professionals with tools to operate from an antiracist approach. Appropriate cultural considerations should be incorporated in every presentation to reinforce the necessary skills to work with clientele. Faculty may also consider offering university-sponsored trainings and invite local practitioners, contribute to local trainings (such as school district level professional development workshops for school counselors), or collaborate with state professional associations to co-host continuing education events. Additionally, antiracist considerations can be implemented into the supervisor training required for practicum and internship site supervisors.

While supervisor training has traditionally focused on supervision models, program faculty may introduce culturally responsive supervision into these workshops. The authors define culturally responsive supervision as an approach to supervision in which supervisees are given opportunities to reflect on their way of being with clients, while also considering how their identities impact and are impacted by marginalized communities. Site supervisors should be taught how to integrate conversations about race, ethnicity, and cultural backgrounds into supervision sessions during the training process. Additionally, supervisors should receive guidance on strategies designed to create opportunities for CITs to explore how their intersecting identities influence their clinical work. Although supervisors work to mitigate some of their power in the room, culturally competent supervisors are obligated to directly address areas of need. Upshaw et al. (2020) suggested providing space to promote trust in the supervisory relationship; this approach creates a supportive environment to grapple with complex cultural issues. It is also important to note that some supervisors may be uncomfortable delivering negative feedback. As such, counselor educators should prepare them for these difficult conversations. The use of role-plays during training may be a beneficial strategy to practice these scenarios. The combination of counselor educator antiracist publications, presentations, and professional development trainings provide a variety of opportunities to reach practitioners.

Skills

As leaders within the field, counselor educators are uniquely positioned to link pedagogy to the world of praxis and bridge education with civic engagement and public service (Gibson & Sandifer, 2020). Community outreach initiatives could serve as an avenue to build relationships between communities and the academy. Grounding antiracist education in the practice of community engagement allows counselors-in-training (CITs) and practitioners to observe collaboration and advocacy in action. This civic engagement may produce mutual benefits and create an enhanced sense of connection. The authors also noted that this engagement contributes to the greater good and supports community well-being.

The following case example illustrates program efforts of the authors and provides a model for consideration. The goal of the project was to provide a small group counseling intervention with a mentoring component for Black boys demonstrating difficulty in middle school. The project was a collaboration between two middle school counselors (one male and one female), a female counselor educator, a female counseling graduate student, and four Black male mentors. The mentors represented a diverse array of perspectives to include: two undergraduate students, one recent college graduate, and a military service member. With the exception of the female school counselor, all members of the team identified as Black. As a collective, the facilitators designed and implemented the six-week intervention created to enhance success skills for Black middle school boys. The facilitators intentionally selected culturally relevant activities, discussion topics that integrated the complexities of the Black male experience, and materials that mirrored the culture of the participants. The project concluded with a culminating mentor/mentee breakfast. Facilitators also planned an all-expense-paid field trip to the local university, but the visit was canceled due to COVID-19. In lieu of this trip, facilitators created video messages for the group participants. This project aligned with the ACA Advocacy Competencies, specifically within the Client/Student Empowerment and Community Collaboration domains, as partners assisted participants in the process of developing approaches to address systemic barriers while utilizing support systems (Toporek & Daniels, 2018). Results of this collaborative project were shared with school system leaders and other counselors within the area. This project not only provided a meaningful learning experience for CITs, but community-based practitioners also gained additional resources for working with Black students. While the majority of facilitators in this example were Black and worked with Black students, the lack of diversity in the counseling field results in a high likelihood of white counselors/CITs working with Black students. It is important to note that these types of interactions may inadvertently reinforce stereotypes and a deficit perspective with white practitioners viewing themselves as saviors (Gibson & Sandifer, 2020). For this reason, it is important that white counselors/CITs are well-prepared to work with Black clients and disrupt racist practices at the micro and macro levels. This approach may also be applied to research. While training programs often engage in and consume research concerning historically oppressed groups, it is important to align with ethical research practices while working with these populations so that marginalized communities are not misrepresented. For example, McCracken (2020) described considerations for community-based participatory research that protects participants and operates from a positivist approach. Her work outlined a process that serves to create partnerships, examine the role of power, foster strengths, and contribute to community growth. This article posed policy considerations and opportunities for improvement. The author recommended additional requirements for the Institutional Review Board process for researchers working with historically oppressed groups. In addition to the routine procedures, researchers should also submit information about their identity and their relationship to the topic or targeted community as well as a report of how the target group has been involved in the research design, development of questions, and ethical procedures.

Intentional collaborations with site supervisors may also serve as an effective method to cultivate antiracist CITs. Typically, Black practitioners actively work to build a more inclusive, antiracist program that benefits its students, but should not be required to engage in this work solely. As co-conspirators in a shared fight toward equity, white counseling professionals are called to act as well. In fact, Janet Helms asserts that white people are directly responsible for ending racism (2020). Mitigating anti-Blackness is not an inherent approach of white counseling educators; therefore, it is important that white colleagues intentionally and consistently interrupt status quo paradigms and activities that cause harm to Black bodies. White professionals can amplify the initiatives that serve to better Black communities by working collaboratively with Black professionals.

Clinical coordinators in counseling programs are encouraged to seek out practicum and internship sites that represent diverse communities and employ culturally diverse practitioners. Students learning in these environments are exposed to a variety of people and are motivated to conceptualize their cases from a multicultural framework, thus benefiting the clients they serve. Cultural competence is something to develop over time and not a matter of achievement. Supervision at these diverse sites provides an optimal time to provide clear feedback about competence and model a sense of accountability. Additionally, communication between the site supervisor and university supervision provides a comprehensive picture of CIT development.

As CITs develop a lens that promotes justice and advocacy, their efforts are not just within the classroom or through interpersonal relationships with clients. Rather, CITs are encouraged to join professional organizations within the appropriate domain (e.g., rehabilitation, addictions, etc.), to learn the value of leadership and policy development that directly impact their historically oppressed clients. CITs can be impactful in their communities by creating opportunities to organize individuals around a shared or common goal. For example, individuals with mental health conditions or addictions often experience heightened surveillance and punishment, especially in historically oppressed communities. This is important to keep in mind if a client voices frustrations about racial profiling in his neighborhood where a disproportionate amount of people lack access to resources and supports. With this knowledge, the CIT can meet with the client and others with like-minded interests in a shared space to address concerns. The CIT (through leadership in their organization and appropriate supervision) can formulate a task force designed to advocate for policies to foster safe and supportive communities. The CIT could advocate for officers to complete de-escalation training or the CIT's organization could develop workshops to ensure that police officers understand the unique needs of individuals with co-occurring diagnoses.

Faculty members must stress the importance of early engagement in advocacy at state and local levels to sustain positive community connections. Advocacy may require policy change and grassroots community organizing to disrupt inequitable systems. Through actionable steps, social justice becomes more than a buzzword, but an extension of their career as a professional counselor.

Advocacy Recommendations for Professional Practice

Scholars have noted the need for practitioners to balance counseling with social justice advocacy (Ratts et al., 2016). In fact, ACA adopted advocacy as one of the strategic drivers of the counseling profession (Toporek & Daniels, 2018). As such, counseling training programs are tasked with the responsibility to cultivate antiracist counselors who understand the complexities of multiculturalism, recognize the influence of diversity on the counseling relationship, acknowledge the adverse impact of oppression on mental health, comprehend the context of the social environment, and engage in social justice advocacy. While this process is ongoing and requires a life-long commitment, training programs begin this journey by connecting advocacy to the development of attitudes/beliefs, knowledge, and skills. Specific recommendations for action are embedded in each component.

Attitudes and Beliefs

As competence begins with knowing oneself, counselors who evaluate their own attitudes and beliefs are better suited to deliver effective services and support marginalized clients (Ratts et al., 2016). Practitioners increase their self-awareness by identifying the ways they perceive client's problems and learning to reframe those experiences from the "person" of the client. Counselors learn to dispel stereotypes commonly held toward marginalized populations rather than viewing the client as resistant or oppositional. Combs and Freedman (2012) considered this change in thought patterns as an act of social change. Counselor educators must introduce CITs to the concept and purpose of practitioner reflection as training programs seek to engage graduate students in understanding cultural similarities, differences, cultural norms and values.

Faculty members can provide students with self-assessments to evaluate their status and progress. One scale, the *Multicultural Counseling Self-Efficacy Scale-Racial Diversity Form* (Sheu & Lent, 2007) is a 37-item self-report instrument that assesses perceived ability to perform various counselor behaviors in counseling a racially diverse client population. Some questions on this form address confidence to work with someone from a racially different background to a person's understanding of culture-bound symptoms. Utilizing this form could give students a preliminary introduction to the types of presentations they might experience working with Black clients. The *Personal Self-Assessment of Anti-Bias Behavior* is also a helpful tool adapted by Dr. Beverly Tatum and Andrea Ayvazian (as cited in Katz, 1978) to identify personal strengths, areas of growth, and future goals. Checking one's bias is the first step in being able to improve skills to help others. The *Self-Assessment Checklist for Personnel Providing Behavioral Health Services and Supports to Children, Youth and their Families* is a 40-item checklist designed for practitioners to self-assess their awareness and sensitivity to the importance of cultural diversity and cultural competence surrounding behavioral health issues for children, youth, and their families (Goode, 2009). Practitioners can only effectively use culturally appropriate interventions if they have first evaluated their own skills in this area and developed strategies to strengthen areas of need. If CITs are not taught this concept early then they will struggle with skill application and miss the mark when working with culturally diverse clients.

Knowledge

While balancing counseling with social justice advocacy, it is critical for practitioners to be knowledgeable about resources that may support marginalized clients. The Client/Student Empowerment domain of the ACA Advocacy Competencies addressed the need for counselors to aid clients through the process of identifying strengths and resources (Toporek & Daniels, 2018). Counselor educators may encourage informal research into community capital in an effort to help students become aware of the existing resources within the Black community. Community asset mapping may be a valuable class activity to achieve this goal. This activity may be used to identify assets within the local community to include individual citizen abilities and talents, community organizations, and formal institutions of support (Griffin & Farris, 2010). CITs can create resource toolkits for future use with diverse clients by identifying what is currently available.

Training programs may also consider framing culturally responsive supervision and consultation as a necessary component in the CIT's toolkit. As the ACA Advocacy Competencies (Ratts et al., 2016) called for counselors to be knowledgeable of how oppression impacts marginalized clients, the ongoing use of culturally responsive supervision and consultation provides a resource for practitioners as they strive to meet this expectation. Research indicates that effective supervision positively impacts counselor competency as well as client outcomes (Falender et al., 2013). Supervisors who utilize an antiracist lens demonstrate culturally responsive conceptualizations throughout the supervision process and provide opportunities for supervisees to reflect on beliefs, attitudes and behaviors that may inform work with diverse clients. Supervisors may also utilize the *Cross-Cultural Counseling Inventory-Revised* as an assessment tool to evaluate trainee competency and provide feedback on development (Chung & Bemak, 2012). Correspondingly, trainees should seek the advice of their supervisor, applying feedback and developing a process of accountability moving forward toward competence. This could be as simple as carving out time in supervision regarding growth specific to competence, reviewing recorded sessions (as applicable) to review potential areas of concern or missed opportunities to address something culturally relevant within the session. Training programs may integrate these strategies into the supervision process and promote the use of ongoing culturally responsive supervision as CITs transition into professional practice. Clinicians may also choose to utilize culturally responsive consultation if they are experiencing difficulty while working with a client of a diverse background. Consultation varies from supervision in that it is freely sought and initiated on an as-needed basis (Bernard & Goodyear, 2004). Research indicates that cultural consultation may enhance therapeutic alliance and promote positive outcomes for clients (Kirmayer et al., 2003). Training programs that introduce and promote this practice help prepare antiracist counselors that are equipped to face challenges and disrupt barriers.

Skills

Research indicates that the use of culturally responsive approaches to counseling positively impacts the counseling process and client outcomes (Benish et al., 2011; Lopez et al., 2014). However, clinicians must first understand contextual factors that might negatively impact engagement with clients throughout their professional practice prior to the implementation of services. The Client/Student Advocacy domain of the ACA Advocacy Competencies addressed the need for counselors to identify client barriers and negotiate relevant services (Toporek & Daniels, 2018). Scholars Fripp and Carlson (2017) illustrated the importance of this strategy in their research. Their findings indicated that stigma and negative attitudes toward the counseling process limit Black clients from help-seeking and participation in counseling. This resistance may partially be attributed to cultural mistrust as many clinicians are White. This psychological reaction may be experienced by Black persons in response to historical and personal oppression (Neville et al., 2009; Vontrees & Epp, 1997). Consequently, Black individuals often do not engage in counseling to reduce potential encounters with stereotyping, microaggressions, discrimination, and marginalization (Sandifer et al., 2021). Practitioners and CITs must understand these barriers to counseling and work to deconstruct these obstacles.

One strategy in particular that may be beneficial employs the integration of cultural practices inherent to the communities they serve. For example, within the Black community spirituality serves as a form of coping. According to Avent et al. (2015), Black persons prefer to seek support from religious communities; thus, clinicians and CITs must consider these implications in practice. Incorporating religious elements could serve useful to maintain engagement and promote buy-in with participation. Additionally, collaborations between stakeholders and Black churches are mutually beneficial, as members of the church receive mental health counseling from trained professionals, while those counselors take a stance of unknowing, gaining knowledge and wisdom from pastors who have counseled the community for some time (Avent-Harris et al., 2019). Brokering these relationships can improve trust between mental health systems and the Black community, but counselors must understand the level of difficulty ahead of them to develop meaningful connections as an outsider. However, when approached intentionally, sustaining a strong relationship proves to be an important first step to engage Black persons in the counseling process.

The use of culturally appropriate techniques from the onset of the therapeutic relationship is critical for effective outcomes. Zigarelli et al. (2016) provided recommendations to integrate cultural considerations throughout the experience. In an effort to gain a foundational understanding of cultural factors, the authors encouraged the use of clinical interviewing tools such as the Jones Intentional Multicultural Interview Schedule (JIMIS) or the Cultural Formulation Interview. These tools help the clinician and client explore and discuss cultural factors. The authors also advocated for the application of a culturally responsive model, such as the ADDRESSING Framework. This particular framework facilitates the clinician's ability to attend to cultural influences. As these tasks may cause discomfort, especially for cross-cultural dyads, the authors emphasized the importance of maintaining momentum and pushing through feelings of personal unease. It is crucial that clinicians directly address the culturally unique challenges and strengths created by ecological systems. In line with the previously mentioned research by Kirmayer et al. (2003), the recommendation of consultation with a cultural broker may also be advantageous if the counseling process appears to be impaired by relationship dynamics (Zigarelli et al., 2016). The final recommendation acknowledged the need to address counseling themes with an intersectional lens and recognize that systems of oppression are maintained if they are not actively disrupted.

Another skill that could serve beneficial to professional counselors looking to engage marginalized clients is the use of counter-narratives and storytelling. As clients of underrepresented groups are provided the opportunity to challenge hegemonic narratives historically maintained by dominant groups, this allows them to be the expert of their life experiences. Storytelling promotes dialogue with clients regarding their experiences from institutions and individuals of power. According to Duke and Fripp (2020), exposing individuals to counter-narratives disrupts biases and weakens negative perspectives. This is true for the client and the counselor. This experience could be difficult for a novice counselor as well as seasoned practitioners. Counselors should actively work to build rapport and consistency with clients as a means to facilitate this process. To establish trust and maintain engagement, the counselor should avoid using language that challenges the stories as untrue; furthermore, White counselors should resist the impulse to express "common ground" by self-disclosing personal anecdotes of personal injustice. This ensures the client's story is not co-opted by the counselor's personal accounts in which their experience becomes the dominant experience in the room. As noted in the ACA Advocacy Competencies, when counselors recognize their position and facilitate effective partnerships with clients, the clients experience more empowerment and enhanced outcomes (Toporek & Daniels, 2018). A continued focus on these goals contributes to a stronger collective well-being.

Conclusion

This chapter is a call to action for counselor educators. As the profession begins to acknowledge the impact of systemic oppression and social injustice, obligations to the field have evolved to reflect the need for counselors who boldly embrace antiracism and advocate on behalf of marginalized groups. Preparation programs have a professional responsibility to prepare counselors to do this work. As previously noted, an intentional antiracist approach is required to facilitate meaningful change and disrupt oppressive systems and practices. As such, counselor education programs should embed consistent opportunities for students to develop antiracist attitudes/beliefs, knowledge, skills, and actions. This entails the use of deliberate programming that is culturally responsive and integrates social justice constructs throughout the preparation process. The recommendations presented in this chapter addressed methods to incorporate antiracist strategies into graduate programming, develop and sustain community connections, and refine advocacy efforts for professional practice. Programs that attend to these issues cultivate antiracist counselors committed to social justice.

While this chapter is targeted to counselor education programs, some of the information presented here may be helpful for other helping professions. Similar to the recommendations for counseling programs, other helping professions, like allied health training programs, may benefit from an early introduction to social justice approaches. Training programs may require students to examine their beliefs and create plans to address racist ideologies. Programs should be intentional in the development of their curriculum and include issues that impact historically marginalized communities. Additionally, universities should develop relationships with community groups and organizations and connect students to community resources. Most helping professionals have professional standards they are expected to align with. Many of these guiding documents address cultural considerations. Practitioners must pay close attention to these recommendations and adhere to these expectations while utilizing culturally-relevant techniques. Furthermore, helping professionals need to be prepared to engage in advocacy work and continued education. In an ever-diversifying world, it is critically important that helping professionals center culturally-affirming practices and adopt an antiracist approach.

Guiding Questions

1. As course content and activities should be intentional and focus on equity, what specific classroom activities would support the development of antiracist counselors?
2. How can counselor educators provide meaningful mentorship to underrepresented professionals?
3. In what other ways can our current systems be reconstructed to dismantle oppressive policies and practices?

Quiz Questions

1. This serves to provide feedback to counselors-in-training on traits not measured in classroom assignments:

   (a) comprehensive exams
   (b) oral exams

(c) formal assessment and review of dispositions
(d) client evaluations

2. Antiracist discussions within the classroom should allow for:

(a) a safe space
(b) critical inquiry into social justice issues
(c) a focus on intent
(d) apology and explanation

3. The _____sets the tone for each class.

(a) syllabus
(b) seating arrangement
(c) accrediting standards
(d) campus climate

4. The gatekeeping process begins:

(a) during the diversity class
(b) during disposition assessment
(c) during fieldwork
(d) before the first class

5. Civic engagement may:

(a) produce mutual benefits and create an enhanced sense of connection
(b) may inadvertently reinforce stereotypes and a deficit perspective without adequate preparation
(c) both A & C
(d) none of the above

References

American Counseling Association. (2014). *ACA code of ethics*. Author.

Arredondo, P., D'Andrea, M., & Lee, C. (2020, September). Unmasking white supremacy and racism in the counseling profession. *Counseling Today, 63*(3), 40–42.

Avent, J. R., Cashwell, C. S., & Brown-Jeffy, S. (2015). African American pastors on mental health, coping, and help-seeking. *Counseling and Values, 60*, 32–47. https://doi.org/10.1002/j.2161-007X.2015.00059.x

Avent-Harris, J. R., Garland-McKinney, J. L., & Fripp, J. A. (2019). "God is a keeper": A phenomenological investigation of Christian African American women's experiences with religious coping. *The Professional Counselor, 9*(3), 157–170. https://doi.org/10.15241/jrah.9.3.171

Bal, A. S., Grewal, D., Mills, A., & Ottley, G. (2015). Engaging students with social media. *Journal of Marketing Education, 37*(3), 190–203. https://doi.org/10.1177/0273475315593380

Bandura, A. (1971). *Social learning theory*. General Learning Press.

Benish, S. G., Quintana, S., & Wampold, B. E. (2011). Culturally adapted psychotherapy and the legitimacy of myth: A direct-comparison meta-analysis. *Journal of Counseling Psychology, 58*, 279–289. https://doi.org/10.1037/a0023626

Bernard, J. M., & Goodyear, R. K. (2004). *Fundamentals of clinical supervision*. Pearson.

Brown-Rice, K., & Furr, S. (2015). Gatekeeping ourselves: Counselor educators' knowledge of colleagues' problematic behavior. *Counselor Education and Supervision, 54*, 176–188. https://doi.org/10.1002/ceas.12012

Chew, S., Houston, A., & Cooper, A. (2020). The anti-racist discussion pedagogy. *Packback*. https://www.packback.co/resources/anti-racist-discussion-pedagogy-guide/

Chung, R. C., & Bemak, F. (2012). *Social justice counseling: The next steps beyond multiculturalism*. SAGE.

Combs, G., & Freedman, J. (2012). Narrative, poststructuralism, and social justice: Current practices in narrative therapy. *The Counseling Psychologist, 40*(7), 1033–1060. https://doi.org/10.1177/0011000012460662

Duke, A. M., & Fripp, J. A. (2020). Examining youth participatory action research as a context to disrupt implicit bias in African American adolescent girls. *Educational Action Research*, 1–15. https://doi.org/10.1080/09650792.2020.1774404

Falender, C. A., Burnes, T. R., & Ellis, M. V. (2013). Multicultural clinical supervision and benchmarks: Empirical support informing practice and supervisor training. *The Counseling Psychologist, 41*(1), 8–27. https://doi.org/10.1177/0011000012438417

Foster, V. A., & McAdams, C. R. (2009). A framework for creating a climate of transparency for professional performance assessment: Fostering student investment in gatekeeping. *Counselor Education and Supervision, 48*, 271–284. https://doi.org/10.1002/j.1556-6978.2009.tb00080.x

Fripp, J. A., & Carlson, R. (2017). Exploring the influence of attitude and stigma on participation of African American and Latino populations in mental health services. *Journal of Multicultural Counseling and Development, 45*(2), 80–94. https://doi.org/10.1002/jmcd.12066

Fuentes, M. A., Zelaya, D. G., & Madsen, J. W. (2021). Rethinking the course syllabus: Considerations for promoting equity, diversity, and inclusion. *Teaching of Psychology, 48*(1), 69–79. https://doi.org/10.1177/0098628320959979

Gibson, E. M., & Fripp, J. A., Moore, C. R., Shepard, D. L. & Campbell, S. M. (2021). *More than talking the talk: Counselor educators as models of anti-racist work.* Southern Association for Counselor Education and Supervision. http://www.saces.org/resources/Documents/Fall%202020%20Newsletter.pdf

Gibson, E. M., & Sandifer, M. C. (2020). It takes a village: Service learning as our social responsibility in higher education. In P. Blessinger & E. Sengupta (Eds.), *Civil society and social responsibility in higher education: International perspectives on curriculum and teaching development* (pp. 93–108). International Higher Education Teaching and Learning. https://doi.org/10.1108/S2055-364120200000021008

Goode, T. D. (2009). *Promoting cultural diversity and cultural competency: Self-assessment checklist for personnel providing behavioral health services and supports to children, youth, and their families.* National Center for Cultural Competence. https://nccc.georgetown.edu/documents/checklistbehavioralhealth.pdf

Griffin, D., & Farris, A. (2010). School counselors and collaboration: Finding resources through community asset mapping. *Professional School Counseling, 13*(5), 248–256. https://doi.org/10.1177/2156759X1001300501

Helms, J. E. (2020). *A race is a nice thing to have: A guide to being a white person or understanding the white persons in your life* (3rd ed.). Cognella Academic Publishing.

Henderson, K. L., & Dufrene, R. L. (2011). *Student remediation: Practical considerations for counselor educators and supervisors.* https://www.counseling.org/resources/library/vistas/2011-V-Online/Article_45.pdf

Janoske, M., Byrd, R., & Madden, S. (2019). One liners and catchy hashtags: Building a graduate student community through twitter chats. *Journal of Public Relations Education, 5*(1), 70–100.

Katz, J. (1978). *White awareness: Handbook for anti-racism training.* The University of Oklahoma Press.

Kendi, I. X. (2019). *How to be an antiracist.* Random House.

Kirmayer, L. J., Groleau, D., Guzder, J., Blake, C., & Jarvis, E. (2003). Cultural consultation: A model of mental health service for multicultural societies. *The Canadian Journal of Psychiatry, 48*(3), 145–153. https://doi.org/10.1177/070674370304800302

Littleford, L. N., Ong, K. S., Tseng, A., Milliken, J. C., & Humy, S. L. (2010). Perceptions of European American and African American instructors teaching race-focused courses. *Journal of Diversity in Higher Education, 3*(4), 230–244. https://doi.org/10.1037/a0020950

López, C. M., Shealy, K. M., & Rheingold, A. A. (2014). Empirically supported trauma treatment for an adult Latino man diagnosed with PTSD: Overcoming barriers to engagement. *Clinical Case Studies, 13*, 436–452. https://doi.org/10.1177/1534650114521282

McCracken, J. (2020). Ethics as obligation: Reconciling diverging research practices with marginalized communities. *International Journal of Qualitative Methods, 19*, 1–11. https://doi.org/10.1177/1609406920964336

Neville, H. A., Tynes, B. M., & Utsey, S. O. (2009). *Handbook of African American psychology*. Sage.

Ratts, M. J., Singh, A. A., Nassar-McMillan, B., & S. K., & Rafferty McCullough, J. (2016). Multicultural and social justice counseling competencies: Guidelines for the counseling profession. *Journal of Multicultural Counseling and Development, 44*(1), 28–48. https://doi.org/10.1002/jmcd.12035

Roblyer, M. D., McDaniel, M., Webb, M., Herman, J., & Witty, J. V. (2010). Findings on Facebook in higher education: A comparison of college faculty and student uses and perceptions of social networking sites. *Internet and Higher Education, 13*(3), 134–140. https://doi.org/10.1016/j.iheduc.2010.03.002

Sandifer, M. C., Gibson, E. M., & Brant-Rajahn, S. N. (2021). WOKE: Advocacy for African American students. In M. A. Rausch & L. L. Gallo (Eds.), *Strengthening school Counselor advocacy and practice for important populations and difficult topics* (pp. 19–40). IGI Global. https://doi.org/10.4018/978-1-7998-7319-8.ch002

Sheu, H. B., & Lent, R. W. (2007). Development and initial validation of the multicultural counseling self-efficacy scale – Racial diversity form. *Psychotherapy, 44*(1), 30–45. https://doi.org/10.1037/0033-3204.44.1.30

Swain, R. D. (2018). Negative Black stereotypes, support for excessive use of force by police, and voter preference for Donald Trump during the 2016 presidential primary election cycle. *Journal of African American Studies, 22*(1), 109–121. https://doi.org/10.1007/s12111-018-9398-4

Tatum, B. (1997). *"Why are all the Black kids sitting together in the cafeteria?" and other conversations about race*. Basic Books.

Toporek, R. L., & Daniels, J. (2018). *American counseling association advocacy competencies: Updated*. https://www.counseling.org/docs/default-source/competencies/aca-advocacy-competencies-may-2020.pdf?sfvrsn=85b242c_4

Upshaw, N. C., Lewis, D. E., & Nelson, A. L. (2020). Cultural humility in action: Reflective and process-oriented supervision with Black trainees. *Training and Education in Professional Psychology, 14*(4), 277–284. https://doi.org/10.1037/tep0000284

Verduzco-Baker, L. (2018). Modified brave spaces: Calling in brave instructors. *Sociology of Race and Ethnicity, 4*(4), 585–592. https://doi.org/10.1177/2332649218763696

Vontrees, C. E., & Epp, L. R. (1997). Historical hostility in the African American client: Implications for counseling. *Journal of Multicultural Counseling and Development, 25*(3), 170–184. https://doi.org/10.1002/j.2161-1912.1997.tb00327.x

Washington, A. R., & Henfield, M. S. (2019). What do the AMCD multicultural and social justice counseling competencies mean in the context of Black lives matter? *Journal of Multicultural Counseling and Development, 47*, 148–160. https://doi.org/10.1002/jmcd.12138

Zigarelli, J. C., Jones, J. M., Palomino, C. I., & Kawamura, R. (2016). Culturally responsive cognitive behavioral therapy: Making the case for integrating cultural factors in evidence-based treatment. *Clinical Case Studies, 15*(6), 427–442. https://doi.org/10.1177/1534650116664984

Zinga, D., & Styres, S. (2019). Decolonizing curriculum: Student resistances to anti-oppressive pedagogy. *Power and Education, 11*(1), 30–50. https://doi.org/10.1177/1757743818810565

12

Examining Multicultural Pedagogy in Counselor Programs: Recommendations for Enhanced Clinical Competency

Taylor J. Irvine, Adriana C. Labarta, and Danna Demezier

Introduction

> There must exist a paradigm, a practical model for social change that includes an understanding of ways to transform consciousness that are linked to efforts to transform structures (bell hooks)

Among the counseling profession, the inclusion of antiracist pedagogy and multicultural training is integral to culturally responsive practice. The American Counseling Association (ACA) Code of Ethics (2014) mandates counseling programs to integrate multicultural and diversity issues into all courses to develop culturally responsive counselors (ACA, 2014, F.7.c.). As helping professionals, counselors are also called to demonstrate cultural sensitivity, honor clients' cultural identities and

T. J. Irvine (✉) • A. C. Labarta
Florida Atlantic University, Boca Raton, FL, USA
e-mail: tirvine1@fau.edu; alabarta2018@fau.edu

© The Author(s), under exclusive license to Springer Nature Switzerland AG 2022

K. Johnson et al. (eds.), *Developing Anti-Racist Practices in the Helping Professions: Inclusive Theory, Pedagogy, and Application*,
https://doi.org/10.1007/978-3-030-95451-2_12

contexts, and critically examine multicultural issues in diagnosis, assessment, and treatment (ACA, 2014). However, counselors-in-training (CITs) frequently report a lack of self-efficacy in essential multicultural competencies upon graduating (Flasch et al., 2011), leaving them ill-equipped to effectively treat and address diverse clients (Barden et al., 2017; Bidell, 2012). Given the recent increase in culturally diverse populations and the continued sociopolitical unrest across the United States, there is an increased need to equip CITs with multicultural knowledge and skills. An educational paradigm shift is needed across counselor education (CE) programs to accomplish this task, centralizing equity and social justice throughout the curriculum. Failure to prioritize these tenets serves to perpetuate a hegemonic educational culture that, in effect, cultivates an oppressive and inequitable training environment (Gorski & Goodman, 2016; Haskins & Singh, 2015).

In 2015, the Association for Multicultural Counseling and Development (AMCD) endorsed the Multicultural and Social Justice Counseling Competencies (MSJCC) to address the unique needs of marginalized group members, or "those who are oppressed in society and lack the systemic advantages bestowed on privileged groups" (Ratts et al., 2016, p. 36). Marginalized group members include but are not limited to women; Black, Indigenous, and People of Color (BIPOC); LGBTQQIA+ persons; those that are poor or are of lower socioeconomic status; individuals with (dis) abilities; and undocumented immigrants and refugees (Lee, 2019). The revised MSJCC includes a social justice component that is critical to the dismantling of decolonizing practices in counseling. For instance, studies examining multicultural competence among CE programs reveal that CITs are more actively engaged in social justice and advocacy work if their program infuses multiculturalism throughout the training experience (Beer et al., 2012; Gonzalez-Voller et al., 2020; Presseau et al., 2018). As such, the onus of responsibility falls on CE programs to create an equitable and social justice-focused training environment. Further, counselor educators are called to facilitate awareness of the institutionalized structures and sociopolitical factors that uphold colonizing educational practices. Goodman et al. (2016) operationally define *colonizing practices* as:

D. Demezier
Barry University, Miami, FL, USA

> educational practices that reproduce the existing conditions of oppression by failing to challenge the hegemonic views that marginalize groups of people, perpetuate deficit-based ideologies, and continue to disenfranchise the diverse clients and communities with whom our students will work. (p. 148)

This chapter will review current training standards across CE programs, examine deficits and ineffective pedagogical practices in multicultural education, and provide recommendations to address these issues. Table 12.1 provides a chart that outlines definitions used throughout this chapter.

Multicultural Education Pedagogy: Examining Current Practices and Gaps

The United States is steadily becoming a more culturally pluralistic society. According to a report by the U.S. Census Bureau, roughly one in seven people in the U.S. was born in a different country, with this number projected to increase by approximately 15% come the year 2028 (Vespa et al., 2020). This same report revealed that by the year 2060, multiracial persons in the U.S. are expected to grow by a rate of 200% (Vespa et al., 2020). Now more than ever, CITs' attainment of multicultural competence is crucial as the prospect of encountering a culturally diverse client is becoming increasingly likely. However, CITs continue to report a lack of preparedness to treat clients from culturally diverse backgrounds upon graduating from their programs (Barden et al., 2017; Bidell, 2012); they also note diminished self-efficacy in essential multicultural competencies (Flasch et al., 2011). This issue is attributable to ineffective pedagogical practices and delivery methods across CE programs (Killian & Floren, 2020). Therefore, CE programs must draw upon pedagogical strategies rooted in a multicultural education framework. Gorski (2010) provides a robust interpretation of multicultural education as:

Table 12.1 Definitions chart (Definitions for this chapter are as follows:)

Term	Definition
Broaching	A counselor's ability to acknowledge their sources of privilege and various sociopolitical factors that may serve to disempower diverse clients, minimize their presenting concerns, and negatively impact the therapeutic alliance (Day-Vines et al., 2007, 2017; Gorski & Goodman, 2016).
Colonizing practices	"educational practices that reproduce the existing conditions of oppression by failing to challenge the hegemonic views that marginalize groups of people, perpetuate deficit-based ideologies, and continue to disenfranchise the diverse clients and communities with whom our students will work" (Goodman et al., 2016, p. 148).
Multicultural education	"A progressive approach for transforming education that holistically critiques and responds to discriminatory policies and practices in education. It is grounded in ideals of social justice, education equity, critical pedagogy, and a dedication to providing educational experiences in which all students reach their full potentials as learners and as socially aware and active beings, locally, nationally, and globally" (Gorski, 2010, para. 6).
Critical consciousness	The process of actively fostering awareness of sociopolitical and structural factors that have served to disenfranchise marginalized group members, with the aim of liberating and empowering a sense of agency among these persons (Freire, 1972).
Banking model of education	A traditional paradigm of education whereby teachers view students as containers to transmit (or deposit) information; ultimately, proponents of this model believe that students will compliantly absorb the information without any critical thinking or pushback (Freire, 1972).
Intersectionality	A theory that considers the multidimensional identities in individuals not limited to nationality, color, age, social status, cultural background, ethnicity, history, physical location, language, migratory status, sexual orientation, gender, religion, spirituality, disability status, etc. while considering interlinking oppression and privilege across numerous contexts (Crenshaw, 1993; Samuels & Ross-Sheriff, 2008).

a progressive approach for transforming education that holistically critiques and responds to discriminatory policies and practices in education. It is grounded in ideals of social justice, education equity, critical pedagogy, and a dedication to providing educational experiences in which all students reach their full potentials as learners and as socially aware and active beings, locally, nationally, and globally (para. 6).

The following section will examine existing deficits and ineffective pedagogical practices in multicultural education.

Ineffective Pedagogical Strategies

The multicultural education research literature has seen an increase in scholarship written on theoretical models to improve CE programs' pedagogical practices. Despite this upsurge, CE programs continue to only superficially address matters of equity and diversity, thus perpetuating a colonized and oppressive learning environment (Goodman et al., 2016). One suggested source of this colonizing and superficial classroom environment is that many CE programs tend to rely on a single-course model, which inadequately addresses the depth of multiculturalism. Recommendations to address this challenge will be explored later on in this chapter. Another reason for this issue is the delivery method through which multicultural skills and knowledge are transmitted. For instance, in his seminal book *Pedagogy of the Oppressed*, Paulo Freire (1972) asserted that oppressive educational practices could be facilitated through a *banking model of education*, epitomizing an oppressive society. This educational concept can be operationally defined as a traditional paradigm of education whereby teachers view students as containers to transmit (or deposit) information; ultimately, proponents of this model believe that students will compliantly absorb the information without any critical thinking or pushback (Freire, 1972). This colonizing model takes a top-down didactic approach to teaching, which inherently disempowers CITs from engaging in the process of critical thinking (Goodman et al., 2016), thereby viewing students as incapable of engaging in higher-order thinking. In this regard, Suárez-Orozco et al. (2015) conducted a study of 60 diverse college campus classrooms which revealed that undermining students' intellect and competence emerged as the most common form of microaggressions, globally impacting about 30% of all sampled college classrooms. Instead, counselor educators are encouraged to embrace a more constructivist teaching style that challenges colonizing educational practices while also promoting an antiracist learning environment.

A constructivist educational paradigm draws upon collaborative pedagogical strategies such as promoting open discussions, encouraging critical thinking, and broaching difficult conversations. *Broaching* is operationally defined as a counselor's ability to acknowledge their sources of privilege and various sociopolitical factors that may serve to disempower diverse clients, minimize their presenting concerns, and negatively impact the therapeutic alliance (Day-Vines et al., 2007; Day-Vines et al., 2017; Gorski & Goodman, 2016). Counselor educators who embrace a constructivist teaching style may also foster critical consciousness in CITs by encouraging students to reflect on how their prejudices, expectations, and cultural worldviews influence their perception of diversity and power roles on a personal basis (Pitner & Sakamoto, 2005). Developed by Paulo Freire (1973), *critical consciousness* is defined as the process of actively fostering awareness of sociopolitical and structural factors that have served to disenfranchise marginalized group members, with the aim of liberating and empowering a sense of agency among these persons. With critical consciousness, CITs can surrender their urge to maintain the expert role in helping and instead join with their clients (Pitner & Sakamoto, 2005). Further, CITs can use critical consciousness not only to recognize differences and injustices but also to work to rectify presenting inequalities (Pitner & Sakamoto, 2005). Furthermore, a constructivist pedagogical approach is more congruent with current recommendations outlined in the Multicultural and Social Justice Competencies (MSJCC; Ratts et al., 2016), which underscore the roles of social justice, cultural humility, and intersectionality in counseling and counselor education.

Multicultural and Social Justice Competencies (MSJCC)

In 1992, Sue, Arredondo, and McDavis developed the Multicultural Counseling Competencies (MCC), which became the guiding document to assist counseling professionals in their work with culturally diverse populations. Since that time, the MCC were integrated into many facets of the profession, including the *ACA Code of Ethics* (2014), and have played a pivotal role in centering multicultural counseling issues and facilitating paradigm shifts that allowed for more meaningful integration into theory and practice. Since the development of the MCC, social justice has emerged as a crucial component of the multicultural counseling literature, thus prompting the development of revised competencies, known as the MSJCC (Ratts et al., 2016).

The MSJCC address current practices and gaps, provide guidelines to enhance accreditation and training and describe the relationships between various multicultural and social justice constructs (Ratts et al., 2016). Rooted in multicultural and social justice scholarship, the MSJCC acknowledge the dynamics of power and privilege within the counseling relationship, the negative impact of oppression on mental health in marginalized populations, and the integration of social justice advocacy to enhance culturally responsive practice beyond the counseling room. Furthermore, counselors do not "achieve" competence; rather, the MSJCC advocate for counselors and counselor educators to practice cultural humility by approaching their work as an ongoing, lifelong process (Ratts et al., 2016). Four developmental domains describe the process of moving towards multicultural and social justice practice, including counselor self-awareness, client worldview, the counseling relationship, and counseling and advocacy interventions (Ratts et al., 2016). The MSJCC further expand upon the original MCC's (Sue et al., 1992) developmental stages (i.e., attitudes and beliefs, knowledge, and skills) by including an additional aspirational and developmental competency: action. Despite the evident call for culturally responsive, socially just, and advocacy-informed practices, the Council for Accreditation of Counseling and Related Professions (CACREP) 2016 Standards appear to lack guidance for educators to effectively integrate MSJCC into counseling curricula.

CACREP Standards

CACREP serves as an accrediting body for master's and doctoral counseling programs across the U.S. and worldwide. The *2016 CACREP Standards* outline eight common core areas, including social and cultural diversity (CACREP, 2015). Regardless of specialty area (i.e., school counseling, clinical mental health counseling, etc.), CITs are expected to learn about the effective implementation of multicultural counseling competencies (CACREP, 2015). Although CACREP (2015) underscores the need to incorporate diversity into pedagogy, the *2016 Standards* appear ambiguous and lack specific guidelines to effectively infuse multicultural matters and competencies throughout the counseling curriculum. Arguably, this allows CE programs to decide what is deemed "important," which may perpetuate colonizing and oppressive pedagogical practices, thereby inadvertently sending the message that multiculturalism is not central to developing competent counselors. Alternatively, CE programs may wish to foster more equitable learning environments but may feel stuck on how to implement necessary changes. Therefore, it is essential for CE programs to move beyond the *2016 Standards* (CACREP, 2015) and to support CITs with becoming more culturally competent counselors by integrating the MSJCC into the counseling curriculum. We believe that the integration of the MSJCC is essential to working towards antiracist pedagogy across counseling curricula. We provide an overview of the conceptual integration of the MSJCC across CACREP-required courses in Table 12.2 before moving on to recommendations for best practice.

Recommendations for Best Practice

This section follows up our discussion of ineffective pedagogical practices by providing recommendations to address these issues. We begin by examining the effectiveness of a single-course versus an infusion-based model for multicultural education, followed by theoretical frameworks that align with antiracist pedagogy.

Single Course Versus Infusion-Based Model

The *CACREP Standards* (2015) and the *ACA Code of Ethics* (2014) require that CE programs examine multicultural considerations throughout the curricula (Wagner, 2015). To date, much of the available literature on CE

Table 12.2 MSJCC and CACREP infusion-model chart

MSJCC-CACREP infusion model	Attitudes & beliefs	Knowledge	Skills	Action
Professional counseling orientation and ethical practice	CITs examine their attitudes and beliefs about ethics and multicultural competence.	CITs learn the *ACA Code of Ethics* (2014) and the relevance of diversity, social justice, and advocacy in counseling.	CITs apply ethical decision-making skills from a multicultural model (e.g., Toporek & Reza, 2001) when working with diverse clients.	CITs incorporate advocacy as a crucial component of being an ethical counselor and helping professional.
Social and cultural diversity	CITs examine their positionality and intersecting marginalized and privileged identities.	CITs learn about the implementation of culturally responsive, decolonizing theories.	CITs practice broaching and engaging in conversations about power, privilege, and oppression.	CITs identify immersion experiences and advocacy initiatives to engage beyond the classroom.
Human growth and development	CITs understand their biases and assumptions about multicultural issues in human growth and development.	CITs recognize systemic factors that impact human development and functioning.	CITs apply culturally relevant interventions to promote resilience and wellness for diverse individuals across the lifespan.	CITs become involved in a community setting that serves persons across the lifespan and engage in active reflection of learned experiences (e.g., Lee & Kelley-Petersen, 2018)
Career development	CITs gain awareness of their cultural beliefs that impact career counseling processes with diverse students, clients, and colleagues.	CITs learn about the roles of identity and diversity in career development.	CITs integrate culturally informed career counseling strategies.	CITs engage in community service learning and provide outreach to marginalized persons needing resources for career development (e.g., Goodman et al., 2016)

(*continued*)

Table 12.2 (continued)

MSJCC-CACREP infusion model	Attitudes & beliefs	Knowledge	Skills	Action
Counseling and helping relationships	CITs recognize the inherent power differential within the counseling relationship.	CITs learn about multicultural and social justice-oriented counseling theories.	CITs build on basic counseling skills to incorporate strengths-based approaches for diverse clients.	CITs examine the social, cultural, and political systems that influence the counseling relationship.
Group counseling	CITs recognize various power differentials that exist within a group counseling context.	CITs learn about culturally informed group counseling theories and interventions.	CITs incorporate inclusive and affirming group facilitation skills.	CITs actively create a safe group space and recognize that this setting may serve to empower marginalized individuals
Assessment and testing	CITs reflect on their assumptions regarding assessment with diverse populations.	CITs learn competencies for culturally responsive assessment in counseling (e.g., O'Hara et al., 2016).	CITs practice ways to conduct assessments in a culturally informed manner.	CITs enhance the assessment process by considering culturally relevant systemic variables that impact marginalized clients.
Research and program evaluation	CITs examine their own biases regarding counseling research and program evaluation.	CITs learn competencies for culturally responsive counseling research (e.g., O'Hara et al., 2016).	CITs critically examine research studies to understand applicability and relevance to diverse populations.	CITs conduct research using culturally informed, equitable research methodologies and approaches.

pedagogy has reviewed the use of a single course approach to relay multicultural and social justice competencies to CITs. Although a single course has demonstrated some efficacy with fostering higher levels of openness and comfort in counseling trainees, it remains insufficient regarding multiculturalism's depth and scope (Celinska & Swazo, 2016; Presseau et al., 2018). To this effect, we recommend an infusion-based model across CE programs.

An infusion-based model to multicultural education entails examining matters of diversity and equity throughout the curriculum. In doing so, CE programs send the message that multiculturalism is a necessary component of CITs' training experience and indispensable to developing competent multicultural counselors (Gorski & Goodman, 2016). In this regard, the *ACA Code of Ethics* (2014) mandates professional counselors to promote diverse clients' wellbeing, which becomes jeopardized when counselors are unwilling to routinely engage in difficult conversations about privilege, inequity, and oppression. Thus, an infusion-based approach encourages CITs to become actively involved in advocacy and social justice endeavors that extend beyond a single course and continue throughout their professional careers.

There remains a lack of research conducted on infusion-based models in CE programs, with some studies having previously noted contradictory findings. For instance, Celinska and Swazo (2016) conducted a study examining a single multicultural course's impact versus an infusion-based model on trainees' openness and comfort levels. Findings from this study revealed that CITs reported similar levels of openness and comfort before the course began; conversely, a single-course (explicit approach) demonstrated a more significant effect on increasing CITs' overall level of openness and comfort than the infusion-based model (implicit approach) at post-test (Celinska & Swazo, 2016). However, this study posed generalizability concerns such as low sample size and only sampling one university (Celinska & Swazo, 2016). Although research on infusion-based models is still in its infancy, several studies have established the efficacy of this approach, with CITs having shown higher degrees of involvement in social justice and advocacy endeavors when training programs implemented this pedagogical practice (Beer et al., 2012; Gonzalez-Voller et al., 2020; Presseau et al., 2018). Additional strategies to enhance MSJCC among CITs are reviewed below.

Strategies to Enhance MSJCC across CE Programs

Counselor educators play an essential role in fostering the MSJCC in CITs by adopting this framework to enhance diversity training (Ratts et al., 2016). Strategies may include modeling cultural humility, infusing the MSJCC in their course work and syllabi, conducting research informed by the competencies, and advocating for the integration of socially just practices in counseling programs and training sites. Despite the importance of the MSJCC, Melamed et al. (2020) have drawn attention to the CE literature's minimal guidance to infuse them into counseling programs. Although empirical research appears to be lacking, various scholars have suggested pedagogical models, frameworks, and strategies that may help enhance MSJCC in CITs (e.g., Melamed et al., 2020; Singh et al., 2020). These will be explored further in the next section.

Moving Towards a Community Service Learning (CSL) Standard of Practice

An essential aspect of CITs' development into culturally competent clinicians is the attainment of multicultural counseling knowledge, skills, and personal awareness, which first get cultivated in a classroom setting. Although various means for imparting multicultural knowledge and skills are available, experiential learning activities and open discussions about cultural and diversity matters have demonstrated efficacy in bolstering trainees' clinical knowledge, skills, and attitudes (Collins & Arthur, 2010; Wagner, 2015). A form of experiential learning that integrates these components is *community service learning* (CSL). Within the context of CE programs, CSL is an inherently decolonizing pedagogical practice that prepares CITs to become multicultural and social justice clinicians by exposing them to conditions of inequity and oppression faced by marginalized group members. Through this experience, CITs encounter the opportunity to critically examine the structural factors that maintain these institutionalized barriers.

Research on CSL has demonstrated its effectiveness in developing multicultural counseling competency and self-efficacy among CITs

(Burnett et al., 2004; Keller-Dupree et al., 2014; Midgett et al., 2016). CSL accomplishes this by providing trainees with opportunities to actively learn about marginalized persons' cultural backgrounds and lived experiences in a community setting. However, it is essential to note that the effective implementation of CSL requires that CITs engage in a self-reflective process, entailing a critical examination of their own power and privilege, group identity, and personal biases before engaging in CSL. For instance, in a qualitative study that examined the impact of CSL on white students' racial attitudes, Houshmand et al. (2014) found that the experience did not enhance students' level of contextual awareness or multicultural sensitivity as they were unable to see past their own biases and examine socio-structural factors that negatively impacted the community residents. The authors suggested that this outcome was attributable to the lack of antiracist discussions in graduate training programs which must entail conversations about power, privilege, negative stereotyping, color-blind racial views, and patronizing (or paternalistic) beliefs of helping (Houshmand et al., 2014). This form of self-awareness is crucial to CITs' and counselors' effective implementation and development of the MSJCC (Midgett et al., 2016; Ratts et al., 2016). Ultimately, CITs engage in critical consciousness when they cultivate an awareness of power imbalances and oppression needed to competently conceptualize and treat diverse clients. Antiracist pedagogical frameworks that promote this form of self-awareness are examined in the next section.

Antiracist Pedagogical Frameworks

Enhancing counseling trainees' multicultural and social justice competency requires that CE programs consider ways to engage in multicultural training that is inclusive, antiracist, and socially just. It is also crucial that these efforts do not ignore the perspectives and injustices experienced by marginalized trainees from diverse backgrounds, who feel underprepared and not well represented while being trained (Haskins & Singh, 2015). This section offers suggestions and practical ways in which CE programs and educators may go beyond the traditional multicultural training format and embrace contemporary theoretical frameworks such as broaching, critical race theory, intersectionality, and relational cultural theory. Educators can integrate these four frameworks within their curricula and pedagogical practices to enhance the clinical effectiveness of counseling trainees who work with diverse populations, regardless of their own cultural background.

These theories acknowledge the impact of race, culture, racism, oppression, and injustices while simultaneously making room to recognize how these issues impact presenting problems in people of color and marginalized individuals. This list of theories is by no means exhaustive. Still, it is merely an introduction to different models that may be utilized to promote culturally relevant counseling practice for students training to become professional counselors in schools, the community, hospitals, private practice, or other professional settings. This section concludes with a case example that offers practical suggestions on how each identified theory may be used to support CITs in developing an antiracist and multicultural approach in their work.

Broaching

Infusing multicultural and social justice counseling competencies in CE programs is essential to fostering quality multicultural training and education. One proposed strategy to help promote culturally relevant counseling involves an organized framework that explores matters of race, ethnicity, and culture during the counseling process, otherwise known as broaching (Day-Vines et al., 2007). *Broaching* is empirically tested and is supported as a multicultural counseling competency that considers the role of diversity in counseling (Day-Vines et al., 2007; Day-Vines et al., 2017). It enables CITs to engage in ethical behavior and fulfill CACREP standards as they self-reflect on their own attitudes, biases, and assumptions and consider how all these factors influence their responses and interactions with clients who are ethnically or lingually different than them (Day-Vines et al., 2017). Counseling trainees who develop broaching skills acknowledge, rather than ignore or undermine, the sociopolitical issues which influence the client's presenting issues (Day-Vines et al., 2007) by maintaining critical consciousness of the issues at hand.

As part of their pedagogical practice, counselor educators may utilize specific strategies to develop their students' broaching skills. Day-Vines et al. (2017) have suggested five different broaching techniques to develop multicultural competence in CITs. The first involves improving one's racial self-awareness by reviewing one's attitudes, biases, and assumptions when confronting racial topics. A second example is attending to cultural factors during treatment planning to ensure culturally relevant techniques are applied. A third way is to use case studies with racial and ethnic minorities to allow trainees to examine cultural issues and develop their multicultural competency. Another technique is incorporating media and film with unbiased depictions of individuals from different cultural groups to practice how to go about broaching emerging cultural issues. Finally, Day-Vines et al. (2017) suggested using counseling simulations to enable students to explore multicultural issues, create multicultural case conceptualizations, and address their attitudes, biases, and assumptions, which surfaced during the therapeutic process. CITs may process and review this information in supervision with peers and with their instructors to receive useful feedback on their efforts.

Critical Race Theory and Intersectionality Theory

Critical race theory (CRT) explores race, racism, and power relations in larger contexts and social structures (Anderson, 2020; Delgado & Stefancic, 2017). CRT attends to the prevalence of racism in society by critically reviewing the role of power and oppression and their intersection with race (Anderson, 2020). In CRT, the primary themes are the normalcy of racism, material determinism, the social construction of race, differential racialization, intersectionality and anti-essentialism, and the voices of people of color (Delgado & Stefancic, 2017). Since CRT's essential purpose is to attend to racism and unjust traditions that suppress the voices of traditionally disregarded and marginalized groups of people, CRT is amenable and applies to different fields such as the legal system and education sector (Haskins & Singh, 2015). For the purpose of this chapter, tenets of CRT guide pedagogical practices to center an antiracist approach.

Many scholars describe the perpetuity of race and racism in everyday life on different levels, lawfully, socially, and mentally, which traverse social classifications of race, economic status, nationality, and sexual orientation, to name a few (Bell, 1995; Crenshaw, 1993; Haskins & Singh, 2015; Solórzano, 1997). From a counselor education stance, CRT considers the role of institutional racism in removing power and silencing the voices of those without privilege while also inflicting feelings of isolation and anguish onto those with various intersecting marginalized identities (Haskins & Singh, 2015). The normalcy of racism and intersectionality is observed in the negative experiences of traditionally marginalized persons. A second CRT principle relevant to CE is counter storytelling, which is the process whereby marginalized individuals' experiences and truths challenge and work against dominant discourses and beliefs (Delgado & Stefancic, 2017; Ladson-Billings, 1999; Solórzano & Yosso, 2001) such as meritocracy or colorblindness (Haskins & Singh, 2015). As part of their pedagogical practice, counselor educators can apply all CRT principles by (1) reviewing their curriculum to explore how their race and intersecting identities impact them and their curriculum development; (2) investigating the influence of colorblindness in their teaching practice by acknowledging that Whiteness functions to benefit certain groups of people and is present within the curriculum; and (3) applying a culturally sensitive approach that is untraditional yet all-encompassing (Haskins & Singh, 2015).

Relational Cultural Theory

Relational Cultural Therapy (RCT; Miller, 1976) is a feminist counseling theory developed by Jean Baker Miller, Irene Stiver, Judith Jordan, and Janet Surrey in 1977. RCT posits that isolation is the primary source of suffering for humans; therefore, mutually empowering, growth-fostering relationships allow for healing to occur (Jordan, 2010). Since RCT challenges traditional counseling theories developed from Westernized frameworks, it is a decolonizing, social justice theory that can help counselors integrate the MSJCC into practice (Singh et al., 2020). Specifically, RCT recognizes how oppressive systems perpetuate experiences of isolation for marginalized populations, thus leaving individuals feeling disconnected and disempowered (Jordan, 2010). To dismantle inequitable systems, RCT emphasizes the role of therapist authenticity to repair relational ruptures and foster mutual empowerment within the counseling relationship (Jordan, 2010).

RCT's inherent multicultural focus makes it suitable for application in CE programs, especially to advance the provision of culturally informed pedagogy (Dorn-Medeiros et al., 2020; Lertora et al., 2020). Using an RCT lens, the learning environment is co-constructed by the counselor educator and CITs. RCT may help examine classroom relational dynamics and minimize the power differential between instructors and students (Miller, 1976). This process can be facilitated when counselor educators demonstrate honesty and openness with their students (Dorn-Medeiros et al., 2020). For example, educators can model authenticity through self-disclosure of their own multicultural and social justice competency journey (Reynolds, 2011), thus demonstrating cultural humility to effectively implement the MSJCC (Ratts et al., 2016). Through this process, CITs may feel more willing to self-reflect, take relational risks, and engage, versus withdraw, from challenging conversations on power, privilege, and oppression (Dorn-Medeiros et al., 2020).

Concerning practical strategies and techniques, counselor educators may incorporate RCT-informed activities to enhance multicultural and social justice pedagogy with CITs, including developing a shared mission and vision statement for the course, creating social location maps and completing weekly reflective journals (Dorn-Medeiros et al., 2020). Counselor educators may assign social location maps during the middle of the semester to encourage CITs to individually select various social locations and consider the interplay of power, privilege, and oppression (Dorn-Medeiros et al., 2020). Ideally, the self-reflection journals are conducted by both CITs and instructors to help counselor educators model self-reflection, transparency, and cultural humility to CITs. In addition, counselor educators can use role-plays to demonstrate RCT principles to students, such as creating an environment conducive to authenticity and growth-fostering relationships; this may occur by having CITs simulate a counselor-client relationship and acting out learned RCT principles under the supervision of the counselor educator (Lertora et al., 2020).

Summary

This section outlined antiracist pedagogical approaches rooted in constructivist philosophy that can help enhance counseling trainees' multicultural and social justice competency. Ultimately, CE programs and educators are encouraged to implement a constructivist approach to teaching, which is necessary to fostering critical consciousness in CITs. The following case illustration depicts a typical presentation (i.e., limited cultural knowledge and awareness) of CITs before engaging in clinical work. This case provides insight into CE programs' role in facilitating critical consciousness in CITs and how this preparation is crucial for trainees to approach their work from an antiracist lens, thus operating competently and ethically when working with clients.

Case Illustration

Angelique is a second-year master's-level student in a CACREP-accredited counselor education (CE) program and is excited to begin an internship at a community mental health agency (CMHA) situated in an urban area. Angelique selected this placement because they wanted to challenge themselves, sharpen their foreign language skills, and become more culturally competent. Although Angelique is a quick learner, they admit to having limited knowledge of other cultures and share that they do not think they will face any issues because they are a "people person." Angelique has developed critical consciousness and established a working plan to confront personal biases and assumptions of individuals from diverse populations who may present at the CMHA for counseling. Angelique has committed to prepare for sessions by conducting a multicultural case conceptualization, as learned in counseling theories, for each diverse client and will apply a multicultural ethical decision-making model to navigate ethical dilemmas which present during the counseling process. Even as a novice counselor, Angelique recognizes the importance of engaging in a strengths-based approach to highlight each client's individual strengths. Table 12.3 outlines theoretical interventions that counselor educators can incorporate when CITs, like Angelique, are confronted with similar multicultural training challenges.

Table 12.3 Common challenges and theoretical interventions

Common challenges	Theory	Intervention examples
Lack of self-awareness *Personal biases*	Broaching	Assign CITs to watch a movie with individuals from another culture and select someone to serve as her client. Have CITs maintain a journal that reviews her attitudes, biases, and assumptions about individuals of a different race. Have CITs create a multicultural case conceptualization and simulate an actual session that addresses issues of race with the client.
Single focus of people's social identity *Separates people's oppressive experiences from their social identities* (Chen et al., 2020)	Critical race theory/ intersectionality theory	Assign CITs to explore intersections for marginalized that are not readily noticeable Help CITs identify aspects of power and privilege which impact clients in CMHA Instruct CITs to consider how intersectionality applies to them (Chen et al., 2020)
Failure to consider the impact of marginalization *Misunderstanding of cultural differences*	Relational-cultural theory	Model authenticity and cultural humility by recounting and processing a personal experience where marginalization was overlooked. Engage in role-plays to demonstrate ways to address and repair relational ruptures through mutual empathy and empowerment, thereby moving towards connection.

Conclusion

Multicultural and social justice competency is an essential component of CE training programs due to the rise in diverse populations that CITs may encounter during their matriculation in school or their professional practice. As the profession and world are becoming more inclusive and socially just, CE programs must also shift from traditional, ineffective pedagogical practices by implementing MSJCC throughout the curriculum. We have offered suggestions on ways to incorporate the MSJCC competencies within CACREP's curriculum to help CITs develop these skills throughout their training instead of learning them in a single course. A case illustration was also offered, which demonstrated decolonizing practical strategies and techniques to help counselor educators transform their pedagogical approach through an antiracist framework, thereby increasing cultural responsiveness in trainees. Ultimately, an antiracist and constructivist pedagogical style is crucial to facilitating culturally responsive teaching and MSJCC competence in trainees.

The information outlined in this chapter poses relevance to all helping professionals, extending beyond the field of counseling. Readers can use the knowledge acquired from this chapter to enhance current training and educational standards across other helping fields, including but not limited to psychology, education, and social work. Specifically, readers can apply learned strategies to decolonize their educational programs, helping to illuminate current programmatic deficits and deconstruct ineffective pedagogical practices in multicultural education and training. In addition, the multicultural and social justice competencies discussed in this chapter are critical to developing a culturally responsive approach across professions. Finally, readers will walk away with useful antiracist pedagogical practices that can be implemented to enrich their personal and professional development.

Guiding Questions

As a current trainee or counselor educator…

1. What are biases that I hold about antiracist pedagogy? Did they shift after reading this chapter? If so, how?

2. How is my counseling or teaching orientation aligned with the Multicultural and Social Justice Counseling Competencies (MSJCC)? What are the gaps or limitations of my orientation that may impact the way I engage with culturally diverse clients or trainees?
3. What are ways that I have challenged colonizing practices in my teaching or counseling practice? How can I begin or continue to integrate socially just approaches (such as CRT, intersectionality, RCT, and broaching) to decolonize counseling pedagogy?

Quiz Questions

1. Which of the following is a characteristic of colonizing educational practices?

   (a) Perpetuates hierarchical power dynamics
   (b) Utilizes deficit-based frameworks
   (c) Fails to recognize the impacts of marginalization
   (d) All of the above

2. True or False? Although much of the current literature has focused on a single-course approach to multicultural education, it continues to remain insufficient to address the breadth and depth of multicultural and social justice issues in counseling.

   (a) True
   (b) False

3. What is the fourth aspirational and developmental competency that was recently incorporated into the MSJCC?

   (a) Action
   (b) Attitudes and beliefs
   (c) Knowledge
   (d) Skills

4. Which of the following does **not** demonstrate the application of Relational-Cultural Theory into pedagogy?

   (a) Modeling authenticity to students
   (b) Addressing relational ruptures

   (c) Counterstorytelling
   (d) Growth-fostering relationships

5. How does broaching help CITs and counselors when working with diverse clients?
   (a) Initiate and continue discussions on power, privilege, and oppression
   (b) Self-reflect on personal biases
   (c) Examine the intersecting roles and identities within the counseling relationship
   (d) All of the above

References

Anderson, B. N. (2020). "See Me, See Us": Understanding the Intersections and Continued Marginalization of Adolescent Gifted Black Girls in U.S. Classrooms. *Gifted Child Today, 43*(2), 86–100. https://doi.org/10.1177/1076217519898216

American Counseling Association. (2014). *ACA code of ethics*. Author.

Barden, S. M., Sherrell, R. S., & Matthews, J. J. (2017). A national survey on multicultural competence for professional counselors: A replication study. *Journal of Counseling & Development, 95*, 203–212. https://doi.org/10.1002/jcad.12132

Beer, A. M., Spanierman, L. B., Greene, J. C., & Todd, N. R. (2012). Counseling psychology trainees' perceptions of training and commitments to social justice. *Journal of Counseling Psychology, 59*(1), 120–133. https://doi.org/10.1037/a0026325

Bell, D. (1995). Who's afraid of critical race theory? *University of Illinois Law Review, 1995*(4), 893–910.

Bidell, M. P. (2012). Examining school counseling students' multicultural and sexual orientation competencies through a cross-specialization comparison. *Journal of Counseling & Development, 90*(2), 200–207. https://doi.org/10.1111/j.1556-6676.2012.00025.x

Burnett, J. A., Hamel, D., & Long, L. L. (2004). Service learning in graduate counselor education: Developing multicultural counseling competency.

Journal of Multicultural Counseling and Development, 32(3), 180–191. https://doi.org/10.1002/j.2161-1912.2004.tb00370.x

Celinska, D., & Swazo, R. (2016). Multicultural curriculum designs in counselor education programs: Enhancing counselors-in-training openness to diversity. *Journal of Counselor Preparation and Supervision, 8*(3). https://doi.org/10.7729/83.1124

Chen, S. Y., Basma, D., Ju, J., & Ng, K. M. (2020). Opportunities and challenges of multicultural and international online education. *Professional Counselor, 10*(1), 120–132. https://doi.org/10.15241/syc.10.1.120

Collins, S., & Arthur, N. (2010). Culture-infused counselling: A model for developing multicultural competence. *Counselling Psychology Quarterly, 23*(2), 217–233. https://doi.org/10.1080/09515071003798212

Council for Accreditation of Counseling and Related Educational Programs. (2015). *2016 CACREP standards* [Accreditation standards]. Retrieved from https://www.cacrep.org/for-programs/2016-cacrep-standards/

Crenshaw, K. (1993). Mapping the margins: Intersectionality, identity politics, and violence against women of color. *Standard Law Review, 43*, 1241–1299.

Day-Vines, N. L., Booker Ammah, B., Steen, S., & Arnold, K. M. (2017). Getting comfortable with discomfort: Preparing counselor trainees to broach racial, ethnic, and cultural factors with clients during counseling. *International Journal for the Advancement of Counselling, 40*(2), 89–104. https://doi.org/10.1007/s10447-017-9308-9

Day-Vines, N. L., Wood, S. M., Grothaus, T., Craigen, L., Holman, A., Dotson-Blake, K., & Douglass, M. J. (2007). Broaching the subjects of race, ethnicity, and culture during the counseling process. *Journal of Counseling & Development, 85*(4), 401–409. https://doi.org/10.1002/j.1556-6678.2007.tb00608.x

Delgado, R., & Stefancic, J. (2017). *Critical race theory: An introduction* (3rd ed.). New York University Press. https://doi.org/10.2307/j.ctt1ggjjn3

Dorn-Medeiros, C. M., Christensen, J. K., Lértora, I. M., & Croffie, A. L. (2020). Relational strategies for teaching multicultural courses in counselor education. *Journal of Multicultural Counseling and Development, 48*(3), 149–160. https://doi.org/10.1002/jmcd.12174

Flasch, P., Bloom, Z., & Holladay, K. (2011). Self-efficacy of counselor trainees in pre-practicum: A phenomenological study. *Journal of Counselor Practice*. https://doi.org/10.22229/sft309871

Freire, P. (1972). *Pedagogy of the oppressed*. Herder and Herder.

Freire, P. (1973). *Education for critical consciousness*. Seabury Press.

Gonzalez-Voller, J., Crunk, A. E., Barden, S. M., Harris, S., & Belser, C. T. (2020). A preliminary longitudinal study of multicultural competence in counselor education. *Journal of Counseling & Development, 98*(3), 308–318. https://doi.org/10.1002/jcad.12325

Goodman, R. D., Williams, J. M., Chung, R. C., Talleyrand, R. M., Douglass, A. M., McMahon, H. G., & Bemak, F. (2016). Decolonizing traditional pedagogies and practices in counseling and psychology education: A move towards social justice and action. In R. D. Goodman & P. C. Gorski (Eds.), *Decolonizing "multicultural" counseling through social justice* (Ser. International and cultural psychology) (pp. 147–164). Springer.

Gorski, P. C. (2010). *The challenge of defining "multicultural education"*. Retrieved from http://www.edchange.org/multicultural/initial.html

Gorski, P. C., & Goodman, R. D. (2016). Introduction: Toward a decolonized multicultural counseling and psychology. In R. D. Goodman & P. C. Gorski (Eds.), *Decolonizing "multicultural" counseling through social justice* (Ser. International and cultural psychology) (pp. 1–10). Springer.

Haskins, N. H., & Singh, A. (2015). Critical race theory and counselor education pedagogy: Creating equitable training. *Counselor Education and Supervision, 54*(4), 288–301. https://doi.org/10.1002/ceas.12027

Houshmand, S., Spanierman, L. B., Beer, A. M., Poteat, V. P., & Lawson, L. J. (2014). The impact of a service-learning design course on white students' racial attitudes. *Journal of Higher Education Outreach and Engagement, 18*(2), 19–48.

Jordan, J. V. (2010). *Theories of psychotherapy. Relational – Cultural therapy.* American Psychological Association.

Keller-Dupree, E. A., Little, M. L., Hagman, A. G., & Deckert, J. J. (2014). *Collaborative learning: The effects of service learning on personal and professional development for school counselors-in-training.* https://www.counseling.org/docs/default-source/vistas/article_07.pdf?sfvrsn=fa020a65_12

Killian, T., & Floren, M. (2020). Exploring the relationship between pedagogy and counselor 'trainees' multicultural and social justice competence. *Journal of Counseling & Development, 98*, 295–307. https://doi.org/10.1002/jcad.12324

Ladson-Billings, G. (1999). Preparing teachers for diverse student populations: A critical race theory perspective. *Review of Research in Education, 24*, 211–247.

Lee, C. C. (2019). Multicultural competency: A conceptual framework for counseling across cultures. In C. C. Lee (Ed.), *Multicultural issues in counsel-*

ing: New approaches to diversity (5th ed., pp. 3–14). American Counseling Association.

Lee, K., & Kelley-Petersen, D. (2018). Service learning in human development: Promoting social justice perspectives in counseling. *The Professional Counselor, 8*(2), 146–158. https://doi.org/10.15241/kal.8.2.146

Lertora, I. M., Croffie, A., Dorn-Medeiros, C., & Christensen, J. (2020). Using relational cultural theory as a pedagogical approach for counselor education. *Journal of Creativity in Mental Health, 15*(2), 265–276. https://doi.org/10.1080/15401383.2019.1687059

Melamed, L., Casado Pérez, J. F., & Hunt, B. (2020). Teaching strategies for incorporating the multicultural and social justice counseling competencies. *Journal of Counselor Preparation and Supervision, 13*(2). https://doi.org/10.7729/42.1350

Midgett, A., Hausheer, R., & Doumas, D. M. (2016). Training counseling students to develop group leadership self-efficacy and multicultural competence through service learning. *Journal for Specialists in Group Work, 41*(3), 262–282. https://doi.org/10.1080/01933922.2016.1186765

Miller, J. B. (1976). *Toward a new psychology of women*. Beacon Press.

O'Hara, C., Clark, M., Hays, D. G., McDonald, C. P., Chang, C. Y., Crockett, S. A., Filmore, J., Portman, T., Spurgeon, S., & Wester, K. L. (2016). AARC standards for multicultural research. *Counseling Outcome Research and Evaluation, 7*(2), 67–72. https://doi.org/10.1177/2150137816657389

Pitner, R. O., & Sakamoto, I. (2005). The role of critical consciousness in multicultural practice: Examining how its strength becomes it limitation. *American Journal of Orthopsychiatry, 75*(4), 684–694. https://doi.org/10.1037/0002-9432.75.4.684

Presseau, C., Luu, L. P., Inman, A. G., & Deblaere, C. (2018). Trainee social justice advocacy: Investigating the roles of training factors and multicultural competence. *Counselling Psychology Quarterly, 32*(2), 260–274. https://doi.org/10.1080/09515070.2018.1476837

Ratts, M. J., Singh, A. A., Nassar-McMillan, S., Butler, S. K., & McCullough, J. R. (2016). Multicultural and social justice counseling competencies: Guidelines for the counseling profession. *Journal of Multicultural Counseling and Development, 44*(1), 28–48. https://doi.org/10.1002/jmcd.12035

Reynolds, A. L. (2011). Understanding the perceptions and experiences of faculty who teach multicultural counseling courses: An exploratory study. *Training and Education in Professional Psychology, 5*, 167–174. https://doi.org/10.1037/a0024613

Samuels, G. M., & Ross-Sheriff, F. (2008). Identity, oppression, and power: Feminisms and intersectionality theory. *Journal of Women and Social Work, 23*(1), 5–9. https://doi.org/10.1177/0886109907310475

Singh, A. A., Appling, B., & Trepal, H. (2020). Using the multicultural and social justice counseling competencies to decolonize counseling practice: The important roles of theory, power, and action. *Journal of Counseling and Development, 98*(3), 261–271. https://doi.org/10.1002/jcad.12321

Solórzano, D. (1997). Images and words that wound: Critical race theory, racial steoreotyping, and teacher education. *Teacher Education Quarterly, 24*(3), 5–19.

Solórzano, D. G., & Yosso, T. J. (2001). Critical race and LatCrit theory and method: Counter-storytelling. *International Journal of Qualitative Studies in Education, 14*(4), 471–495.

Suárez-Orozco, C., Casanova, S., Martin, M., Katsiaficas, D., Cuellar, V., Smith, N. A., & Dias, S. I. (2015). Toxic rain in class: Classroom interpersonal microaggressions. *Educational Researcher, 44*(3), 151–160. https://doi.org/10.3102/0013189x15580314

Sue, D. W., Arredondo, P., & McDavis, R. J. (1992). Multicultural counseling competencies and standards: A call to the profession. *Journal of Multicultural Counseling and Development, 20*, 64–88. https://doi.org/10.1002/j.2161-1912.1992.tb00563.x

Toporek, R. L., & Reza, J. V. (2001). Context as a critical dimension of multicultural counseling: Articulating personal, professional, and institutional competence. *Journal of Multicultural Counseling and Development, 29*(1), 13–30. https://doi.org/10.1002/j.2161-1912.2001.tb00500.x

Vespa, J., Medina, L., & Armstrong, D. M. (2020). *Demographic turning points for the United States: Population projections for 2020 to 2060.* https://www.census.gov/content/dam/Census/library/publications/2020/demo/p25-1144.pdf

Wagner, T. M. (2015). *Addressing multicultural issues in the counselor education classroom: A phenomenological analysis* (publication no. 10075971). Doctoral dissertation, University of North Texas. ProQuest dissertations and theses global.

13

Strategies for Implementing Antiracist Frameworks in Teaching Materials for Health Professions

Sarah E. LaFave, Lea A. Marineau, Keilah A. Jacques, Cassidy Griffith, Ruth-Alma Turkson-Ocran, Mona Shattell, Sarah L. Szanton, and Lucine Francis

Introduction

Racism is an organized system of dominance and subordination, premised on the arbitrary categorization and ranking of social groups into races. It devalues, disempowers, disembodies, and differentially allocates desirable opportunities and resources to groups regarded as racially inferior (Williams & Mohammed, 2013). Antiracism is an educational and organizing framework that seeks to confront and eradicate racism and racialized privilege (Came & Griffith, 2018). Although methods to analyze the impact of racism have existed for some time, methods to

S. E. LaFave (✉) • L. A. Marineau • K. A. Jacques • C. Griffith •
R.-A. Turkson-Ocran • S. L. Szanton • L. Francis
Johns Hopkins University, Baltimore, MD, USA
e-mail: sarah.lafave@jhu.edu; lmarine1@jhmi.edu; keilah.jacques@jhu.edu; cgriff37@jhmi.edu; rturkso1@jhmi.edu; sarah.szanton@jhu.edu; lfranc12@jhu.edu

© The Author(s), under exclusive license to Springer Nature Switzerland AG 2022

K. Johnson et al. (eds.), *Developing Anti-Racist Practices in the Helping Professions: Inclusive Theory, Pedagogy, and Application*,
https://doi.org/10.1007/978-3-030-95451-2_13

educate and organize people to achieve health equity in the context of racism are less well established (Ford & Airhihenbuwa, 2018).

In health professions education, examination of racial disparities is limited, and in some cases, misleading. Course content often focuses on describing race-based differences in health conditions and outcomes without providing context on the social and political structures that contribute to those differences. This focus on *race*, as opposed to *racism*, perpetuates misinterpretation of race as a biological, rather than a social construct (Amutah et al., 2021). As educators in the health professions, we need to adopt antiracist pedagogy. We have a responsibility to prepare our students to analyze and re-design systems and structures based on their impact on marginalized groups. In this chapter, we describe the current landscape of teaching on race and racial disparities in health professions and present strategies to address current issues at the classroom, institutional, and professional practice levels as part of a necessary shift to antiracist practice.

Race & Racial Disparities in Health Professions Teaching Materials: Current State

Authors and editors inadequately represent and contextualize race and racial health disparities in health professions' textbooks and teaching materials (Amutah et al., 2021; Burnett et al., 2020). Much of the literature evaluating the state of framing disparities focuses on medical and nursing education, and these studies show that teaching materials often pathologize race by presenting disparities without social context, ascribe biological differences between racial groups, inappropriately conflate race and ethnicity, and lack representation of People of Color (Acquaviva & Mintz, 2010; Amutah et al., 2021; Byrne, 2001; Curry, 2001; Louie & Wilkes, 2018; Martin et al., 2016; Massie et al., 2020; Sheets et al., 2011; Tsai et al., 2016).

Health professions instructors often inaccurately portray race as biologic. We teach students to pathologize race by associating specific diseases with race, rather than historical and contemporary inequities

---

M. Shattell
University of Central Florida, Orlando, FL, USA
e-mail: mshatte1@jhu.edu

(Amutah et al., 2021; Tsai et al., 2016). Tsai et al. (2016) examined all lecture slides mentioning race in first- and second-year preclinical lecture materials at one medical school. Most slides that included information about a racial disparity excluded any context or justification. Only 4% of the slides acknowledged social determinants as the cause for racial and ethnic health disparities; 96% of slides suggested biological differences as risk factors for racial and ethnic health disparities, of which 38% listed specific biological differences and 58% implied biological differences. In further analysis, the researchers found that 50% of slides linked race with the epidemiology of diseases without context, 42% demonstrated race as a risk, diagnostic, or treatment factor, 6% included race as part of a vignette or case study, and 2% described race as an indication for adjustment of a physiologic measurement. In another study, Byrne (2001) reviewed textbooks and found text that "minimized the concept of racism."

Researchers have also found issues with how authors cite racial disparities in health professions textbooks (Sheets et al., 2011). In one study, researchers searched a medical pathology book for statements claiming African Americans have different disease profiles than other races, examined references cited, and if a statement was not supported or was unconfirmed by the reference cited, the researchers searched the literature for evidence supporting or contradicting the statements. Sheets et al. (2011) found that two-thirds of the statements claiming differences in risk factors for African Americans compared to other races were not supported by published literature. Researchers have also found that textbooks overgeneralize sociocultural differences and include stereotypical content, such as outlining racial differences in beliefs about matriarchy, nutrition, territoriality, and the importance of time (Byrne, 2001).

Medical literature and educators teach students that race is an important factor to consider when diagnosing and treating patients (Acquaviva & Mintz, 2010). Race *is* an important epidemiologic category to consider within the context of social and political structures, including structural discrimination; however, teaching racial disparities without this context inaccurately suggests biological differences between groups of people as the cause (Tsai et al., 2016).

Teaching race as a risk factor for disease dangerously implies that disparities are inevitable, which can lead to healthcare providers expecting and accepting them. Teaching race as a risk factor can also lead to underdiagnosis in racial groups not traditionally associated with a disease, such as misdiagnosis of hemoglobinopathies in White people because curricula depict the diseases as "Black" diseases (Louie & Wilkes, 2018).

In addition to pathologizing race, medical and nursing teaching materials often conflate race and ethnicity, failing to present them as distinct constructs (Acquaviva & Mintz, 2010). Ethnicity is defined as the shared heritage or origin and culture of a group of people, while race is one of several markers of ethnicity that persons within a particular ethnic group may use to identify themselves (Eriksen, 2012). The conflation of race and ethnicity is not specific to health professions teaching materials. The United States federal government's categorization of people has even reinforced it by creating five categories for race (American Indian or Alaska Native, Asian, Black or African American, Native Hawaiian or Other Pacific Islander, and White) and a dichotomous category for ethnicity (Hispanic or Latino; Not Hispanic or Latino). These categories ignore a much broader classification of ethnicity and disconcertingly include both racial and ethnic terms as options for race (Acquaviva & Mintz, 2010).

While it is important that we examine content that is included in teaching materials, it is just as important that we examine the content that is *excluded*. Almost 40% of Americans identify as People of Color (Frey, 2020), yet in the vast majority of textbook images, People of Color are neither depicted alone nor along with White people (Massie et al., 2019; Nolen, 2020). Textbook images can include both those that authors use to bring content to life, such as photographs of people exercising, as well as technical drawings and photographs that help students gain assessment skills for certain health conditions. Martin et al. (2016) reviewed lecture slides from 33 preclinical courses at the University of Washington School of Medicine and found that of 5230 human images, only 22% included People of Color. In a sub-analysis of images based on course topics, only 7% of the images covering anatomy and embryology included People of Color, 17% of the images covering topics in reproduction included People of Color, and 27% of the images covering topics on hormones and nutrients included People of Color. Similarly, Massie et al. (2020) studied 1381 published images from 1992 to 2017 in the *New England Journal of Medicine's Images in Clinical Medicine* and found that only 18% of the images included People of Color. Researchers also examined the depiction of race and skin tone in a sample of four preclinical textbooks commonly used in medical schools (Louie & Wilkes, 2018). The overall representation of racial groups in three of the four textbooks was proportional to the population of the United States; however, light skin tones were consistently overrepresented in those textbooks, across racial groups. Additionally, distribution of race and skin tone at the chapter and topic levels demonstrated omission of People of Color in several chapters (Louie & Wilkes, 2018). In a content analysis of 3000 images in nine nursing health assessment textbooks, only 6% of nurse images included Black nurses (Curry, 2001). The authors noted that newer textbooks included more Black nurses, while textbooks published before 1998 rarely included Black nurses. Only 12% of patient images included Black patients.

In addition to a lack of representation of People of Color in images, textbooks also problematically exclude racial groups in written text. In clinical textbooks, authors often describe both normal and abnormal signs and symptoms in ways that are specific to White people. For example, Byrne and colleagues found that textbooks described Eurocentric physical characteristics as normal, e.g., stating that normal mucous membranes should be "pink." In that study, researchers also found that authors of three nursing fundamentals textbooks rarely included the accomplishments and contributions of prominent Black nurses and did not reference books authored by important Black scholars when discussing the history of nursing (Byrne, 2001). Representation in teaching materials is important for urgent safety reasons, such as preparing future healthcare providers to recognize signs and symptoms of disease on all skin tones and hair textures, and for broader cultural reasons including the ability of our professions to attract and support a diverse workforce.

Health professions students are increasingly concerned regarding the inaccurate teaching on race and the problematic absence of context surrounding racial disparities. A survey of medical students at the Warren Alpert Medical School of Brown University found that 76% of students believed that the medical school curriculum did not adequately prepare them to address racial and ethnic health disparities, and 89% of students supported curriculum reform to better educate on race and racial and ethnic health disparities (Tsai et al., 2016).

Researchers need to examine the depiction of race and racial disparities in health professions teaching materials more thoroughly. Most studies examining lecture materials only include materials from one school, limiting the generalization of results. Researchers typically analyze one topical area rather than including all the textbooks from a health profession program. In addition, although the studies analyzing depictions of race and skin tone in images provide important information, researchers do not typically accompany that analysis with an analysis of context or content surrounding the images. Because the current literature is limited, and because each health profession program may have specific challenges that are most important to address in their own materials, administrators and faculty should consider systematically evaluating their own course materials and textbooks.

Case Study: Evaluation of One Nursing Program's Textbooks

To provide a practical example of how to systematically evaluate and critique depiction of race and disparities in teaching materials, we will share a case study of a project we conducted at Johns Hopkins University School of Nursing to understand how authors discuss race and ethnicity in relation to health disparities in Master's-level pre-licensure nursing textbooks. We will present the methods of this project, the results it produced, and how educators can tailor these methods to uncover challenges in their school's curriculum and materials to create an antiracist future for health professions.

Planning

In the planning phase, a group of our faculty, doctoral students, and master's students met to define the purpose and aims of the textbook evaluation project. In those meetings, we standardized several components of the systematic evaluation including which texts constituted the "core curriculum" and the methods the team would use for extraction and analysis. Our three aims were:

1. Determine the frequency and language with which authors present racial and ethnic disparities in health outcomes within our program's nursing textbooks
2. Assess what kind of context (e.g., social, geographic, biological), if any, authors provide for racial and ethnic disparities in our program's nursing textbooks
3. Quantify the extent to which authors provide racial and ethnic disparity statistics and cite context for disparities in our program's nursing textbooks

Next, we defined which textbooks of the pre-licensure curriculum to include in the systematic evaluation. We chose the fourteen textbooks associated with required courses that students in all American Association of Colleges of Nursing (AACN) pre-licensure programs take. In addition, we defined a list of 125 search terms from the census list specific to racial and ethnic (including ancestral and religious) groups. We included the roots of terms in our terms list to ensure we would fully capture a term (e.g., we searched "America-" to capture "America," "American," "Americans," and so on). We then defined exclusion and inclusion criteria. We included excerpts if they named a difference in a health outcome between two or more racial or ethnic groups in the United States. We excluded excerpts if they named a difference between two or more global populations, or if they identified a process outcome, perception, belief, behavior, or practice without identifying a difference in health.

Extraction

Following the planning phase, we used the search/find function in digital versions of textbooks to search each book for each of the search terms. We then recorded each incidence in written narratives, lists, and tables and analyzed all text within three sentences of the terms for the presence or absence of a citation for the disparity, presence or absence and type of context presented for the disparity (e.g., socioeconomic disparities, genetics, geographic ancestry, environment, etc.), and whether authors provided a citation for the context. We evaluated whether authors presented race as a social construct or as a biological construct. We first completed data extraction using a copy of the extraction spreadsheet on our own computers and then met to compare and discuss results to check for reliability. We iteratively refined inclusion and exclusion criteria until all our team members were consistent in data extraction. Then, we transitioned to using a shared cloud-based spreadsheet. One team member completed data extraction for a term, and a second team member checked each excerpt. If the two researchers disagreed about whether the excerpt met inclusion criteria, the entire team reviewed, discussed, and came to consensus on that excerpt during team meetings.

Findings

We analyzed findings to understand how many claims about disparities among racial and ethnic groups authors included, cited, and contextualized and to determine common issues with the presentation of disparities. Several themes emerged from the analysis: authors often used racial and ethnic terms interchangeably, they often listed race and ethnicity as an inevitable risk factor for morbidity and mortality, and context provided for disparities differed based on the population and the type of health outcome. For example, authors might provide ample context about the predisposition of Jewish Americans to breast cancer due to genetic mutations that are associated with Ashkenazi ancestry. In contrast, they might present Black Americans' heightened risk for cardiovascular disease without any context. Authors almost always omitted important events and circumstances, including slavery, redlining, racism, segregation, discrimination, colonialism, and oppression, from the discussion of the origins and trends of health disparities. Authors of chapters and books on topics commonly associated with public health were more likely to include social context. For example, authors provided ample detail about the relationship between lack of access to healthcare services and heightened risk for sexually transmitted infection. In contrast, authors of chapters and books largely focused on physiology were least likely to present disparities as manifestations of social inequities. In general, we found a scarcity of context provided for statements made about health disparities between racial and ethnic groups. Though we identified an abundance of tables, lists, and excerpts detailing prevalence rates between minorities, we found little discussion framing how social determinants of health contribute to the differences, and even less framing how structural and societal forces contribute to social determinants of health. Surprisingly, we identified an overall lack of citation for disparities. Our team is currently developing reports for internal and external use that detail the findings from this evaluation, which will serve as the basis for antiracist curricular modifications in the school.

Race & Racial Disparities in Health Professions Teaching Materials: Future State

Our professions have much work to do to ensure that our students enter the workforce prepared for antiracist practice. The literature, as well as discussions with students and colleagues, suggests that the issues presented here are not isolated to one health profession nor to one type of teaching material, course, or program of study. We need systemic and coordinated change.

Recommendations for Textbook Editors and Authors

Textbook editors should improve content on race and racial disparities for all future editions. Editors should ensure that all chapter authors frame health disparities through the historical, structural, sociopolitical, and racial discrimination lens, and attribute racialized differences in health to the social construct of race rooted in racism. When discussing the role of individual behaviors in disparities, authors should provide context for how oppression and unjust systems contribute to differences in behavior (e.g., historical redlining contributing to contemporary lack of access to fresh foods which can influence a person's diet and thereby influence risk for disease) (Amutah et al., 2021). Authors should write case studies and practice questions so that race and ethnicity are not inappropriately included as "clues" for disease risk (Lim et al., 2021).

Editors and authors need to ensure that every time a disparity is stated, it is adequately supported by rigorous and thoughtful peer-reviewed research (Lim et al., 2021). Currently, authors often leave disparities and stereotypical information about racial or ethnic groups entirely uncited, or they cite misleading research. For example, a textbook might state that smoking rates are higher among Black Americans than non-Hispanic White Americans, without acknowledging that smoking rates are actually higher among White Americans when comparing Black and White people who live in the same neighborhoods (LaVeist et al., 2011). Authors must critically examine research methods before citing studies in textbooks, as many studies inappropriately control for race or inaccurately conclude that race, rather than racism, is a risk factor for disease (Boyd et al., 2020). In general, authors and editors should provide more information on the limitations of evidence provided (e.g., a study only included low-income people, or a study was cross-sectional) and should be specific about to whom the cited evidence does and does not apply. If a study only included Mexican Americans, authors should not extrapolate the information to all Latinx Americans, or if citing a study that included participants who identified as Black, the authors should not make a general statement about "minorities" or a specific statement about "African Americans."

Editors and authors should adopt consistent, accurate, and precise language regarding race, ethnicity, ancestry, and geography (Amutah et al., 2021). Currently, they use these identifiers seemingly interchangeably, such as using the term "Black" when a health outcome is actually attributed to geographic ancestry and should use a term such as "people with West African ancestry" instead. The Census Bureau recently adjusted its survey to allow participants to check "all that apply," when identifying their race which importantly recognizes that many people do not identify as a single race. The survey also now asks participants to write in their origins (e.g., Black and Jamaican rather than Black alone) (United States Census Bureau, n.d.). However, many people still feel excluded due to conflation of race and ethnicity, such as people who identify as White whose families came to the United States from the African continent, people of Middle Eastern descent who do not identify with any of the listed racial or ethnic groups, and those who identify Jewish as their ethnicity which the Census Bureau does not list as an option (Parvini & Simani, 2019; Wang, 2017). Textbooks should use racial and ethnic terms precisely and should support the movement toward patients and research participants identifying their race and ethnicity without the limitations of pre-defined categories.

Textbook editors should adopt standards outlining the issues described here and should hold individual authors to those standards. In introductory courses and entry-level programs, textbooks serve as an irreplaceable source of clinical knowledge. Until our textbooks meet equity standards, we cannot fully engage in antiracist education and practice.

Recommendations for Professional Organizations and Societies

Although we desperately need changes to course textbooks, this need for change is a symptom of a broader challenge. Each health profession has a responsibility to set educational standards and to hold institutions of higher education accountable for meeting those standards.

Social work has long been centered on advancing human rights, social and economic justice and we can look to it as an example for other professions that are newer to centering anti-oppressive frameworks in curricula. The social work field has a history of advancing its pedagogy around social justice, race, and racism, embracing "radical, critical, structural, Afrocentric, and feminist" frameworks focused on anti-oppression (Abrams & Moio, 2009; Gil, 2013). The Council on Social Work Education includes educational policies and accreditation standards that state "content on diversity and economic justice needs to be applied in practical curriculum materials across all competency areas" (Council of Social Work Education, 2015). Despite its success in centering social work pedagogy around social justice and antiracism, social work continues to challenge its current educational practices to improve approaches (Abrams & Moio, 2009; Davis, 2016; Wagaman et al., 2019).

Professional organizations such as the American Medical Association (AMA), American Nurses Association (ANA), and National Association of Social Workers (NASW) publish and distribute codes of ethics for their professions. The NASW Code of Ethics states that social workers have a responsibility to understand the role of oppression in society and to "pursue social change with our efforts focused primarily on issues of poverty, unemployment, discrimination, and other forms of social injustice" (National Association of Social Workers, 2017). In June of 2020, in the wake of George Floyd's murder by police, the ANA published a statement pledging to "oppose and address all forms of racism and discrimination" (American Nurses Association, 2020). The AMA also adopted policies in 2020 such as, "Recognize that race is a social construct and is distinct from ethnicity, genetic ancestry or biology. Support ending the practice of using race as a proxy for biology or genetics in medical education, research and clinical practice" (O'Reilly, 2020). In 2021, the ANA, the National Black Nurses Association (NBNA), the National Coalition of Ethnic Minority Nurse Associations (NCEMNA), and the National Association of Hispanic Nurses (NAHN) also launched the National Commission to Address Racism in Nursing (American Nurses Association, 2021). As part of these new efforts, professional organizations and societies should amend their codes of ethics to ensure that principles of "justice" or "equity" explicitly include a call for antiracist teaching and practice. Codes of ethics should include permanent, clear language stating that their profession understands racism and discrimination as fundamental causes of health disparities and has a responsibility to address those fundamental causes through education and practice.

To concretely address the current inadequacy of education on racial and ethnic health disparities, accrediting and testing bodies also need to act. Accrediting bodies dictate the clinical and classroom content and structure that a program must teach to affiliate itself with a profession. For example, just as accreditors require nursing schools to demonstrate that their students practice essential tracheostomy skills, they should also require nursing schools to demonstrate that their teaching on racial and ethnic health disparities is factual and thorough.

Accrediting bodies should require institutions to demonstrate that they have instituted long-term processes for reviewing course materials to ensure that they present disparities with adequate citations and social context and that teaching materials represent diverse populations. In addition, professional bodies should lead the way in amending admissions and licensing exams such as the NCLEX, LCSW exam, and medical school board examinations to include antiracist content and to ensure that the exams do not reinforce racist content, such as alluding to race as a biological construct.

Professional organizations and societies should also wield their power to influence improvements in clinical textbooks and other teaching materials. Professional organizations should set standards for the representation of race and racial disparities in textbooks and publish a list of textbooks that meet these standards. Because schools base their program objectives on accrediting body frameworks, professional organizations should be explicit about accreditation requirements for antiracist content. They should make antiracist content mandatory in continuing education requirements, to ensure that health professionals engage in this work for the duration of their careers and to ensure that updated content reaches existing professionals in the field. Without a central body building momentum for a cultural shift, institutions will continue to depend on individual editors, authors and faculty creating only a trickle of change over time.

Recommendations for Universities and Academic Programs

While professional organizations make systemic changes, individual institutions and programs should take positive steps on their own. First, schools should conduct or solicit third-party evaluations, to understand the current attitudes and understandings of their faculty regarding race as a social construct and the contribution of racism to health disparities. Schools should fund faculty development to help ensure that faculty feel prepared to address semantics and context issues in their teaching materials and to facilitate antiracist discussion in courses. All faculty need to be prepared and expected to contribute to this work, especially White faculty. It is problematic when we assume that this work is best and only done by racial minority faculty because this assumption places undue pressure on minority faculty and gives faculty and students the impression that racism and racial disparities are not of general concern (Smith et al., 2007).

As part of larger efforts to address equity issues within the school, faculty, staff, and students should work together to adopt a set of equity standards, including a statement of commitment on teaching about race as a social construct, and providing social and structural context for disparities in teaching materials. Administrators should work with faculty and students to develop program objectives to ensure that each course meets those standards. Some courses, particularly elective courses on topics such as health equity, social determinants of health, and medical anthropology, more appropriately teach about the roles of race and ethnicity in a person's intersectional identity. However, faculty need to review lectures and readings for core courses, including basic science, clinical and biomedical courses, to ensure that all students receive factual education on disparities in all their classes, including the role that race and ethnicity each does and does not play in contributing to disparities. This content needs to reach not just those students who self-select into relevant electives (Amutah et al., 2021). Administrators should convene program- or school-wide course material equity review committees with responsibility to assess new materials for the issues described above using a systematic process. This committee could make recommendations to faculty on whether proposed materials meet the school's equity standards. The committee should also maintain a library of supplementary course materials addressing race as a social construct, such as journal articles and case studies, that faculty can use instead of or along with course textbooks until adequate textbooks are more widely available. The University of California San Francisco School of Medicine's "Anti-Racism and Race Literacy: A Primer and Toolkit for Medical Educators," available online, is an example of the types of resources that programs should maintain for faculty (O'Brien et al., 2021).

We need to improve course materials to better prepare our next-generation health professionals, but the work is not possible if faculty are unprepared. Health professional schools must institute ongoing education and re-education for faculty on race as a social construct and racism and discrimination as fundamental causes of disparities. Administrators should include this content in required events such as new faculty orientation and routine faculty meetings. Finally, programs should adopt new sections in their midterm and final course review forms specific to equity issues in course content. Programs should invite specific feedback from students on course materials that they find offensive, misleading, or inadequate related to disparities; the equity content committee should review this feedback and incorporate it into course material improvements and faculty education.

Institutions should fund this proposed process (e.g., award involved faculty teaching time for committee involvement, provide credit in promotion and tenure processes for their involvement, etc.). Institutions should also make the process required and permanent to ensure that as faculty develop new course materials over time, and as the school hires new faculty, teaching materials continue to meet equity standards.

Recommendations for Faculty

As we work to improve our curricula for future students, we cannot neglect the immediate need to support our current students. It may not be logistically or financially feasible to adopt all new textbooks immediately, so faculty should be transparent with students about any inadequacies in their existing materials. Faculty should include statements on course websites and syllabi acknowledging that course content may inadequately address race and racial disparities. Such a statement should acknowledge that current course materials do not meet the program's equity standards, should outline efforts underway to address those issues, and should invite students to contribute to or provide feedback on those efforts. For example, a statement might read, *"The School of XXX is committed to preparing future [nurses, social workers, physicians] to provide equitable and inclusive care and to contribute to dismantling racist and unjust systems. As part of our efforts, we are engaged in a formal course material review process to ensure that we accurately represent health disparities as the result of associated societal inequities, rather than biological inevitabilities. We encourage dialogue on this topic between students and course faculty and invite suggestions for improving our course materials for future semesters."*

Faculty can also incorporate critical reflection into their courses as an immediately actionable practice to support students' development as antiracist practitioners. Critical reflection is an approach to learning that questions both social arrangements and the structures that marginalize groups of people and identifies methods to address them across systems (Diemer et al., 2016). While general reflection is an awareness-building practice, critical reflection provides instructors an opportunity to actively work with students to develop structural competence and transform systems outside of themselves as well as inside of themselves (Mitchell et al., 2015; Owen, 2016). As a practice, critical reflection generates knowledge through an excavation of history, unmasking the role of power, illuminating the social construction of privilege, and inspecting the role that systemic, institutional, interpersonal and internalized racism play in the social determinants of health (Blanchet Garneau et al., 2018).

Critical reflection is a valuable component of transformative learning as a tool to examine structural bias and social inequities, and to explicitly address the role of racism in practices as well as in health outcomes (Blanchet Garneau, 2016; Mezirow, 1997). We should examine racism as a social *determinant* of health meaning people do not experience discrimination in isolation. Rather, their experiences of discrimination are amplified by the structural violence of poverty, substance use, chronic conditions, mental health issues, and other factors (Varcoe et al., 2014).

Critical reflection provides health professional students the opportunity to examine the social and political underpinnings of racism and other forms of discrimination, within the context of healthcare practice and systems (Blanchet Garneau et al., 2018). Although empirical studies assessing the impact of reflective practice on health professions students is lacking, studies in the field of social justice education, critical service learning, and cultural pedagogy conclude that reflection is necessary for deconstructing the role of racism in systems and structures and that it empowers learners to engage in praxis to employ social justice orientation in their personal and professional lives (Mitchell et al., 2015; Owen, 2016; Schuessler et al., 2012; Snyder, 2014). Health professions have historically presented discrimination as individual-level biases, overlooking systemic and institutional level racism (Blanchet Garneau et al., 2018). Critical reflection differs from other pedagogical approaches because of its intentional focus on systems change as a critical practice. Critical reflection can build epistemological shifts and student praxis due to the commitment to contextualize power, creating an opportunity for systems-level change (Snyder, 2014).

As a practice, critical reflection includes three distinct elements in the teaching and learning environment: (1) learn to question social arrangements and structures that marginalize groups of people, (2) develop authentic relationships in the classroom and the community, by understanding systems and power, and (3) work from a social change perspective to redistribute power at all systems levels (Mitchell et al., 2015; Owen, 2016).

1. *Learn to question social arrangements and structures that marginalize groups of people:*

   Health professional students should have the opportunity to understand their own social position in both a national and international context, as well as the skills and knowledge needed to contextualize how social identity is constructed through policy, practice, and procedure, and reinforced through power and privilege. In clinical and classroom settings, faculty should guide students to examine social norms and to question the root causes of variance in the social determinants of health. For students in clinical rotations or field placements, this could look like a post-conference that names the impact of specific policy over generations in the geographic locations of the clinical setting. For example, students could explore the history of Redlining in the closest city and examine how that policy influenced community development, job creation, and school resource allocation. This practice would bring context to the social determinants of health, examine power structures, and hold space for discussion on intersectional identity as it pertains to burden of disease and intentionally equitable plans of care. Following this exercise, students should consider key questions to trace health issues and inequities in the social determinists of health to specific structural and systemic causes.

2. *Developing authentic relationships in the classroom and the community, by understanding systems and power*
   The faculty member should engage students on the topic of power structures in systems.
   Bronfenbrenner's Ecological Systems Theory (Bronfenbrenner, 1992) or the public health nursing Intervention Wheel can serve as reflection and application tools (Bronfenbrenner, 1992; Minnesota Department of Health, 2019). This step allows students to map social and political context across systems and examine themselves as a system socialized and influenced by outside elements including policy and social norms. Instructors can utilize resources like the invisible knapsack as a tool for reflective dialogue to examine the power and privilege they hold as individuals and practitioners (McIntosh, 2005; McIntosh, 2015). Students can consider the community and personal impacts as they plot policy and social norm impacts, such as the sterilization of low-income women of color through federally qualified health providers or the disproportionate death of Black mothers and babies due to the hegemonic belief of higher pain tolerance (Washington, 2006). Students can apply anti-oppressive frameworks and structural competency to interventions, advocacy, and actions. Faculty can help students develop a new epistemological perspective of socialization patterns, social norms, and the ways policy, practices, and procedures generated and perpetuated by systems of power reinforce stigmas.
3. *Working from a social change perspective to redistribute power at all systems levels*

Critical reflection also provides the opportunity to strategize approaches to personal and structural shifts that redistribute power and support antiracist results in care, services, and collegiality. Critical reflection is a tool to accomplish deeper awareness and insight through building a practice of thinking with intentionality and mindfulness. It can be a tool for designing actions with a significant appreciation for human dignity and equitable societal change. Through critical reflection, we can address misconceptions that we as students and faculty have about the world, and develop strategy to change behaviors, attitudes, language, and systems accordingly. Working to redistribute power through critical reflection can be as practical as intentional examination and strategizing of new methods for improving bedside manner, to advocating for historical considerations of the neglect and coercion of minority populations in clinical trials or the intentional examination of COVID-19 vaccine messaging and distribution for equity.

Health professions have experienced a major shift towards addressing social determinants of health, yet still shy away from naming racism as a fundamental cause of disparities (Blanchet Garneau et al., 2018). Critical reflection serves to enhance the didactic and practice learning space by incorporating antiracism and anti-oppressive pathways to transform education.

Conclusion

Students can not engage in an opportunity to develop antiracist practice and address the root causes of racialized health disparities if educators do not invite learning around the role of racism and discrimination in inequity and health disparities. We have shared our perspective on the importance of this work in nursing education, but these issues persist across health professions. We invite our colleagues from all disciplines to examine the representation of race and the role of racism in producing racial disparities in their course materials. Naming, questioning, and addressing racism in our course materials and discussions means that we, as students and faculty, must grapple with our own positionality and power. Shifting our practice to focus on these topics will cause discomfort. Still, this challenge is necessary for the advancement of our professions, alignment with our codes of ethics, and to meet our responsibility in contributing to a more just society.

Guiding Questions

1. How do your institution's course materials present race and racial disparities? Do your course materials ask students to critically examine the role of racism in producing health disparities? Does the presentation of race, racism, and health disparities differ among types of materials (e.g., lecture slides versus textbooks) or types of courses?
2. What institutional processes and procedures could your institution implement or enhance to ensure that your faculty are presenting on race and racial disparities with appropriate context?
3. Beyond your own institution, what steps can you take to advocate for change within your profession related to teaching on race and racial disparities?

Quiz Questions

1. How should textbook authors present racial disparities in textbooks? *select all that apply*

   (a) Authors should avoid presenting on racial disparities whenever possible because race is a social construct.
   (b) Each example of a disparity should be cited with recent, accurate data that supports a specific disparity being attributed to a specific population.
   (c) Context should be provided for disparities to help students understand how social, historical and political factors, rather than biology, contribute to disparities.
   (d) Disparities should be presented objectively and with as little detail as possible such as in a table of statistics unaccompanied by narrative.

2. Which of the following strategies should textbook authors *not* use to make their content more inclusive?

   (a) Ensure that images depict people who represent the intended patient population, including people of all skin tones.

(b) Avoid presenting normal and abnormal signs and symptoms in ways that are specific to White skin and other physiology that is not universal.
(c) When attributing disparities to groups of people, use specific and accurate terms as opposed to interchangeably using racial and ethnic terms (e.g., "Black," "dark-skinned," "African American," "of African ancestry").
(d) When writing case studies and practice questions, use race and ethnicity as "clues" for heightened disease risk, common health behaviors, and typical cultural practices.

3. Which of the following statements is correct?

(a) Faculty of all races and ethnicities should be involved in antiracist curricular changes to ensure that changes are supported and implemented across the institution and to ensure that the burden of the work does not fall entirely to faculty of color.
(b) Faculty of color should be charged with leading and executing all antiracist curricular changes to ensure that their voices are heard.
(c) White faculty should lead and execute all antiracist curricular changes because courses taught by White faculty tend to be most problematic.
(d) Institutions should contract with external consultants to lead and execute all antiracist curricular changes, rather than relying on faculty, so that the process is as objective as possible.

4. Which of the following are key elements of critical reflection? *select all that apply*

(a) Learn to question social arrangements and structures that marginalize groups of people.
(b) Develop authentic relationships in the classroom and the community, by understanding systems and power.
(c) Reflect on one's own life experiences to determine how best to care for people in a marginalized group.
(d) Work from a social change perspective to redistribute power.

5. Accrediting bodies should require antiracist content be included in which of the following?
   (a) Teaching materials in each of a program's courses
   (b) Professional examinations
   (c) Continuing education courses
   (d) All of the above

References

Abrams, L. S., & Moio, J. A. (2009). Critical race theory and the cultural competence dilemma in social work education. *Journal of Social Work Education, 45*(2), 245–261. https://doi.org/10.5175/JSWE.2009.200700109

Acquaviva, K. D., & Mintz, M. (2010). Perspective: Are we teaching racial profiling? The dangers of subjective determinations of race and ethnicity in case presentations. *Academic Medicine : Journal of the Association of American Medical Colleges, 85*(4), 702–705. https://doi.org/10.1097/ACM.0b013e3181d296c7

American Nurses Association. (2020). *ANA's membership assembly adopts resolution on racial justice for communities of color.* Nursing World. https://www.nursingworld.org/news/news-releases/2020/ana-calls-for-racial-justice-for-communities-of-color/

American Nurses Association. (2021). *Leading nursing organizations launch the national commission to address racism in nursing.* ANA Enterprise. https://www.nursingworld.org/news/news-releases/2021/leading-nursing-organizations-launch-the-national-commission-to-address-racism-in-nursing/

Amutah, C., Greenidge, K., Mante, A., Munyikwa, M., Surya, S. L., Higginbotham, E., Jones, D. S., Lavizzo-Mourey, R., Roberts, D., Tsai, J., & Aysola, J. (2021). Misrepresenting race – The role of medical schools in propagating physician bias. *New England Journal of Medicine, 384*, 872–878. https://doi.org/10.1056/NEJMms2025768

Blanchet Garneau, A. (2016). Critical reflection in cultural competence development: A framework for undergraduate nursing education. *The J ournal of Nursing Education, 55*(3), 125–132. https://doi.org/10.3928/01484834-20160216-02

Blanchet Garneau, A., Browne, A. J., & Varcoe, C. (2018). Drawing on antiracist approaches toward a critical antidiscriminatory pedagogy for nursing. *Nursing Inquiry, 25*(1), e12211. https://doi.org/10.1111/nin.12211

Boyd, R. W., Lindo, E. G., Weeks, L. D., & McLemore, M. R. (2020, July 2). On racism: A new standard for publishing on racial health inequities. *Health Affairs Blog*. https://doi.org/10.1377/hblog20200630.939347

Bronfenbrenner, U. (1992). Ecological systems theory. In R. Vasta (Ed.), *Six theories of child development: Revised formulations and current issues* (pp. 187–249). Jessica Kingsley Publishers.

Burnett, A., Moorley, C., Grant, J., Kahin, M., Sagoo, R., Rivers, E., Deravin, L., & Darbyshire, P. (2020). Dismantling racism in education: In 2020, the year of the nurse & midwife, "it's time". *Nurse Education Today, 93*, 104532. https://doi.org/10.1016/j.nedt.2020.104532

Byrne, M. M. (2001). Uncovering racial bias in nursing fundamentals textbooks. *Nursing and Health Care Perspectives, 22*(6), 299–303.

Came, H., & Griffith, D. (2018). Tackling racism as a "wicked" public health problem: Enabling allies in anti-racism praxis. *Social Science & Medicine, 199*, 181–188. https://doi.org/10.1016/j.socscimed.2017.03.028

Council on Social Work Education. (2015). *Educational policy and accreditation standards.* Council on Social Work Education. https://www.cswe.org/getattachment/Accreditation/Accreditation-Process/2015-EPAS/2015EPAS_Web_FINAL.pdf.aspx

Curry, M. D. (2001). Patterns of race and gender representation in health assessment textbooks. *Journal of National Black Nurses' Association: JNBNA, 12*(2), 30–35.

Davis, L. E. (2016). Race: America's grand challenge. *Journal of the Society for Social Work and Research, 7*(2), 395–403. https://doi.org/10.1086/686296

Diemer, M. A., Rapa, L. J., Voight, A. M., & McWhirter, E. H. (2016). Critical consciousness: A developmental approach to addressing marginalization and oppression. *Child Development Perspectives, 10*(4). https://doi.org/10.1111/cdep.12193

Eriksen, T. H. (2012, February 29). *Ethnicity*. The Wiley-Blackwell Encyclopedia of Globalization. https://doi.org/10.1002/9780470670590.wbeog179.

Ford, C. L., & Airhihenbuwa, C. O. (2018). Commentary: Just what is critical race theory and what's it doing in a progressive field like public health? *Ethnicity & Disease, 28*(Suppl 1), 223–230. https://doi.org/10.18865/ed.28.S1.223

Frey, W. H. (2020, July 1). *The nation is diversifying even faster than predicted, according to new census data*. Brookings. https://www.brookings.edu/research/new-census-data-shows-the-nation-is-diversifying-even-faster-than-predicted/

Gil, D. G. (2013). *Confronting injustice and oppression: Concepts and strategies for social workers*. Columbia University Press.

LaVeist, T., Pollack, K., Thorpe, R. J., Fesahazion, R., & Gaskin, D. (2011). Place, not race: Disparities dissipate in Southwest Baltimore when blacks and whites live under similar conditions. *Health Affairs, 30*(10), 1880–1887. https://doi.org/10.1377/hlthaff.2011.0640

Lim, G. H. T., Sibanda, Z., Erhabor, J., & Bandyopadhyay, S. (2021). Students' perceptions on race in medical education and healthcare. *Perspectives on Medical Education, 10*, 130–134. https://doi.org/10.1007/s40037-020-00645-6

Louie, P., & Wilkes, R. (2018). Representations of race and skin tone in medical textbook imagery. *Social Science & Medicine, 202*, 38–42. https://doi.org/10.1016/j.socscimed.2018.02.023

Martin, G. C., Kirgis, J., Sid, E., & Sabin, J. A. (2016). Equitable imagery in the preclinical medical school curriculum: Findings from one medical school. *Journal of the Association of American Medical Colleges, 91*(7), 1002–1006. https://doi.org/10.1097/ACM.0000000000001105

Massie, J. P., Cho, D. Y., Kneib, C. J., Burns, J. R., Crowe, C. S., Lane, M., Shakir, A., Sobol, D. L., Sabin, J., Sousa, J. D., Rodriguez, E., Satterwhite, T., & Morrison, S. D. (2019). Patient representation in medical literature: Are we appropriately depicting diversity? Plastic and Reconstructive Surgery. *Global Open, 7*(12), e2563–e2563. https://doi.org/10.1097/GOX.0000000000002563

Massie, J. P., Cho, D. Y., Kneib, C. J., Sousa, J. D., Morrison, S. D., & Friedrich, J. B. (2020). A picture of modern medicine: Race and visual representation in medical literature. *Journal of the National Medical Association, 113*(1), 88–94. https://doi.org/10.1016/j.jnma.2020.07.013

McIntosh, P. (2005). White privilege: Unpacking the invisible knapsack. In M. B. Zinn, P. Hondagneu-Sotelo, & M. A. Messner (Eds.), *Gender through the prism of difference* (pp. 278–281). Oxford University Press.

McIntosh, P. (2015). Extending the knapsack: Using the white privilege analysis to examine conferred advantage and disadvantage. *Women & Therapy, 38*(3–4), 232–245. https://doi.org/10.1080/02703149.2015.1059195

Mezirow, J. (1997). Transformative learning: Theory to practice. In P. Cranton (Ed.), *Transformative learning in action: Insights from practice – New directions for adult and continuing education* (pp. 5–12). Jossey-Bass.

Minnesota Department of Health. (2019). *Public health interventions: Applications for public health nursing practice.* Minnesota Department of Health. https://www.health.state.mn.us/communities/practice/research/phncouncil/docs/PHInterventions.pdf

Mitchell, T. D., Richard, F. D., Battistoni, R. M., Rost-Banik, C., Netz, R., & Zakoske, C. (2015). Reflective practice that persists: Connections between reflection in service-learning programs and in current life. *Michigan Journal of Community Service Learning, 21*(2), 49–63.

National Association of Social Workers. (2017). *Code of ethics.* National Association of Social Workers. https://www.socialworkers.org/About/Ethics/Code-of-Ethics

Nolen, L. (2020). How medical education is missing the bull's-eye. *New England Journal of Medicine, 382*(26), 2489–2491. https://doi.org/10.1056/NEJMp1915891

O'Brien, M., Fields, R., & Jackson, A. (2021). *Anti-racism and race literacy: A primer and toolkit for medical educators.* University of California San Francisco. https://medschool.ucsf.edu/differences-matter/action-groups/focus-area-3

O'Reilly, K. B. (2020). *AMA: Racism is a threat to public health.* Amazoniana. https://www.ama-assn.org/delivering-care/health-equity/ama-racism-threat-public-health

Owen, J. E. (2016). Fostering critical reflection: Moving from a service to a social justice paradigm. *New Directions for Student Leadership, 2016*(150), 37–48. https://doi.org/10.1002/yd.20169

Parvini, S., & Simani, E. (2019). Are Arabs and Iranians white? Census says yes, but many disagree. *Los Angeles Times.* https://www.latimes.com/projects/la-me-census-middle-east-north-africa-race/

Schuessler, J. B., Wilder, B., & Byrd, L. W. (2012). Reflective journaling and development of cultural humility in students. *Nursing Education Perspectives, 33*(2), 96–99. https://doi.org/10.5480/1536-5026-33.2.96

Sheets, L., Johnson, J., Todd, T., Perkins, T., Gu, C., & Rau, M. (2011). Unsupported labeling of race as a risk factor for certain diseases in a widely used medical textbook. *Journal of the Association of American Medical Colleges, 86*(10), 1300–1303. https://doi.org/10.1097/ACM.0b013e31822bbdb5

Smith, W. R., Betancourt, J. R., Wynia, M. K., Bussey-Jones, J., Stone, V. E., Phillips, C. O., Fernandez, A., Jacobs, E., & Bowles, J. (2007). Recommendations for teaching about racial and ethnic disparities in health and health care. *Annals of Internal Medicine, 147*(9), 654–665. https://doi.org/10.7326/0003-4819-147-9-200711060-00010

Snyder, M. (2014). Emancipatory knowing: Empowering nursing students toward reflection and action. *The Journal of Nursing Education, 53*(2), 65–69. https://doi.org/10.3928/01484834-20140107-01

Tsai, J., Ucik, L., Baldwin, N., Hasslinger, C., & George, P. (2016). Race matters? Examining and rethinking race portrayal in preclinical medical education. *Journal of the Association of American Medical Colleges, 91*(7), 916–920. https://doi.org/10.1097/ACM.0000000000001232

United States Census Bureau. (n.d.). *2020 census*. United States Census Bureau. https://2020census.gov/en/about-questions/2020-census-questions-race.html

Varcoe, C., Browne, A. J., & Cender, L. M. (2014). Promoting social justice and equity by practicing nursing to address structural inequities and structural violence. In P. N. Kagan, M. C. Smith, & P. L. Chinn (Eds.), *Philosophies and practices of emancipatory nursing: Social justice as praxis* (pp. 266–284). Routledge.

Wagaman, M. A., Odera, S. G., & Fraser, D. V. (2019). A pedagogical model for teaching racial justice in social work education. *Journal of Social Work Education, 55*(2), 351–362. https://doi.org/10.1080/10437797.2018.1513878

Wang, H. L. (2017). *2020 census may ask white people to get specific about their ethnicity*. NPR. https://www.npr.org/2017/11/30/566975742/2020-census-may-ask-white-people-to-get-specific-about-their-ethnicity

Washington, H. A. (2006). *Medical apartheid: The dark history of medical experimentation on black Americans from colonial times to the present*. Doubleday Books.

Williams, D. R., & Mohammed, S. A. (2013). Racism and health I: Pathways and scientific evidence. *The American Behavioral Scientist, 57*(8). https://doi.org/10.1177/0002764213487340

Section III

Antiracist Helping Professions in Application

14

Breaking Strongholds: Equity Centering in Helping Approaches

Brittany G. Suggs, Lauren B. Robins, Janelle L. Jones, and Dana L. Brookover

Equity-centered care heralds a rising topic of intersectionality due to the biopsychosocial impact and overlapping sociocultural dimensions of health equity (López & Gadsen, 2016; Robins et al., 2021). Persisting inequities in the access and affordability of basic needs and quality health

B. G. Suggs (✉)
Regent University, Virginia Beach, VA, USA
e-mail: britsug@mail.regent.edu

L. B. Robins
Old Dominion University, Norfolk, VA, USA
e-mail: lrobins@odu.edu

J. L. Jones
University of Alabama, Birmingham, AL, USA
e-mail: jljones30@crimson.ua.edu

D. L. Brookover
The University of Scranton, Scranton, PA, USA
e-mail: dana.brookover@scranton.edu

© The Author(s), under exclusive license to Springer Nature Switzerland AG 2022

K. Johnson et al. (eds.), *Developing Anti-Racist Practices in the Helping Professions: Inclusive Theory, Pedagogy, and Application*,
https://doi.org/10.1007/978-3-030-95451-2_14

care echo the prevailing cry against societal reinforcers of discrimination that disproportionately affect certain ethnic and racialized groups (Satcher, 2010; Williams & Cooper, 2019). Helping professionals seek to enhance personal power and promote sociopolitical change that addresses client needs while aiding persons to challenge barriers to holistic development (Kiselica & Robinson, 2001; Ratts, 2009). Given that "racism is an organized societal system" (Williams & Cooper, 2019 p. 606), equity-centered care displays the interconnection between social justice and the alleviation of health burdens among racialized groups.

Within the helping professions, counseling studies primarily focus on increasing awareness, emphasizing counselors' responsibility to address inequalities, developing competency to address inequalities, and helpful strategies to do so (Fong, 2015; Ratts et al., 2016). A focus on anti-racist practices among the helping professions necessitates an interprofessional approach to achieve equitable care that supersedes existing racial disparities and inequities in health and well-being. The inclusion of equity-centered approaches in practice is relatively new. While helping professions view this as a pertinent and undeniable social justice issue (American Counseling Association [ACA], 2014; Lee et al., 2018), the process for minimizing sociocultural inequities with the goal to engage in anti-racist interprofessional practices is still undetermined, however, should be prioritized.

Historically and in the present day, adverse race-related experiences trickle into a domino effect of winding systemic and structural disparities not limited to racial contexts, albeit disproportionately impeding the quality of life for diverse ethnic communities (Harrell et al., 2011; Williams et al., 2019). Within the United States, the searing societal wound of racial trauma seeps into modern ethnic schisms and racially charged rifts, compounded by the seeming unawareness or blindness to the humanity of each individual (Tourse et al., 2018). Could it be that a new narrative, consciousness, and strategies for anti-racist practices call and beckon from the cries of societal pains? Such a call to interprofessional approaches to anti-racist practices is not dismissive, obscuring, nor retorting the realities of race-based traumatic stress (RBTS) and health inequities precipitated by historical adverse racial centering (Bryant-Davis, 2007). Rather, the new paradigm of anti-racist approaches seeks to unravel or unwind the historical ails of adverse racial centering through a cross-sectional awareness of the innate personhood of each individual, family, and community. Thus, the premise of the chapter seeks to explore equity-based frameworks as holistic approaches towards a multi-dimensional helping paradigm across ethnic groups.

Setting the Stage: What Is Equity-Centered Care?

The compass towards equity-centered care points us in the direction of a timeless question, "What is equity?" For starters, the Oxford English Dictionary (n.d.) defines equity as "the quality of being equal or fair; fairness, impartiality; even-handed dealing." In contrast, true equity does not place an emphasis on even-handed dealing when the societal cards of care for marginalized communities historically have been unjustly dealt. Equity at its core acknowledges that individuals experience different circumstances due to their identities and systemically have varying levels of access because of marginalized identities (Legha & Miranda, 2020).

Introducing equity into the conceptualization of care centralizes the individual and their needs, while simultaneously working toward dismantling the very systems that oppress marginalized communities. Equity-centered care seeks to allocate the appropriate, targeted, and culturally relevant resources and care needed to address the unique circumstances of individuals and communities.

Achieving equity-centered care necessitates anti-racist practices in helping professions. Racism is one of the ways communities have been marginalized and denied quality care for centuries (Purnell et al., 2016). Race acts as a social determinant of health that has disproportionately impacted racialized communities in obtaining access to services, thus, having both mental and physical consequences for the client (Legha & Miranda, 2020; Paradies et al., 2015). Interpersonal racial microaggressions that occur in clinical settings often deter individuals from seeking and utilizing health services (Gonzales et al., 2014). Equity-centered care must seek to end all interpersonal microaggressions while also advocating for anti-racist policies within health care systems (Chin, 2014).

Equity-centered care charges helping professionals to identify, reduce, and eliminate disparities in care while protecting the client from racism deeply rooted in the health care system. Eliminating care disparities involves professionals first identifying which care disparities exist for communities while acknowledging that care has not always been optimal for all (Chin, 2014). Equity-centered care calls for clinicians to be anti-racist, identify the racism that is occurring within care systems, and take action to dismantle racism and race-related disparities. Further, this direction calls for professionals to identify the ways in which racism has been entrenched within their field's ideology and practice, coupled with remaining mindful of how it presents in pathology, diagnosis, and resource allocation for clients.

Promoting the Avenue: An Introduction to Interprofessional Collaboration

When considering equity-centered care, interprofessional collaboration is imperative to acknowledge and include. Interprofessional collaboration has been defined as "a partnership between a team of health professionals and a client in a participatory, collaborative and coordinated approach to shared decision-making around health and social issues" (Bainbridge et al., 2010, p. 58). The core concept of interprofessional collaboration is the creation of a trusting and respectful team of professionals that successfully integrate the perspectives of each profession into a collaborative effort to address the unique and complex needs of the client (D'Amour et al., 2005). When engaging in interprofessional collaboration, it is important to realize the attitudes and perceptions of each health care professional are essential. Research has generally found that providers' perceptions and attitudes are a determining factor of a successful or unsuccessful approach (D'Amour et al., 2005; Johnson & Mahan, 2019). A recent study investigating behavioral health care providers' perceptions of interprofessional collaboration found that providers express many benefits of interprofessional collaboration for the clients (i.e., helps achieve client goals and best approach for client) and for the profession (i.e., professional development and overall benefits; Johnson & Mahan, 2019). Additively, this study also found that providers engage in interprofessional collaboration through collaborative efforts, referrals, consultation, and an overall holistic approach (Johnson & Mahan, 2019).

Interprofessional collaboration is useful for many reasons. Specific to equity-centered care, a common factor between interprofessional collaboration and anti-racist practices is the chief goal of instilling structural competency and approaches (Cahn, 2020). These practices require an overarching understanding and perspective of the systems that impact the clients served. To engage in an equity-centered approach, the helping professional must put the client at the center of their care, which ultimately includes having a thorough understanding of the systems that collectively impact the client (Cahn, 2020). Intentionally combining interprofessional collaboration and anti-racist approaches require a shift in emphasis and core competencies (Cahn, 2020). In fact, the interprofessional collaboration core competencies have been revised and improved to provide recognition of the wider contextual factors that can potentially impact individual health. For example, the following core competencies are addressed: (a) values/ethics, (b) roles/responsibilities, (c) interprofessional communication, and (d) teams/teamwork (Interprofessional Education Collaborative, 2016). Interprofessional collaboration paired with anti-racist and equity-centered practice will serve as a foundation in which various frameworks can be used to help individuals achieve optimal mental health.

Achieving Anti-Racist Practices: Equity-Centered Interprofessional Frameworks

As the helping professions strive to advance beyond the historical missteps of adverse race-centered practices into the progressive dimensions of equity-centered care, we encourage helping professionals to tailor care and advocacy approaches around an actionable equity commitment. In congruence with the recommendations of Reid (2020), a transparent equity-centered action plan speaks volumes to extending equity approaches beyond the realm of individualized practice. A multi-tiered equity commitment framework, engaging a diverse network of clients, helping providers, staff, leadership teams, and community collaborators, raises inter-and intra-personal professional standards for creating anti-racism environments parallel to equity-centered care aims. Several helping professions operationalize programmatic initiatives to decolonize care approaches and address long-standing racialized health disparities (Corneau & Stergiopoulos, 2012; Crear-Perry et al., 2020; Gamby et al., 2021; Jones, 2018; Svetaz et al., 2020). This section introduces adaptable interprofessional frameworks for equity-centered care.

Wellness Care

In seeking to achieve equity-centered care, helping professionals can consider and incorporate the tenets of wellness counseling. Professional counselors seek to promote wellness (i.e., a positive state of well-being), rather than strictly eliminate disease (Myers & Sweeney, 2008). Thus, wellness-enhancing care is preventative and developmental in nature (Myers & Sweeney, 2008). Promoting wellness can help to ensure equitable, positive development of all humans, in addition to eliminating adverse outcomes, thus mirroring a recognizable goal among helping professionals. The Indivisible Self Model of Wellness (IS-Wel; Myers & Sweeney, 2005) is a widely studied model of wellness (e.g., Gill et al., 2015; Myers & Sweeney, 2008; Watson, 2017). The subsequent lines explore the IS-Wel in more detail.

As the name suggests, the theoretical basis of the IS-Wel is a holistic, indivisible view of wellness (Wolf et al., 2012) based on Adlerian theory and individual psychology (Adler, 1954). Within the IS-Wel, there are five second-order factors of the self: Creative, Coping, Social, Essential, and Physical. Within those factors, the model demonstrates 17 third-order factors covering a wide range of wellness factors, from positive humor and love to cultural identity (Myers & Sweeney, 2005). Also important is the ecological emphasis in the model. IS-Wel presents four contexts as integral to the self, including local, institutional, global, and chronometrical contexts (Myers & Sweeney, 2008). Proposed steps to wellness counseling encompass: (a) introducing the IS-Wel wellness model to clients, (b) assessment of wellness, (c) developing and implementing a personal wellness plan with clients, and (d) evaluating and following up (Shannonhouse et al., 2015).

It is imperative to note that Gamby et al. (2021) provide an important commentary on the colonization of wellness. Their manuscript contains an overview of wellness, its connection to colonization, and suggestions for how counselors (and other helping professionals) can decolonize wellness. Their article details the history of wellness, including Eastern healing practices and Afro-Native Indigenous Folk Medicine, as the current counseling literature often does not provide the history of wellness practices prior to the 1980s. Further, the authors provide recommendations for decolonizing wellness when working with historically marginalized groups (Gamby et al., 2021). The authors synthesize the IS-Wel (Myers & Sweeney, 2005) with historical and current contexts of colonization. They call for helping professionals to (a) decolonize wellness education, (b) acknowledge context, (c) integrate individualistic and collectivistic aspects of wellness, and (d) increase equity and access to wellness/self-care practices (Gamby et al., 2021). Thus, while existing wellness frameworks can provide a starting point for anti-racist practices in the helping professions, all helping professionals must remain critical and address the four above-mentioned calls for action reflected by Gamby and colleagues. Relatedly, holistic care is another framework helping professionals can utilize when striving for equity-centered collaborative care.

Holistic Care

On the journey of exploring equity-centered care, holistic care carries an enduring legacy with an adaptable paradigm buildable towards a complementary framework for anti-racist practices. The concept of holistic care, originating from holistic medicine, spans centuries with historical beginnings around 400 B.C. (Mantri, 2008; Ventegodt et al., 2007). Within the helping professions, holistic care applications branch into traditional

Eastern healing practices and Western scientific-driven medical practices: each branch reflecting a specific school of thought or worldview on pathology, healing, wellness, and recognition of the whole individual towards the path of improved quality of life and well-being (Mantri, 2008). Integrative holistic care bridges the Eastern and Western approaches by balancing a scientific consciousness with client-centered compassion in care perspectives (Mantri, 2008; Riley et al., 2016). The Mantri (2008), Riley et al. (2016), and Ventegodt et al. (2007) articles referenced in this chapter further introduce the histories of holistic and integrative care beyond the scope of this mild summary.

In nursing and medicine, evolving principles of holistic care outstretch beyond a particular school of thought. Instead, the emphasis on "holistic" seeks to promote "the treatment of the whole person, taking into account mental and social factors, rather than just symptoms of an illness" (Lexico, n.d.). Foundational to holistic care is a comprehensive helping approach that accounts for the physical, mental, emotional, spiritual, sociocultural, and familial dimensions of an individual's well-being. In congruence with the mental health theoretical orientation of person-centered therapy (Raskin & Rogers, 2005), holistic care strives for empirically-based, person-centered practices that exhibit empathy, respect, and dignity for the whole person (Riley et al., 2016). Now, let us more closely examine the connection between holistic care as an equity-centered pathway to anti-racist helping practices.

Across Boundaries, an ethnoracial mental health center in Ontario, Canada, provides a window into a practical example for implementing holistic care as an equity-centered approach. The work of Across Boundaries (2021) promotes a vision and diligence for "equitable, inclusive, and holistic mental health" for racialized communities in Toronto, Ontario (n.p.). A review of the agency's anti-oppression service delivery model begins with a posture of genuine curiosity, open learning, and information sharing on the dynamic ethnoracial experiences of each client. Through the years of learning, Across Boundaries (2007) adopted the framework language of "racialized" (versus "racial minority") person or groups to account for the social, structural, and systemic complexities that reinforce racial-centralized viewpoints, inequities, and marginalization. Across Boundaries (2007) tailors their holistic helping strategies, staff practices, and agency support choices on three chief principles:

1. That racism and oppression have profound negative effects on the health and mental health of racialized people
2. That clients need to heal in ways that are meaningful and relevant to them
3. That racism and oppression can occur at individual, organizational and systemic levels; intervention is needed at all levels. (p. 6)

The core agency values transfer into equity-centered care through a three-pronged holistic approach: (a) client-paced adaptations to service delivery; (b) integrative service responsiveness to client needs; and (c) inclusion of client-considerate, culturally representative healing preferences (Across Boundaries, 2007). The agency welcomes fellow mental health and broader helping professions to adaptively leverage the framework in the interest of cultivating a whole-person care perspective. Across Boundaries nurtures an example of an ongoing amplification and advocacy towards equity-centering in helping practices.

As an interprofessional approach, adopters of holistic care acknowledge that no one profession holds the key to understanding the intricate tapestry of human experiences that impact quality-of-life composites and outcomes. Rather, holistic care embraces interprofessional collaboration as vital for optimizing services delivery, facilitating client empowerment, and prioritizing diverse perspectives in comprehensive client care (Riley et al., 2016). When following the holistic care line into equity-centered practices, holistic care deconstructs the historic voiding of cultural differences through revering complementary therapies in healing approaches. Additively, holistic care professionals favor a helping vantage point that (a) demonstrates respect and responsiveness towards the client as a unique individual; (b) embraces the client, regardless of socio-cultural background, as a valued co-collaborator in achieving optimal health outcomes; and (c) values relationship-centered practices that competently consider the biopsychosocial needs of each client (Jasemi et al., 2017). This biopsychosocial emphasis converges with social determinants of health as a social justice framework for propelling equity-centered collaborative care.

Social Determinants of Health

While there are various frameworks to explore and utilize when focusing on equity-centered care, helping professionals can consider a comprehensive framework that contributes to optimal health in all individuals. Optimal health is a consistent state of well-being when the individual can realize their own abilities, properly cope with normal stressors of life, work productively, and adequately contribute to their family (World Health Organization [WHO], 2014). To achieve and maintain optimal health, an equity-centered and comprehensive treatment approach is necessary. Helping professionals can utilize the social determinants of health framework (Office of Disease Prevention and Health Promotion [ODPHP], 2020).

Social determinants of health (SDOH) are biopsychosocial and environmental conditions in which people live and develop (WHO, 2008). These conditions and determinants largely shape individuals' physical and mental health (WHO, 2008). While the majority of research and practice has focused on the physical aspects of health regarding SDOH, mental health has been deemed an essential part of overall health. The federal government developed a prevention agenda entitled *Healthy People 2020,* to assist with recognizing, understanding, and treating adverse SDOH. *Healthy People 2020* suggested five categories of SDOH: (a) economic stability (e.g., employment, poverty, food insecurity, and housing instability); (b) health and health care (e.g., access to health care, access to primary care, health insurance, and health literacy); (c) social and community context (e.g., social support/cohesion, incarceration, and discrimination); (d) education (e.g., early childhood education, high school enrollment, graduation rates, and literacy); and (e) neighborhood and built environment (e.g., quality of housing, neighborhood crime, environmental conditions, and access to food) (Office of Disease Prevention and Health Promotion, 2020).

Social determinants of health can positively and negatively influence mental health and well-being outcomes (Centers for Disease Control and Prevention [CDC], 2020). For instance, if a person has consistent employment and stable housing, this is a positive determinant; however, if a person is unemployed, homeless, and unable to provide enough food for their family, this is an adverse determinant. When considering equity-centered care, it is important to acknowledge the five SDOH domains for determining what adverse determinants are present to ensure all individuals receive the care and resources they need. Additionally, it is imperative that helping professionals assess clients for the resources and services necessary to reach optimal mental health, rather than simply providing individuals resources and care incomparable to biopsychosocial dimensions of varied need presentations.

Using the adverse determinants mentioned above (i.e., an individual being unemployed, homeless, and unable to provide enough food for their family), it is imperative to view these factors through an anti-racist and equity-centered lens. By adopting an anti-racist lens to SDOH, professionals can better visualize and respond to the systemic issues surrounding SDOH. Additively, this lens perspective can be conceptualized and understood by looking at the prevalence of the SDOH factors in underserved communities. In turn, such an equity-centered approach allows the helping professional to get a comprehensive look at the problem and better render client care. The anti-racist lens is imperative, especially in this situation, as racialized persons in the United States often experience greater barriers, mental and physical health concerns, issues with health care access and utilization, and individual discrimination (Legha & Miranda, 2020). Similarly, viewing these factors through an equity-centered lens, as discussed above, will allow the professional to accurately assess and treat each individual based on their circumstance and diagnoses, rather than haphazardly providing each individual with the care and resources deficient in biopsychosocial awareness and sociocultural competence. Relatedly, working from a multicultural perspective will allow helping professionals to provide equity-centered care, while also placing an emphasis on an anti-racist approach.

Multicultural Frameworks

Equity-centered care works to rectify the adverse impact that racism and social injustice have on the health and well-being of all clients. Professional counseling began in the twentieth century, with social justice advocacy rooted in the profession's inception (Kiselica & Robinson, 2001). The political neutrality of counselors was challenged with the seminal call for multicultural counseling competencies. Similarly, the political neutrality of all helping professionals must be challenged to engage in anti-racist practice through equity-centered care (Sue et al., 1982). A multicultural framework aids to further examine systems of oppression tied to client identities, including within health care and clinical services. Many of the themes found in social justice counseling and multicultural counseling, such as acknowledgment of power, privilege, oppression, injustice, and client context, are essential to begin anti-racist equity-centered care.

Currently, the Multicultural and Social Justice Counseling Competencies (MSJCC) act as a merged guide and conceptual framework for counselors to advocate for clients and have a better understanding of the intricacies of client-counselor interactions (Ratts et al., 2016). The MSJCCs assert that multicultural competence must always be contextualized. Equity-centered care takes a paralleled stance to contextualize the unique identities and needs of the client. Utilizing the MSJCC to frame equity-centered care aids helping professionals in viewing identities as intersecting and interconnected aspects of the individual instead of isolated components (Ratts et al., 2016).

In anti-racist practice, clinicians must connect the dots of how racism influences quality of care and the intersectionality dimensions of a person's holistic identity. This approach can also extend from clinical practice into research by ensuring that helping professionals conduct research within the social contexts of the communities the research intends to serve (Ford & Airhihenbuwa, 2010). MSJCC utilizes socioecological models to address interactions between the individual and their environments while addressing the levels of influence. Utilizing an ecological lens is an integral component of engaging in equity-centered work, as racism has infiltrated and remains pervasive in the individual, interpersonal, communal, institutional, and structural domains of our society.

The Ecological Model of Antiracism (Svetaz et al., 2020) asserts that being anti-racist is an active participatory practice and requires deconstructing racism through a socioecological lens. The model suggests that racism first emerges on an individual level through attitudes, beliefs, and behaviors. There are several elements of anti-racism mentioned within this framework for the sake of client health, including defining racism, teaching the history of racism, teaching leadership, and having multidirectional accountability (Svetaz et al., 2020). Multidirectional accountability entails helping professionals become comfortable and intentional in accountability through anti-racism education. Svetaz et al. (2020) share that accountability involves (a) developing community coalitions and alliances, (b) honoring language that does not stigmatize nor assert power dynamics between the helping professional and the client, and (c) respecting the numerous alternative or holistic healing methods of the client and their heritage instead of enforcing a medical model. Additionally, the Ecological Model of Antiracism suggests engagement in advocacy that is anti-oppressive and anti-racist while practicing reflexivity to self-examine the ways we perpetuate and dismantle oppressive care.

Interprofessional Commitment to Equity-Centered Practices

When navigating the spheres of anti-racism motivation to actualized equity-centered practices, the expression "ministry begins at home" is a fitting description for the enduring mind frame, personal inner work, and professional commitment required for sustainable healing and progression. Perceivably, an entrenched viewpoint that can surface about equity-centered action is that pursuing this undertaking in one's life and helping work requires immediate or all-at-once large-scale change for effectiveness. In actuality, movement from adverse race-centering to equity-centering is an ongoing process of steadily, albeit intentionally, peeling back the layers to expose the undercurrents of racialized perspectives and inequities through individual heart work, personal and societal thought renewal, and communal engagement.

A Milwaukee, Wisconsin, interprofessional team of family medicine faculty, residents, medical educators, and pharmacists demonstrates a committed effort to equity-centering through local action. In a concerted response to address the "syndemic problems" (i.e., "synergistic afflictions contributing to excess burden in a population") of racial injustice and COVID-19 pandemic disparities, the interprofessional team formed local partnerships with the YWCA and medical students for an eight-hour virtual anti-racism training (Knox et al., 2021, p. S70). The team adapted the Unlearning Racism training from its original in-person format for safe and suitable online delivery during the COVID-19 pandemic. The training comprised a series of group education sessions, reflective processing, and discussion spanning four hours across two days, permitting a one-week interim between the two training days (Knox et al., 2021). A spectrum of topics, ranging from "privilege and implicit biases" to "race and racism in medicine and research," steered the sessions' focuses (Knox et al., 2021, p. S71). The online Unlearning Racism training received glowing participant feedback, with 96% of surveyed participants denoting the training as valuable and 88% of surveyed participants believing the training will improve their clinical care (Knox et al., 2021). Hence, the described interprofessional training on anti-racism practices captures a grassroots approach to tackling adverse race-centering and transforming helping practices into equitable quality care.

Transforming Holistic Care into Equity-Centered Practices

Amid the effort to present equity-centered interprofessional frameworks, a notable finding in composing this chapter is that the prevailing recommendations and approaches speak to building alliances as an indispensable component of anti-racism and anti-oppression within the helping professions (Corneau & Stergiopoulos, 2012; Crear-Perry et al., 2020; Svetaz et al., 2020). In their recommendations for building alliances,

Corneau and Stergiopoulos (2012) specify three means for building alliances to promote and enhance equity-centered mental health care: (a) cultivate collaborative community alliances, partnerships, and coalitions with racialized groups; (b) build and form networks purposed for working on behalf of oppressed individuals; and (c) promote projects spearheaded by racialized communities. The recommendations with a holistic helping approach embody respect for clients' cultural differences and preferences for receiving care. Notwithstanding, it behooves us to spotlight that several existing equity-centered strategies, noted as interprofessional, rarely detail or actionably model multidisciplinary collaboration beyond the invisible boundaries of like-minded helping professions or associated disciplines. Consequently, an evident limitation to the refinement of helping care in momentum to achieve equity-centered objectives is the very silos and impermeable walls of knowledge-sharing created among the helping professions. Too often, the conditioned response is to retreat to the safety and comfortability of these silos: stunting capacities and directions towards greater professional unity that enable the learning and accountability necessary for equitable holistic care advancements.

Corneau and Stergiopoulos (2012) call to the foreground the pertinence of prioritizing cross-professional collaboration as a standard for equity-centering care: "Building alliances can be a powerful tool in changing perceptions, racist discourses, and practices at multiple levels… Alliances may facilitate the development of services specifically geared towards racialized minorities" (p. 271). Thus, equity-centered care reaches its pinnacle effectiveness when helping professionals extend an invitation for collaborative synergy, information-sharing, services coordination, and empirical engagement while collectively alleviating disparities that impede client well-being. A challenge posed to the helping professions is to continue to devise equity-centered pedagogy and actionable frameworks that motivate cross-professional interactions surrounding anti-racism and anti-oppression competence and care. The effectual local and global aim is to combat adverse racialized care and care inequities across all helping dimensions. If holistic care requires interprofessional approaches to ensure the mind, body, and spirit needs of diverse client presentations, then our reach must extend beyond the helping silos. As stated by Crear-Perry et al. (2020), "This involves training at the interdisciplinary nexus of medicine and the disciplines that highlight how deeply entrenched social dynamics of power, opportunity, and wellness are delineated along racial lines" (p. 453), lest we continue in the perpetual repetition of historical mistakes.

Chapter Summary

This chapter outlines various frameworks helping professionals can utilize towards interprofessional collaboration. From highlighting a critical perspective on wellness (Gamby et al., 2021; Myers & Sweeney, 2008) and utilizing holistic care practices (Mantri, 2008; Ventegodt et al., 2007), to addressing social determinants of health (WHO, 2008) and ensuring multiculturalism tenets in practice, these frameworks can provide both conceptualization and skills needed to intentionally enact anti-racist interprofessional care. Interprofessional teams can work together to learn and utilize the frameworks discussed in this chapter in their practices. Across the frameworks, there is a focus beyond the absence of illness to promote an individual's well-being; the need to take into account multiple dimensions of personhood; an emphasis on environmental and sociocultural characteristics; and the reminder that every individual needs individualized care (Table 14.1). We believe that interprofessional care is crucial due to the varied dimensions of anti-racist care necessary to promote the health of each individual and achieve equitable care that conquers existing racial disparities and inequities in health and well-being.

Guiding Questions

1. Detail your understanding of equity-centered care. How does equity-centered care connect with anti-racist practices within the helping professions?
2. Describe the competencies associated with interprofessional collaboration. How is interprofessional collaboration beneficial within equity-centered care?
3. Discuss the similarities and differences between wellness and holistic care. How can you utilize each of these frameworks to promote equity-centered care in your work with clients?

Table 14.1 Frameworks for Equity-Centered Interprofessional Collaboration

Wellness (Myers & Sweeney, 2008)	Holistic Care (Mantri, 2008; Riley et al., 2016)	Social Determinants of Health (WHO, 2008)	Multiculturalism (Ratts et al., 2016)
• Preventative and developmental in nature • Holistic, indivisible view of wellness with the self in the center • Based on Adlerian Theory and Individual Psychology (Adler, 1954)	• Balancing scientific consciousness with client-centered compassion • Accounts for the physical, mental, emotional, spiritual, sociocultural, and familial dimensions of an individual's well- being	• Biopsychosocial and environmental conditions in which people live and develop • Individual should realize their own abilities, properly cope with normal stressors of life, work productively, and adequately contribute to their family (WHO, 2014)	• Acknowledgment of power, privilege, oppression, injustice, and client context • Viewing identities as intersecting and interconnected aspects of the individual instead of isolated components

Characteristics of anti-racist care across frameworks
1. Helping practices focus beyond the absence of illness to promoting an individual's well-being.
2. Helping approaches take into account multiple dimensions of personhood.
3. Environmental and sociocultural characteristics are of utmost importance.
4. Each individual needs individualized care.
5. Interprofessional care is necessary due to the varied dimensions of anti-racist care necessary to promote the health of each individual.

4. What are social determinants of health (SDOH)? How do the five categories of SDOH positively and negatively influence well-being outcomes?
5. Compare and contrast the Multicultural and Social Justice Counseling Competencies (MSJCC) and Ecological Model of Antiracism frameworks. In your opinion, what makes each framework essential to anti-racism practices and equity-centered care?
6. Corneau and Stergiopoulos (2012) specify three means for building alliances to promote and enhance equity-centered care. Choose one (1) of the alliance-building means and draft an action plan containing

practical steps for incorporating the recommendation into your helping work with clients.

7. After reviewing this chapter, reflect on your progress as an equity-centered helping professional. What are your thoughts and feelings towards the concepts discussed in this chapter? What concepts did you find rewarding or difficult to encounter? What support or additional information would prove helpful in your journey towards equity-centered interprofessional care approaches?

Quiz Questions

1. Race acts as a ________ having both ________ consequences for the client.

   A. Barrier; spiritual and social
   B. Social determinant of health; mental and physical
   C. Advantage; mental and social
   D. Buffer; mitigating and short-term

2. Equity-centered care charges helping professionals to ________ disparities in care while protecting the client from the racism that is deeply rooted in the health care system.

   A. Identify
   B. Reduce
   C. Magnify
   D. A and B

3. The core concept of interprofessional collaboration comprises the creation of teams that embody the following characteristics except:

   A. Silos
   B. Trust
   C. Respect
   D. Integration

4. Across the Boundaries (2007) models a three-pronged holistic approach that includes:

   A. Client-restrictive healing approaches

B. Clinician-paced adaptations to service delivery
C. Integrative service responsiveness to client needs
D. Culturally exclusive therapeutic strategies

5. According to *Healthy People 2020*, the five categories of social determinants of health (SDOH) include the following elements except:

   A. Health care
   B. Climate stability
   C. Discrimination
   D. Housing quality

6. The Ecological Model of Antiracism asserts that being anti-racist is a singular practice and requires deconstructing racism through a socio-ecological lens.

   A. True
   B. False

7. An entrenched viewpoint about equity-centered action is that such action requires immediate or all-at-once large-scale change for effectiveness.

   A. True
   B. False

8. Three means for building alliances towards equity-centered mental health care, offered by Corneau and Stergiopoulos (2012), include:

   A. Cross-reference providers, cultivate coalitions with racialized groups, and promote individual-centered projects
   B. Build networks that aid the oppressed, promote race-centered projects, and cultivate professional-focused partnerships
   C. Cultivate community alliances, build networks that aid the oppressed, and promote projects spearheaded by ethnic communities
   D. Promote projects spearheaded by ethnic communities, cultivate community alliances, and cross-reference providers

9. Equity-centered care heralds a rising topic of ________ due to the ________ impact and overlapping sociocultural dimensions of health equity.

   A. Multiplicity; biopsychosocial
   B. Diversity; targeted
   C. Diversity; intersectional
   D. Intersectionality; biopsychosocial

10. The Multicultural and Social Justice Counseling Competencies (MSJCC) assert that multicultural competence must always be contextualized.

   A. True
   B. False

11. Holistic care embraces interprofessional collaboration as optional for optimizing services delivery, facilitating client empowerment, and prioritizing diverse perspectives in comprehensive client care.

   A. True
   B. False

Column A	Column B
________ 12. Accounts for the physical, mental, emotional, spiritual, sociocultural, and familial dimensions of an individual's well-being	A. Wellness
________ 13. Views identities as intersecting and interconnected aspects of the individual instead of isolated components	B. Social determinants of health
________ 14. Preventative and developmental in nature	C. Holistic care
________ 15. Biopsychosocial and environmental conditions in which people live and develop	D. Multiculturalism

References

Across Boundaries. (2007, May). *How we do it: Across Boundaries' anti-racist, holistic service delivery model.* https://static1.squarespace.com/static/535010aee4b02e8e0e0eb13b/t/5d711255cb38ee0001d3d8eb/1567691354015/How+We+Do+It+Manual.pdf

Across Boundaries. (2021). *What we do.* https://www.acrossboundaries.ca/what-we-do

Adler, A. (1954). *Understanding human nature* (H. Ansbadur, Trans.). Fawcett.

American Counseling Association. (2014). *2014 ACA code of ethics.* https://www.counseling.org/resources/aca-code-of-ethics.pdf

Bainbridge, L., Nasmith, L., Orchard, C., & Wood, V. (2010). Competencies for interprofessional collaboration. *Journal of Physical Therapy Education, 24*(1), 6–11. https://doi.org/10.1097/00001416-201010000-00003

Bryant-Davis, T. (2007). Healing requires recognition: The case for race-based traumatic stress. *The Counseling Psychologist, 35*(1), 135–143. https://doi.org/10.1177/2F0011000006295152

Cahn, P. S. (2020). How interprofessional collaborative practice can help dismantle systemic racism. *Journal of Interprofessional Care, 34*(4), 431–434. https://doi.org/10.1080/13561820.2020.1790224

Centers for Disease Control and Prevention. (2020). *About social determinants of health.* https://www.cdc.gov/socialdeterminants/about.html

Chin, M. H. (2014). How to achieve health equity. *The New England Journal of Medicine, 371*(24), 2331–2332. https://doi.org/10.1056/NEJMe1412264

Corneau, S., & Stergiopoulos, V. (2012). More than being against it: Anti-racism and anti- oppression in mental health services. *Transcultural Psychiatry, 49*(2), 261–282. https://doi.org/10.1177/1363461512441594

Crear-Perry, J., Maybank, A., Keeys, M., Mitchell, N., & Godbolt, D. (2020). Moving towards anti-racist praxis in medicine. *The Lancet, 396*(10249), 451–453. https://doi.org/10.1016/S0140-6736(20)31543-9

D'Amour, D., Ferrada-Videla, M., Rodriguez, S. M., & L., & Beaulieu, M. D. (2005). The conceptual basis for interprofessional collaboration: Core concepts and theoretical frameworks. *Journal of Interprofessional Care, 19*(sup1), 116–131. https://doi.org/10.1080/13561820500082529

Fong, C. (2015). *The systemic perspective approach (SPA) – A multi-cultural model for workplace counseling in the Singapore context,* Doctoral dissertation, University of Southern Queensland. https://eprints.usq.edu.au/27623/1/Fong_DPST_2015.pdf

Ford, C. L., & Airhihenbuwa, C. O. (2010). Critical race theory, race equity, and public health: Toward antiracism praxis. *American Journal of Public Health, 100*(S1), S30–S35.

Gamby, K., Burns, D., & Forristal, K. (2021). Wellness decolonized: The history of wellness and recommendations for the counseling field. *Journal of Mental Health Counseling, 43*(3), 228–245. https://doi.org/10.17744/mehc.43.3.05

Gill, C. S., Barrio Minton, C., & Myers, J. (2015). Poor, rural women: Spirituality, religion, and wellness across the life span. *Adultspan Journal, 14*(2), 66–76. https://doi.org/10.1002/adsp.12005

Gonzales, K. L., Lambert, W. E., Fu, R., Jacob, M., & Harding, A. K. (2014). Perceived racial discrimination in health care, completion of standard diabetes services, and diabetes control among a sample of American Indian women. *The Diabetes Educator, 40*(6), 747–755. https://doi.org/10.1177/0145721714551422

Harrell, C. J. P., Burford, T. I., Cage, B. N., Nelson, T. M., Shearon, S., Thompson, A., & Green, S. (2011). Multiple pathways linking racism to health outcomes. *Du Bois Review: Social Science Research on Race, 8*(1), 143–157. https://doi.org/10.1017/2FS1742058X11000178

Interprofessional Education Collaborative. (2016). *Core competencies for interprofessional collaborative practice: 2016 update*. Interprofessional Education Collaborative. https://hsc.unm.edu/ipe/resources/ipec-2016-core-competencies.pdf

Jasemi, M., Valizadeh, L., Zamanzadeh, V., & Keogh, B. (2017). A concept analysis of holistic care by hybrid model. *Indian Journal of Palliative Care, 23*(1), 71–80. https://doi.org/10.4103/0973-1075.197960

Johnson, K. F., & Mahan, L. B. (2019). A qualitative investigation into behavioral health providers attitudes toward interprofessional clinical collaboration. *The Journal of Behavioral Health Services & Research, 47*, 1–12. https://doi.org/10.1007/s11414-019-09661-9

Jones, C. P. (2018). Toward the science and practice of anti-racism: Launching a national campaign against racism. *Ethnicity & Disease, 28*(Suppl 1), 231–234. https://doi.org/10.18865/ed.28.S1.231

Kiselica, M. S., & Robinson, M. (2001). Bringing advocacy counseling to life: The history, issues, and human dramas of social justice work in counseling. *Journal of Counseling & Development, 79*(4), 387–397. https://doi.org/10.1002/j.1556-6676.2001.tb01985.x

Knox, K., Simpson, D., Bidwell, J., & Lehmann, W. (2021). Implementing an interprofessional anti-racism training with community partners during a pandemic: Outcomes and recommended strategies. *Wisconsin Medical Journal, 120*(S1), S70–S73. https://wmjonline.org/wp-content/uploads/2021/120/S1/S70.pdf

Lee, C. C., Baldwin, R., Mamarà, S. M., & Quesenberry, L. (2018). Counselors as agents of social justice. In C. C. Lee (Ed.), *Counseling for social justice* (3rd ed., pp. 3–20). American Counseling Association. https://doi.org/10.1002/jcad.12298

Legha, R. K., & Miranda, J. (2020). An anti-racist approach to achieving mental health equity in clinical care. *Psychiatric Clinics, 43*(3), 451–469. https://doi.org/10.1016/j.psc.2020.05.002

Lexico. (n.d.). Holistic. In *Lexico.com dictionary*. Retrieved July 12, 2021, from https://www.lexico.com/definition/holistic

López, N., & Gadsden, V. L. (2016, December 5). *Health inequities, social determinants, and intersectionality*. National Academy of Medicine. https://nam.edu/health-inequities-social-determinants-and-intersectionality/

Mantri, S. (2008). Holistic medicine and the western medical tradition. *The Virtual Mentor, 10*(3), 177–180. https://doi.org/10.1001/virtualmentor.2008.10.3.mhst1-0803

Myers, J. E., & Sweeney, T. J. (2005). *Counseling for wellness: Theory, research, and practice*. American Counseling Association.

Myers, J. E., & Sweeney, T. J. (2008). Wellness counseling: The evidence base for practice. *Journal of Counseling & Development, 86*(4), 482–493. https://doi.org/10.1002/j.1556-6678.2008.tb00536.x

Office of Disease Prevention and Health Promotion. (2020). *Social determinants of health*. https://www.healthypeople.gov/2020/topics-objectives/topic/social-determinants-health/interventions-resources

Oxford English Dictionary. (n.d.). Equity. In *Oxford English Dictionary*. Retrieved July 10, 2021, from https://www.oed.com/view/Entry/63838

Paradies, Y., Ben, J., Denson, N., Elias, A., Priest, N., Pieterse, A., Gupta, A., Kelaher, M., & Gee, G. (2015). Racism as a determinant of health: A systematic review and meta- analysis. *PLoS One, 10*(9), e0138511–e0138511. https://doi.org/10.1371/journal.pone.0138511

Purnell, T. S., Calhoun, E. A., Golden, S. H., Halladay, J. R., Krok-Schoen, J. L., Appelhans, B. M., & Cooper, L. A. (2016). Achieving health equity: Closing the gaps in health care disparities, interventions, and research. *Health Affairs, 35*(8), 1410–1415. https://doi.org/10.1377/hlthaff.2016.0158

Raskin, N. J., & Rogers, C. R. (2005). Person-centered therapy. In R. J. Corsini & D. Wedding (Eds.), *Current psychotherapies* (pp. 130–165). Thomson Brooks/Cole Publishing Co.

Ratts, M. J. (2009). Social justice counseling: Toward the development of a fifth force among counseling paradigms. *The Journal of Humanistic Counseling, Education and Development, 48*(2), 160–172. https://doi.org/10.1002/j.2161-1939.2009.tb00076.x

Ratts, M. J., Singh, A. A., Nassar-McMillan, S., Butler, S. K., & McCullough, J. R. (2016). Multicultural and social justice counseling competencies: Guidelines for the counseling profession. *Journal of Multicultural Counseling and Development, 44*(1), 28–48. https://doi.org/10.1002/jmcd.12035

Reid, W. (2020, July 17). *How to promote an anti-racist culture in social work*. CommunityCare. https://www.communitycare.co.uk/2020/07/17/promote-anti-racist-culture-social-work/

Riley, D. S., Anderson, R., Blair, J. C., Crouch, S., Meeker, W., Shannon, S., Sudak, N., Thornton, L., & Low Dog, T. (2016). The academy of integrative health and medicine and the evolution of integrative medicine practice, education, and fellowships. *Integrative Medicine, 15*(1), 38–41. https://www.ncbi.nlm.nih.gov/pmc/articles/PMC4818068/

Robins, L. B., Johnson, K. F., Gant, A. C., Brookover, D. L., Jones, J., Suggs, B. G., & Cannedy, M. (2021). The role of human services providers in addressing social determinants of health. *The Journal of Human Services, 40*(1), 83–101. https://nohs.memberclicks.net/journal

Satcher, D. (2010). Include a social determinants of health approach to reduce health inequities. *Public Health Reports, 125*(Suppl 4), 6–7. https://doi.org/10.1177/00333549101250S402

Shannonhouse, L. R., Myers, J. E., & Sweeney, T. J. (2015). Counseling for wellness. In I. Marini & M. A. Stebnicki (Eds.), *The professional counselor's desk reference* (2nd ed., pp. 617–623). Springer Publishing.

Sue, D. W., Bernier, J. E., Durran, A., Feinberg, L., Pedersen, P., Smith, E. J., & Vasquez- Nuttall, E. (1982). Position paper: Cross-cultural counseling competencies. *The Counseling Psychologist, 10*(2), 45–52. https://doi.org/10.1177/0011000082102008

Svetaz, M. V., Barral, R., Kelley, M. A., Simpson, T., Chulani, V., Raymond-Flesch, M., Coyne- Beasley, T., Trent, M., Ginsburg, K., & Kanbur, N. (2020). Inaction is not an option: Using antiracism approaches to address health inequities and racism and respond to current challenges affecting youth. *Journal of Adolescent Health, 67*(3), 323–325. https://doi.org/10.1016/j.jadohealth.2020.06.017

Tourse, R. W., Hamilton-Mason, J., & Wewiorski, N. J. (2018). *Systemic racism in the United States*. Springer International.

Ventegodt, S., Kandel, I., & Merrick, J. (2007). A short history of clinical holistic medicine. *The Scientific World Journal, 7*, 1622–1630. https://doi.org/10.1100/tsw.2007.238

Watson, J. C. (2017). Examining the relationship between self-esteem, mattering, school connectedness, and wellness among middle school students. *Professional School Counseling, 21*(1), 1096–2409. https://doi.org/10.5330/1096-2409-21.1.108

Williams, D. R., & Cooper, L. A. (2019). Reducing racial inequities in health: Using what we already know to take action. *International Journal of Environmental Research and Public Health, 16*(4), 606–632. https://doi.org/10.3390/ijerph16040606

Williams, D. R., Lawrence, J. A., & Davis, B. A. (2019). Racism and health: Evidence and needed research. *Annual Review of Public Health, 40*, 105–125. https://doi.org/10.1146/annurev-publhealth-040218-043750

Wolf, C. P., Thompson, I. A., & Smith-Adcock, S. (2012). Wellness in counselor preparation: Promoting individual well-being. *Journal of Individual Psychology, 68*(2), 164–181. https://psycnet.apa.org/record/2012-13606-005

World Health Organization. (2008). *Social determinants of health*. http://www.who.int/social_determinants/sdh_definition/en/

World Health Organization. (2014). *Social determinants of health*. https://apps.who.int/iris/bitstream/handle/10665/112828/9789241506809.pdf

15

Voices from the Field of School Counseling: Promoting Anti-Racism in School Settings

Rawn Boulden and Ne'Shaun Borden

Anti-racism in School-Based Mental Health

In recent years there has been a shift in our understanding of the importance of anti-racism in the helping professions (Abrams, 2020; Bussey, 2020; National Association of Social Workers ([NASW]; 2020). Fueled by recent events such as the murders of George Floyd and Breonna Taylor, the Black Lives Matter movement and what has often been referred to as a racial reckoning in the United States (U.S.), the concept of anti-racism is now being highlighted in mainstream media more frequently than before with many declaring that "not being racist" is simply not enough

R. Boulden (✉)
West Virginia University, Morgantown, WV, USA
e-mail: rawn.boulden@mail.wvu.edu

N. Borden
Jacksonville University, Jacksonville, FL, USA
e-mail: nborden@ju.edu

© The Author(s), under exclusive license to Springer Nature Switzerland AG 2022

K. Johnson et al. (eds.), *Developing Anti-Racist Practices in the Helping Professions: Inclusive Theory, Pedagogy, and Application*,
https://doi.org/10.1007/978-3-030-95451-2_15

(Kendi, 2019). Although the foundations of anti-racist work date back hundreds of years, most recently scholar and historian, Ibram X. Kendi has been highly sought after to educate and offer practical solutions for ways to embody antiracism based on his bestselling novel, *"How to be an Antiracist,"* (Kendi, 2019). Considering Kendi's work and the work of countless other anti-racist scholars and activists, we explore the importance of anti-racism for school based mental health professionals (SMHPs) and offer practical ways to incorporate anti-racism into our work as school-based professionals.

Historical Overview of Racism in Education

Racism is defined as "The marginalization and/or oppression of people of color based on a socially constructed racial hierarchy that privileges White people' ('Anti-Defamation League, [ADL], 2020, para. 1). Racism is deeply embedded in the fabric of educational systems around the globe (Barbieri & Ferede, 2020). The groundbreaking work of Ladson-Billings and Tate (1995) focused on Critical Race Theory (CRT) in education and asserted that race is inextricably linked to inequity in education. Believing this fact, we assert that due to sordid history of race relations in the U.S., which include the eradication of indigenous persons, more than 400 years of chattel slavery, and laws that deemed Black, Indigenous, and People of Color (BIPOC) as less than, it would be nearly impossible to have an education system that equitably serves those from all races and ethnicities (Barbieri & Ferede, 2020). It has been 67 years since the historic Brown v. Board of Education of Topeka ruling that determined that racial segregation in public schools is unconstitutional (Bell, 1980). Although the ruling in this case was considered landmark and an important impetus in the civil rights movement, it was a long-fought struggle (Patterson, 2001). There were many cases prior to this ruling (e.g., *Murray v. Maryland, Missouri ex rel Gaines v. Canada, Sweat v. Painter, McLaurin v. Oklahoma Board of Regents of Higher Education*) seeking racial equality in the U.S., with rulings that favored racial segregation in education.

The impact of systemic racism in education can be seen in educational outcomes for students of color in the United States. Even though the demographics of students in the U.S. is changing, BIPOC students still disproportionately represent negative outcomes when compared to White students even with a significant increase in BIPOC students enrolling in U.S. public schools. According to the National Center for Education Statistics [NCES] (NCES, 2019b), between 2000 and 2017, the number of White students enrolled in U.S. public schools decreased from 62% to 51% and the number of Black students decreased from 15% to 14%. During this same time, there was a significant increase in the number of Asian (3–5%), and multiracial students (2–4%) enrolled in U.S. public schools, with the most significant growth among the Hispanic student population (i.e., 16–25%). Even though U.S. public schools are more diverse than in the past as far as racial and ethnic, the achievement gap remains.

The National Center for Education Statistics [NCES] (NCES, 2019b), utilized data from the National Assessment of Educational Progress (NAEP) to evaluate reading and math achievement among U.S. students by race since 1990, with the most recent data being collected in 2017. The NAEP showed that when evaluated in 4th, 8th and 12th grades, White students had higher reading scores than Black and Hispanic students. When evaluating math achievement in the same grades, White students scored higher than Black and Hispanic students. The National Center for Education Statistics [NCES] (NCES, 2016) also evaluated enrollment in Advanced Placement (AP) and International Baccalaureate (IB) courses by race. The results showed that Asian students (45%) were more likely to be enrolled in advanced math courses when compared to White (18%), Black (6%), Hispanic (10%) and multiracial students (11%). When evaluating which students earned the most AP and IB credits by race, NCES found that Asian students (72%) and White students (40%) were most likely to have earned AP and IB credits. For Hispanic and Black students, these numbers were much lower with 23% of Black students and 34% of Hispanic students earning advanced math and science credits. These disparate differences follow students into postsecondary degree attainment.

Although the number of BIPOC students enrolling in college is higher than ever, graduation rates tell a different story. At the 6-year mark, 74% of Asian students complete a 4-year degree program, compared to 64% of White students, 60% of multiracial students, 54% of Hispanic students, 40% of Black students, and 39% of Alaska native/Pacific Islanders (NCES, 2019b). In addition to the connection between race and educational outcomes, there is also a relationship between mental health and educational achievement, with mental stability being related to educational achievement (Murphy et al., 2015).

Voices from the Field

I've had the opportunity to work in various school settings. I have worked more than 16 years in elementary school settings where the population is predominantly African-American. I have also worked in elementary schools where African American students only made up 20% of the school enrollment. I have found that inequities exist across the board. I have found that in schools with a large population of students of color, exceptional education services have not always been equitable. I have worked in schools in which there was no certified exceptional education teacher. The students were being serviced by a substitute teacher. In some cases, the substitute teacher worked really hard to assist the students in meeting the IEP goals. In other cases, the substitute teacher only assisted with a general assignment. In either situation the students were not receiving the specialized attention they needed from a certified exceptional education teacher. These were schools that served mostly African-American students. I have seen where there was a certified exceptional education teacher in place but for various reasons, the teacher resigned. Again, leaving the students without a teacher. I have been a school counselor at two schools that served predominately White students and had not experienced this at either. It has only been the schools that serve predominantly African American students where I have witnessed this "teacher shortage." The result remained the same. The needs of children weren't being met. (MP, School Counselor)

Mental Health in Public Education

The impact of school segregation has led to many inequities, chief among those being a lack of funding for schools that serve mostly BIPOC students compared to schools that serve White students (Baker & Corcoran,

2012; Darling-Hammond, 1998). Yeager et al. (2018) reported that minoritized students receive less mental health care and are more likely to report mental health concerns compared with White students. Locke et al. (2017) utilized Medicaid data of children and adolescents (n = *23,601*), ages 5–17 to examine the use of behavioral healthcare services for diagnosed mental health disorders such as Autism Spectrum Disorders (ASD), Attention Deficit Hyperactivity Disorder (ADHD), Oppositional Defiant Disorder (ODD), and other mental health concerns. The study revealed that Hispanic students utilized the least behavioral care services and that Black students were less likely to receive school-based services when compared to White students.

In the U.S., despite students racial and ethnic demographics, school based mental health professionals (SMHPs) have hundreds of students assigned to their caseload (The National Center for Education Statistics [NCES], 2019a). NCES reported that in public schools where most of the students identified as members of minoritized groups ("*majority-minority*"), the number of at least one full-time or part-time mental health professionals (counselor, social worker, psychologist, any mental health provider) was similar. NCES found that 94% of schools had one mental health professional despite the racial make-up of the school. Similarly, 80% of "*majority-minority*" schools employed a counselor compared to only 82% of White schools, 67% of "majority-minority" schools employed a psychologist compared to 66% of White schools, and 46% of "*majority-minority*" schools employed a social worker compared to 37% of White schools. Although these ratios are similar, the caseloads for SMHPs are highly unrealistic, with the caseload for a mental health provider in a "*majority-minority*" school being 390:1, for psychologists 880:1, and the ratio in schools with any mental health professional being 250:1, respectively. With previous studies showing that students from historically-minoritized backgrounds are more likely to have unmet mental health concerns (Bear et al., 2014; Cook et al., 2017; Marrast et al., 2016), it is important that more SMHPs are available to these populations. Disparities in SMHP and mental health services highlight the need for advocacy and anti-racist paradigms to lead to the provision of equitable services.

Voices from the Field

I had the opportunity to work in an elementary school and high school doing crisis and trauma focused mental health counseling. Both schools brought their own set of challenges; however, there were barriers I was taught about in school, but I had not experienced myself that I was witnessing daily while in the school settings. It was important not to make assumptions or to presume that I knew what a day in the children's shoes was like. Instead, I worked to meet my clients where they were at and ask them to tell me about their experience. Many of my clients had labels put on them by family, friends, teachers, and a lot of what I did was working with them to establish what they wanted to be known for. Also advocating for each client with their teachers and administrators was a big component. (AM, Mental Health Counselor)

Anti-Racism Versus Cultural Competence

While perhaps tempting to use the terms "cultural competence" and "anti-racism" interchangeably, the reality is that these terms have similarities and defining differences. Cultural competence, occasionally used interchangeably with multicultural competence, generally involves being able to interact effectively with individuals with similar and differing identities (Cross et al., 1989). Various helping professionals have interspersed cultural competence mandates in their ethical standards and similar resources germane to their specific discipline. For example, the National Organization for Human Services' ethical standards (2015) assert that human services professionals (1) respect and support clients across all identities, (2) exhibit awareness of cultural identities and issues pertaining to their clientele, (3) exhibit awareness of their own cultural identity, and (4) engage in ongoing professional development to increase cultural competence. The National Association of Social Workers' (NASW) Ethical Standards (2017) also has a multipronged approach to cultural competence; specifically, NASW proclaims that social workers (1) employ a strengths-based lens to similar and different cultural identities, develop a fundamental understanding of their clients' culture, (3) render services that are sensitive to the client's culture, (3) engage in ongoing professional development regarding cultural competence, and (4) consider cultural differences regarding electronic technology in the rendering of social work services. Cultural competence is also highly applicable to school settings, given the diverse world in which we live. In K-12 settings, cultural competence can be operationalized to describe educators' ability to teach students from differing cultural backgrounds (Diller & Moule, 2005). Several scholars note key dimensions of cultural competence among educators. For example, King et al. (2007) provide four key cultural competence domains salient to educators: (1) appreciating and accepting diversity, (2) being aware of one's culture along with their students' unique cultures, (3) understanding the nuanced nature of cross-cultural interactions, and (4) intentionally curating a school environment that affirms students' identities through protocols and sustainable practices. Similarly, Diller and Moule (2005) operationalize the term as developing the knowledge, awareness, and sensitivity of students' cultures that support the effectiveness of cross-cultural teaching.

Most SMHPs obtain some degree of training regarding multiculturalism and cultural competence (e.g., formal coursework, in-service workshops, certifications). While these efforts are certainly commendable, the reality is that merely engaging in training centered on multiculturalism is not sufficient in having the knowledge, skills, and capacity to effect meaningful and sustainable change through anti-racist practices. For example, Lynch (1987) suggested that multiculturalism alone fails to address systemic and institutional issues that oppress students from historically-minoritized backgrounds (e.g., privilege, power, access). The Regional Arts and Culture Center (n.d.) contends that multiculturalism upholds hegemonic practices and teachings that further marginalize non-White students. Plainly put, anti-racism is not an episodic or ad hoc effort—it is a paradigm shift in mindsets, approaches, attitudes, policies, and practices. Regardless of our helping profession (e.g., school counselor, qualified mental health professional, school psychologist, or school based mental health counselor), we have a moral, legal, and ethical obligation to prioritize student wellbeing. Shifting to an anti-racist paradigm reflects a departure from culture competence. As eloquently articulated by *Teaching Tolerance* (2020), anti-racism is a lifelong journey, thus requiring a deep commitment to introspection and critical examination and critique of the status quo related to school norms, values, and practices. Thus, aligned with the theme of this book, this chapter offers strategies SMHPs can employ to promote an anti-racist school community.

Voices from the Field

An anti-racist school climate and culture is inherent to an effective education. As a mental health counselor, I believe that helping to nurture this experience within the academic environment is part of my job. Anti-racist educators must be prepared to address the diversity of student needs within their population. It's important to create opportunities that will develop knowledge, skills, and awareness of anti-racism work. This includes offering professional development, educational resources and efficacious tools that support faculty members in incorporating culturally informed and responsive practices within their curriculum development, academic instruction, and daily interactions. It is equally important to facilitate students' awareness and understanding about anti-racism work. I use individual and group sessions to provide a safe space that encourages open and honest dialogue and support in processing these issues. (KC, Mental Health Counselor)

Systems Thinking

What does it mean to *think systemically*? While numerous definitions exist, this chapter defines "systems thinking" as understanding the interrelationships that exist within systems, and how these interrelationships inform both policy and practice (Stroh, 2015). Systems thinking has been researched in various disciplines, including school and counseling settings. Namely, schools are complex social systems composed of various individuals (e.g., teachers, parents) with established roles and responsibilities; these individuals collaborate to ultimately promote student success and achievement (Bryk et al., 2015). The degree of synergy between these individuals largely informs the system's health; in other words, school systems in which its individuals work harmoniously (e.g., healthy parent—teacher communication and relationships, teachers feeling supported by administrators, a positive school climate) can support improved student outcomes. Conversely, the opposite could stymie student outcomes. This approach represents a stark contrast to "linear thinking," often viewed as an antiquated model of solving today's educational problems (Pisapia et al., 2009; Senge, 2006). Today's educators and SMHPs must understand the interconnectedness of school community members, and how these connections impact students' educational experiences.

As expressed previously, anti-racism involves multiple school-based entities, including school personnel, students, and even community members. Cultivating an anti-racist school environment is truly a collaborative effort, and SMHPs can serve as a critical catalyst in this process. As we continue the conversation on anti-racism in school settings, it is important to highlight a model through which this topic can be further examined. Ecological systems theory, developed by Urie Bronfenbrenner (1979), describes the unique relationships that exist between the individual and environment, and how these relationships can impact the individual's development. Furthermore, it helps illustrate how entities, such as families, schools, and communities, coalesce to impact child development. Bronfenbrenner's model is most often visualized as a series of concentric circles, each representing a unique system that impacts an individual's development. Five systems comprise Bronfenbrenner's theory: microsystem, mesosystem, exosystem, macrosystem, and chronosystem. The succeeding section contextualizes this theory, augmented by examples of each system.

The first system, microsystem, consists of the people and environments closest to the student and, thus, most likely to directly influence development. Bronfenbrenner (1979) expressed that entities within this system tend to have the most frequent interaction and involvement with the individual. For most children, individuals comprising the microsystem often include friends, family, teachers, and siblings. Whereas the microsystem consists of one- on-one interactions (e.g., the student interacting with teachers, the student interacting with a sibling), the next system, mesosystem, entails interactions between the individual's microsystems. In other words, the mesosystem can be viewed as a "system" composed of microsystems. For example, "parents" and "teachers" are two salient microsystems related to student success, development, and wellbeing. A parent—teacher conference, which merges both microsystems, is an example of a mesosystem. Like the microsystem, the mesosystem directly impacts students. Additional examples include (1) birthday parties (family and friends), (2) parents chaperoning a school event (family and school), and (3) a family attending a religious or spiritual event. The preceding layers (i.e., microsystem and mesosystem) directly impact the student. The following layers depart from this characteristic and indirectly impact the student. The next layer is the exosystem; this layer encompasses policies and procedures that indirectly impact an individual. In other words, despite not being directly involved in the setting, the outcomes related to the setting still impact the individual. A school board meeting is an example of an exosystem. Typically, children are unable to formally vote on school board-related issues. Despite not being involved in the decision-making process, the decisions rendered often have some degree of impact on the child.

Parent job loss is another example. While the child did not lose employment, it is highly likely that the parent's loss of employment will negatively impact the child and family. The macrosystem is the penultimate layer. The macrosystem can be described as cultural, geographic, economic, and political variables that indirectly impact the student. Examples of macrosystem variables may include political affiliations, economic recession, and geographic differences (e.g., urban vs. rural vs. suburban environments). Lastly, the outermost layer, the chronosystem, generally refers to how environmental changes spanning one's lifespan impact an individual's development. Examples include divorce, attending school for the first time, and retirement.

Traditionally, Bronfenbrenner's model is utilized to demonstrate the various entities which directly and indirectly impact child development, with the child serving as the "individual" at the core of the model. While this is certainly meritorious, in considering the proliferation of anti-racism in school settings, ecological systems theory is also a viable lens SMHPs can use in strategically supporting efforts to create a sustainable anti-racist school environment for all school community members. Accordingly, in the succeeding section, we discuss strategies SMHPs can employ, stratified by the layers of Bronfenbrenner's seminal model.

Anti-Racist Action Steps for Helping Professionals

For school based mental health professionals (SMHPs) to cultivate an anti-racist environment and improve mental health outcomes, SMHPs must think systemically. Utilizing Bronfenbrenner's (1979) Ecological Systems Theory, we have identified actionable steps that can be taken to address inequity at various levels by targeting the micro, meso, exo, and macrosystems with which SMHPs interact. We begin with steps for the individual, with the belief that much of the work for creating an anti-racist environment begins with an internal desire.

Action Steps for the Individual

Usually in Bronfenbrenner's model the child is in the center; in our plan we have replaced the child with SMHPs and will focus on how individual school based professionals interact with each level of the model (Bronfenbrenner, 1979). SMHPs must **acknowledge the presence of racism and the stronghold of White Supremacist ideology.** To promote anti- racism, one must understand and accept its mere existence. As highlighted in previous sections of this chapter, racism and White supremacist ideology are social constructs that pervade all aspects of our lives; this notion extends to our clients' lives, too. White supremacist ideology and racism are inherently embedded into American schools. Mercifully, schools have employed various methods, including incorporating anti-racism teachings and trainings, to dismantle hegemonic systems of oppressions that are all-too-often present in school settings. Some SMHPs may be tempted to enact an attitude akin to "I don't see color" to perhaps shield themselves of any culpability or accountability. While perhaps tempting to employ a "color-blind" or "color- neutral" lens, doing so (1) invalidates clients' lived experiences and (2) may signal to clients that their culture does not matter. Accepting and understanding the universality of racism and White supremacist ideology can assist helping professionals in recognizing how they manifest in school settings.

This is critical in increasing one's capacity to speak out and move the needle toward meaningful change and anti-racism.

We encourage SMHPs to engage in **personal introspection** and self-reflection. The process of developing multicultural competence has long been touted as multidimensional with a focus on awareness, knowledge, and skills. We encourage SMHPs to continue that interrogation of their values on their anti-racist journey. Anti-racism is a lifelong journey, one that requires vigorous inspecting of one's actions, practices, attitudes, power, and privilege. Within the school context, helping professionals should reflect on their interactions with students, clients and colleagues. Example introspective questions include:

- Do my practices *support* or *dismantle* hegemonic systems of oppression?
- Do my practices *uplift* or *silence* voices and perspectives of students from historically- minoritized backgrounds?
- Are my institution's policies and protocols ethnocentric and/or marginalizing of students of color?
- When rendering services, do I utilize resources (e.g., books, worksheets, examples) that are culturally sustaining and non-stereotypical?

Clearly, this list is not exhaustive; however, it is critical that we engage in introspection, and encourage our school colleagues to do the same.

As anti-racist helping professionals, it is important that we **exercise cultural humility.** Cultural humility reflects an openness to diverse cultures, backgrounds, and perspectives (Worthington et al., 2017). Namely, cultural humility requires awareness of one's worldview, along with possible limitations or "blind spots" that may impede one's ability to understand other cultural backgrounds and lived experiences (Hook et al., 2013). Culturally-humble helping professionals recognize the existence of cultural blind spots, and come to terms with the likelihood of making future mistakes stemming from said cultural blind spots (Fouad & Arredondo, 2007). In other words, the culturally-humble helping professional understands that they have a lot to learn regarding client's worldviews, and this growth process never ceases. While impossible to be "fully competent" in a differing culture, culturally humble helping professionals seek greater understanding through continuous self-reflection, interrogating implicit biases, demonstrating an acceptance of differing cultures, and dismantling oppressive power structures (Minkler, 2012). To help accomplish this, helpers should avoid assuming mastery of a client's cultural background; merely reading a book or engaging in training on a cultural group, while beneficial, it does not equate to obtaining a mastery level of understanding. Employing active listening, unconditional positive regard, and empathy are critical first steps in the journey toward cultural humility. Adopting a culturally humble mindset can augment the helping professional's efforts to promote anti-racism within both oneself and their school community.

Action Steps for the Microsystem

While constantly increasing their knowledge, skills, and awareness and interrogating their actions, practices, and attitudes, power, and privilege, we suggest that SMHPs **thoroughly examine their school environment.** When working in the educational environment it is easy to become overwhelmed and ultimately indifferent to the school environment. As novice and seasoned SMHPs, it is easy to believe that "it's just the way it is" and that it's impossible to overcome systemic barriers that undermine our efforts to create equitable environments for minoritized students. We call on SMHPs not to accept the status quo and to take inventory of their school environments. This inventory includes a needs assessment, meetings with students, teachers, administrators, stakeholders, parents/guardians and other school based mental health professionals. Using the data gathered from these quantitative and qualitative methods, SMHPs can begin to develop a strategic plan to implement anti-racist services that best serve the needs of the school community. As we already mentioned, the ratio of SMHPs compared to students, would make it highly unlikely to provide individualized services to each student. We recommend that SMHPs implement programs that can serve larger groups. This could include anti-racist mental health training for administration and faculty, programs for students, events for the community that educate on anti-racism.

In schools (and most social systems, in some regards) there can often be a toxic "well this is how we have always done things" culture. However, just because certain traditions exist does not mean that they are pardoned from interrogation. In promoting the proliferation of anti- racism, helpers can bring attention to traditions that may be problematic, exclusionary, and even racist. For example, consider an activity such as a "classroom Christmas party." While seemingly innocuous, this tradition inherently excludes students who may not identify with Christianity. An example pertaining to racism consists of teachers directing young children to dress up as Pilgrims and Native Americans to pay homage to the holiday commonly referred to as "Thanksgiving." Credible sources, such as *Teaching Tolerance* (e.g., search "Favorite Holiday Poster Projects Aren't Inclusive"), have a litany of resources designed to help educators and SMHPs critically reflect on these (and others) folkways, and explore ways to supplant these deeply offensive practices with those that are more inclusive and do not degrade individuals from similar and different cultures.

Given the inherently racist paradigm of schooling in the United States, it is logical that most content taught in schools does not adequately reflect the diversity of schools in contemporary America. Often, both written and unwritten school curriculums are centered in Whiteness and Eurocentrism, often "othering" students from non-White cultures. Accordingly, it is important that we **incorporate culturally responsive content** into our work with clients. Gay (2010) defined culturally responsive education as "using the cultural knowledge, prior experiences, frames of reference, and performance styles of ethnically diverse students to make learning encounters more relevant to and effective for them" (p. 31). Truthfully, cultural responsiveness should be a schoolwide aim; in other words, it should be interwoven in all aspects of school settings, such as in teaching (e.g., using culturally relevant books) and administration (e.g., interrogating a school's disciplinary practices to shift to more rehabilitative and restorative practices). To complement this whole-school effort, SMHPs can employ several strategies. For example, consider incorporating books that reflect a broad array of social and cultural identities. Additionally, when facilitating small groups, professionals can help nurture an inclusive and accepting environment, ensuring appropriate representation of diverse perspectives, and lived experiences. It is also important to provide summative and formative feedback to clients regarding their progress in a way that considers cultural preferences. An example, as elucidated by Gersten and Geva (2003), could involve incorporating clients' language, ideas, and responses into our responses pertaining to client goals. Lastly, SMHPs can employ culturally responsive scaffolding techniques, using clients' ideas, culture, and perspectives to help cultivate an increased understanding of relevant topics.

Anti-racism is often a seismic paradigm shift, requiring deep interrogation and challenging of methods, practices, policies, and protocols often deemed as "the norm" or "conventional." Thus, educating school colleagues (e.g., teachers, administrators) is a key step toward affecting change. Once we, helping professionals, develop an appropriate degree of understanding regarding anti-racism, we can **provide meaningful professional development** to help evolve our school community toward being anti-racist. Conversations and professional development centered on anti-racism cannot happen through a staff meeting or a book club alone; professional development must be continuous. Typically, individuals are more likely to attend professional development that (1) is clearly relevant to their work and (2) has an appropriate level of passive and active learning modalities. SMHP can consider partnering with teachers and/or administrators to engage in meaningful professional development that support the development of an anti-racist school community. Incorporating teachers, for example, as co-presenters can help ensure that the professional development clearly speaks to teachers' interests and is digestible to individuals who may not be as far along in their journey toward being anti-racist educators.

The history of conventional clinical assessments in various helping professions is rife with racism, discrimination, prejudice, and bias. Moreover, historically, assessments were commonly used to control access to opportunities, such as jobs and advanced coursework while simultaneously promoting White supremacist ideologies. Schools are certainly complicit in the misuse of assessments, particularly related to students from historically-minoritized communities. While advancements have been made to atone for this checkered history, valid concerns still exist regarding the validity and reliability of assessments used in both clinical and school assessments. Given these contemporary concerns, in promoting **anti-racism, SMHPs should consider the cultural fairness of assessments used in clinical assessments.** Bias generally refers to confounding factors that could obfuscate students' test scores. Recognizing and addressing bias in assessments is a key first step in advancing anti-racism in school settings as helping professionals may not have the liberty to utilize alternative assessments. When critically inspecting test items, SMHPs should consider the presence of content, connotation, and conceptual bias, to name a few. Hayes (2013) offers several additional examples of biases commonly found in assessments. Several ethical codes explicitly address testing and assessment within the context of individualized from historically-minoritized backgrounds. For example, the National Association of Social Workers (2017) assert that "assessments shall use ecological perspectives and functional approaches to enhance understanding of barriers to learning and the interventions that foster improvement of student well-being and academic progress" (p. 9). Similarly, helpers should elicit feedback from various sources, not just assessments, to make an informed decision. For example, if administering a behavioral assessment, it would be wise to employ a holistic approach, considering additional relevant information such as teacher feedback, parent feedback, observations, and perhaps archival data (e.g., test scores, disciplinary history) that may be available. This holistic approach is the norm in modern-day public school settings, most prominently used in the screening and identification process of students with disabilities. While not a perfect process, this process can offer meaningful context not otherwise attainable in an assessment and can counterbalance issues related to cultural fairness in testing and assessment.

Voices from the Field

One of the components of my school counseling program is to teach students to love and care about themselves but also to care about others and accept differences in others. I teach lessons on character traits such as Respect, Kindness, Tolerance, and Responsibility. I teach lessons on just being kind to one another regardless of differences. We talk a lot about how important it is to "treat others the way that you want to be treated". This is a theme that is intertwined throughout all of my lessons. I have not used the term "anti-racism", but we do talk about accepting and respecting others. I talk to students about these character traits with students from PreK through 5th grade. The goal is to prepare our students to become productive, well-adjusted, good citizens. Teaching respect, kindness, tolerance and responsibility puts them on the path to not just being good citizens in society, but just being a good person in general. (MP, School Counselor)

Action Steps for the Mesosystem and Exosystem

While helping professionals can, and should, advocate for students' needs, it's important to **help students develop the agency to lift their voices** when (1) they experience racism, discrimination and/or bias and (2) they notice others experiencing the same issues. In other words, while we can serve as a megaphone for students' needs, we should also help students build their own megaphone and develop their own agency. Students feel hurt when they experience racism, or when their classmates experience racism, but they may not know ways to respond; what's more, students may not feel like it is their place to speak out or actively combat racism. As helping professionals, we employ a strengths-based approach with our clients; we recognize their ability to develop skills and abilities. Thus, we can support our students in developing the vocabulary and action steps to utilize when they experience racism, both in school settings and outside of school. Through building students' self-efficacy and phraseology, they may feel better equipped to speak out against racism.

As Desmond Tutu stated, "if you are neutral in situations of injustice, you have chosen the side of the oppressor." Thus, as helping professionals, it is critical that we use our voice to **speak out** when racism, bias, and discrimination occurs. In fact, many helping professions' ethical codes require this anti-racist practice. SMHPs can immediately condemn racist acts perpetrated by all school community members. Certain situations may necessitate involvement by a school administrator, such as a vice-principal, to ensure the situation is addressed in accordance with school, state, and federal mandates. Inaction is not an answer; in fact, we are truly dis-servicing our clients when we fail to respond.

In our role as SMHPs, we must also ask ourselves, *"who is our client?"* As SMHPs, we have found that not only are students our clients, but also their families and members of the local community that are connected to them. It is important that we offer opportunities for community healing to support our anti-racist environment due to our understanding of the connection between our students and the community. This can be done by creating opportunities for the community to share their voice. SMHPs can collaborate with the Parent Teacher Association (PTA) to connect with parents and guardians that are already really involved with the school community and to recruit those that have the potential and desire to become more involved. SMHPs can host town hall style forums to hear from community members and to provide education on mental health, especially mental health concerns that disproportionately impact minoritized individuals such as race based trauma.

Conclusion

This chapter explored tangible steps SMHPs can employ to promote anti-racism, rooted in Bronfenbrenner's seminal ecological systems theory. Hopefully, the chapter's utility across helping professions is abundantly clear. For example, given school counselors' role in support an equitable school environment, they are well-positioned to collaborate with school stakeholders to integrate anti-racist practices that address longstanding inequities and disparities (e.g., disproportion suspension rates, underrepresentation in advanced coursework and gifted services). School social workers, who often work in tandem with school counselors, would also find the chapter beneficial. Consistent with the National Association of Social Workers' (2002) ethical standards for School Social Work Services, school social workers are committed to ensuring equitable school-based practices and opportunities. Regardless of one's specific subdiscipline, all helping professionals should be attuned to the omnipresence of racism, including in school settings, as highlighted earlier in the chapter. The journey to becoming and embodying the role of an antiracist SMHP is lifelong. We encourage SMHPs to not work in silos, but to form a community with other SMHPs that can help them to enact change individually and systematically.

Guiding Questions

1. What challenges, if any, do you anticipate encountering when promoting antiracism in school settings?
2. Describe the components of Bronfenbrenner's ecological systems theory and explain their similarities and differences.

3. Some school districts and personnel might assert that "cultural responsiveness" is the solution to racism and school-based practices rooted in racism. As a school-based mental health professional, how would you challenge this assertion?
4. Pretend you are a new school-based mental health professional working at a school in a nearby district. Given your understanding of the salience of systemic racism in schools, what initial steps would you take to promote anti-racism in your school environment?

Quiz Questions

1. Which of the following is not an example of an ecological system?
   (a) Mesosystem
   (b) Metasystem
   (c) Microsystem
   (d) None of the Above
2. "Incorporating culturally responsive content" is an example of which system?
   (a) Microsystem
   (b) Microsystem
   (c) Exosystem
   (d) None of the Above
3. Which term requires awareness of one's worldview, along with possible limitations or "blind spots" that may impede one's ability to understand other cultural backgrounds and lived experiences?
   (a) Cultural Humility
   (b) Systems Thinking
   (c) BIPOC
   (d) None of the Above
4. Promoting anti-racist practices in school settings is typically an easy, seamless process.
   (a) True
   (b) False

5. Being anti-racist is not the same as being culturally competent
   (a) True
   (b) False

References

Abrams, Z. (2020). *Working together against racism*. https://www.apa.org/monitor/2020/04/working-against-racism

Anti-Defamation League [ADL]. (2020). *Racism*. https://www.adl.org/racism

Baker, B. D., & Corcoran, S. P. (2012). *The stealth inequities school funding*. https://www.americanprogress.org/issues/education-k-12/reports/2012/09/19/38189/the-stealth-inequities-of-school-funding/

Barbieri, C., & Ferede, M. K. (2020). *A future we can all live with: How education can address and eradicate racism*. UNESCO Futures of Education Ideas LAB. https://en.unesco.org/futuresofeducation/ideas-lab/barbieri-ferede-education-eradic ate-racism

Bear, L., Finer, R., Guo, S., & Lau, A. S. (2014). Building the gateway to success: An appraisal of progress in reaching underserved families and reducing racial disparities in school-based mental health. *Psychological Services, 11*(4), 388–397. https://doi.org/10.1037/a0037969

Bell, D. (1980). Brown vs. Board of education and the interest-convergence principle. *Harvard Law Review, 93*, 518–533.

Bronfenbrenner, U. (1979). *The ecology of human development: Experiments by nature and design*. Harvard University Press.

Bryk, A., Gomez, L., Grunow, A., & LeMahieu, P. (2015). *Learning to improve: How America's schools can get better at getting better*. Harvard Education Press.

Bussey, S. R. (2020). Finding a path to anti-racism: Pivotal childhood experiences of white helping professionals. *Qualitative Social Work, 0(0)*, 1–18. https://doi.org/10.1177/1473325020923021

Cook, B. L., Trinh, N. H., Li, Z., Hou, S. S. Y., & Progovac, A. M. (2017). Trends in racial-ethnic disparities in access to mental health care, 2004–2012. *Psychiatric Services, 68*(1), 9–16. https://doi.org/10.1176/appi.ps.201500453

Cross, T., Bazron, B., Dennis, K., & Isaacs, M. (1989). *Towards a culturally competent system of care* (Vol. 1). Georgetown University Child Development Center, CASSP Technical Assistance Center.

Darling-Hammond, L. (1998). *Unequal opportunity: Race and education.* Washington, D.C. https://www.brookings.edu/articles/unequal-opportunity-race-and-education/

Diller, J. V., & Moule, J. (2005). *Cultural competence: A primer for education.* Thompson.

Fouad, N. A., & Arredondo, P. (2007). *Becoming culturally oriented: Practical advice for psychologists and educators.* American Psychological Association.

Gay, G. (2010). *Culturally responsive teaching: Theory, research, and practice* (3rd ed.). Teachers College Press.

Gersten, R., & Geva, E. (2003). Teaching reading to early language learners. *Educational Leadership, 60*, 44–49.

Hayes, D. (2013). *Assessment in counseling: A guide to the use of physiological assessment procedures.* American Counseling Association.

Hook, J. N., Davis, D. E., Owen, J., Worthington, E. L., & Utsey, S. O. (2013). Cultural humility: Measuring openness to culturally diverse clients. *Journal of Counseling Psychology, 60*(3), 353–366. https://doi.org/10.1037/a0032595

Kendi, I. (2019). *How to be an antiracist.* One World.

King, M. A., Sims, A., & Osher, D. (2007). *How is cultural competence integrated into education.* Center for Effective Collaboration and Practice, American Institutes for Research.

Ladson-Billings, G., & Tate, W. (1995). Toward a critical race theory of education. *Teachers College Record, 97*(1), 47–68.

Locke, J., Kang-Yi, C. D., Pellecchia, M., Marcus, S., Hadley, T., & Mandell, D. S. (2017). Ethnic disparities in school-based behavioral health service use for children with psychiatric disorders. *The Journal of School Health, 87*(1), 47–54. https://doi.org/10.1111/josh.12469

Lynch, J. (1987). *Prejudice reduction and the schools.* Nichols Publishing.

Marrast, L., Himmelstein, D. U., & Woolhandler, S. (2016). Racial and ethnic disparities in mental health care for children and young adults: A national study. *International Journal of Health Services, 46*(4), 810–824. https://doi.org/10.1177/2F0020731416662736

Minkler, M. (2012). *Community organizing and community building for health and welfare* (3rd ed.). Rutgers University Press.

Murphy, J. M., Guzmán, J., McCarthy, A. E., Squicciarini, A. M., George, M., Canenguez, K. M., Dunn, E. C., Baer, L., Simonsohn, A., Smoller, J. W., & Jellinek, M. S. (2015). Mental health predicts better academic outcomes: A longitudinal study of elementary school students in Chile. *Child Psychiatry and Human Development, 46*(2), 245–256. https://doi.org/10.1007/s10578-014-0464-4

National Association of Social Workers. (2002). *Standards for school social work services.* https://aab82939-3e7b-497d-8f30-a85373757e29.filesusr.com/ugd/426a18_a9bc671ba3d54d379163d7e9a541b82b.pdf
National Association of Social Workers. (2017). *Code of ethics.* https://www.socialworkers.org/About/Ethics/Code-of-Ethics/Code-of-Ethics-English
National Association of Social Workers. (2020). *Social workers must help dismantle systems of oppression and fight racism within social work profession.* https://www.socialworkers.org/News/News-Releases/ID/2219/Social-Workers-Must-Help-Dismantle-Systems-of-Oppression-and-Fight-Racism-Within-Social-Work-Profession
National Center for Education Statistics [NCES]. (2016). *Status and trends in the education of racial and ethnic groups: Indicator 14: Advanced placement and international baccalaureate.* https://nces.ed.gov/programs/raceindicators/indicator_RCE.asp
National Center for Education Statistics [NCES]. (2019a). *Mental health staff in public schools by racial and ethnic composition.* https://nces.ed.gov/data-points/2019020.asp
National Center for Education Statistics [NCES]. (2019b). *Status and trends in the education of racial and ethnic groups. Indicator 1: Population distribution.* https://nces.ed.gov/programs/raceindicators/indicator_RAA.asp
National Organization for Human Services. (2015). *Ethical standards for human services professionals.* https://www.nationalhumanservices.org/ethical-standards-for-hs-professionals
Patterson, J. T. (2001). *Brown v. Board of education: A civil rights milestone and its troubled legacy.* Oxford University Press.
Pisapia, J., Pang, N., Hee, T., Lin, Y., & Morris, D. (2009). A comparison of the use of strategic thinking skills of aspiring school leaders in Hong Kong, Malaysia, Shanghai, and the United States: An exploratory study. *International Education Studies, 2*(2), 46–58. https://doi.org/10.5539/ies.v2n2p46
Regional Arts and Culture Center. (n.d.). *Continuum on becoming an anti-racist, multicultural institution.* https://racc.org/wp-content/uploads/building-blocks/foundation/Continuum%20on%20Becoming%20an%20Anti-Racist,%20Multicultural%20Institution.pdf
Senge, P. (2006). *The fifth discipline: The art and practice of the learning organization*. Doubleday.
Stroh, D. P. (2015). *Systems thinking for social change: A practical guide to solving complex problems, avoiding unintended consequences, and achieving lasting results.* Chelsea Green Publishing.

Teaching Tolerance. (2020). *What anti-racism really means for educators.* https://www.tolerance.org/magazine/what-antiracism-really-means-for-educators

Worthington, E. L., Davis, D. E., & Hook, J. N. (Eds.). (2017). *Handbook of humility: Theory, research, and applications*. Routledge.

Yeager, D. S., Dahl, R. E., & Dweck, C. S. (2018). Why interventions to influence adolescent behavior often fail but could succeed. *Perspectives on Psychological Science: A Journal of the Association for Psychological Science, 13*(1), 101–122. https://doi.org/10.1177/1745691617722620

16

"There Isn't a Racist Bone in My Body!": A Case Study on Fostering Anti-Racism in School Counseling

Krystal L. Clemons and Raven K. Cokley

Introduction

During the summer of 2020, there was an influx of invitations for webinars, book clubs, and professional development opportunities, in response to the state-sanctioned murders of Breonna Taylor, Ahmad Arbery, and George Floyd, by police and other White vigilantes. As the Black Lives Matter protests continued to galvanize across the country, the calls for anti-racist education swelled, asking educators (including school counselors, mental health professionals, teachers, and administrators), to question the ways that they have been complicit in upholding White

K. L. Clemons
Liberty University, Lynchburg, VA, USA
e-mail: klfreeman1@liberty.edu

R. K. Cokley (✉)
Clark Atlanta University, Atlanta, GA, USA
e-mail: rcokley@cau.edu

© The Author(s), under exclusive license to Springer Nature Switzerland AG 2022

K. Johnson et al. (eds.), *Developing Anti-Racist Practices in the Helping Professions: Inclusive Theory, Pedagogy, and Application*,
https://doi.org/10.1007/978-3-030-95451-2_16

supremacy in their classrooms, school buildings, and counseling spaces (Mosley et al. 2020).

The fight for Black life was further compounded by the global pandemic, which disproportionately impacted Black people (Yancy, 2020). Another byproduct of the strain of the pandemic included Zoom school, where students were expected to be actively engaged in front of their screens, from their homes. However, the virtual nature of schooling did not disrupt the perpetuation of the school-to-prison pipeline, as Black children were still being punished and disproportionately disciplined, while at home. For example, in May 2020, a 15-year-old Black girl (notoriously known by her middle name, Grace), was sentenced to a juvenile detention center, for failing to complete online course assignments. In July, a family court judge refused to honor the emotional pleas for leniency from Grace's mother and attorney, given the implications of the ongoing pandemic (Watson & Baxley, 2021). In this moment and those that followed, every system that *should* have protected Grace (including the education system), failed her and her family.

In another example, in August 2020, a 12-year-old Black boy was suspended from school for 5 days, after his teacher called the police on him for playing with a colorful toy gun during his virtual art class. Upon their arrival, the police charged this student with bringing a replica of a firearm to school, although he was in his room at the time. This infraction was documented on the student's disciplinary record (Helmore, 2020). Here, again, the education system failed a Black student and his family. A final example occurred in February 2021, when a 9-year-old Black girl was pepper sprayed, handcuffed, and placed in the backseat of a police vehicle, after her mother placed a call to 911 citing "family trouble". Once again, the people that were *charged to care for and protect* this young Black girl, failed her and her family. Each of these harrowing incidents leaves room for us to ask the following questions: "Where was the school counselor? Who is advocating for Black students, in-person and during virtual learning? What is the role of school-affiliated mental health professionals when Black students are in crisis at home? How did every system fail the students and their families?"

As two Black women who practice school counseling and school-based mental health, we are troubled by the lack of critical and timely responses to the questions posed above. Moreover, we feel called to address how failing to address the pressing issues outlined in the introduction further perpetuates anti-Black racism in schools. To that end, we argue that anti-racist education cannot exist without the active practice of anti-racist school counseling. The overarching purpose of this chapter is to place a call to K-12 educators, broadly, and school counselors, more specifically, to engage in anti-racism work to mitigate anti-racist policies and procedures on behalf of all students and families.

The chapter begins by calling out the historically anti-Black and racist underpinnings of the U.S., which is reflected in the anti-Black and systemically oppressive structures within our school systems. We then call attention to the history of anti-Blackness within the school counseling profession, paying attention to the ASCA Ethical Standards and the ASCA National Model. Using a case study, we highlight tangible anti-racist practices for school counselors and other K-12 educators. We conclude the chapter by presenting several implications, including: (1) acknowledging the anti-Black history of the U.S.; (2) acknowledging the anti-Black history of school counseling; (3) centering anti-racist counseling theories in counselor training; (4) moving beyond critical self-reflection; (5) listening to Black students, families, and communities; (6) advocating for anti-racist curricula in schools; (7) deciding what you are willing to risk; and (8) holding yourself and others accountable.

Anti-Black History of Education in the U.S.

The call for anti-racist school counseling practices must be understood within the sociopolitical history of anti-Blackness and anti-Black racism that has undergirded U.S. educational systems, policies, and procedures (Ford & Whiting, 2007; Munroe, 2017). As a theoretical approach, *anti-Blackness* offers a framework for understanding the systemic and structured ways that society refuses to honor the dignity and humanity of Black people across the diaspora (Dumas & Ross, 2016). This framework allows us to explore the anti-Black treatment that Black students experience in schools and in school counseling (Watson & Baxley, 2021). At the same time, the theory of anti-Blackness also allows us to reimagine an educational praxis that sees Blackness and Black children as healthy, capable, lovable, and whole (Watson & Baxley, 2021).

Within U.S. history, Black folks have been the only sociocultural group to be legally and systematically denied access to an equitable education (Ford & Whiting, 2007). Between 1800 and 1835, many southern states established *slave codes* that made it illegal to teach Black children how to read and/or write (Morris, 2001). Specifically, under the Georgia slave codes, Black people who were enslaved were punished with fines or physical violence if it was discovered that they had earned an (informal) education (Morris, 2016). Slave codes delineated the enslaved status of African ascendant people and outlined the unearned privileges of white slave holders (Morris, 2016).

As such, formally educated African ascendant people were (and arguably, still are) perceived as a challenge to oppressive societal structures and systems that relegate Black people to a perceived status of racial inferiority (Campbell, 2012; Morris, 2016). For many African ascendant people, learning to read and write was a political act of resistance and a reclamation of the humanity that Black folks had been denied for centuries (Morris, 2016). Black women in particular, have a demonstrated legacy of risking their lives and livelihood in pursuit of earning a formal education, as Black women who were enslaved developed innovative methods for learning to read and for sharing those skills with others, via informal gatherings or formal schooling (Morris, 2016). As demonstrated by history, Black girls and women continue to push boundaries to foster anti-racist education for all students (Collins, 1989).

Before the passing of Brown v. Board of Education (1954), Black women and girls were underrepresented across multiple levels of education within the U.S. If allowed to attend schools, Black girls were tracked for careers and trades that emphasized domestic labor and home economics, regardless of their academic prowess (Nuamah, 2019). However, only 67 years ago, the Brown vs. Board of Education (1954) decision made segregation and discrimination in education illegal in the United States, overturning the Plessy vs. Ferguson (1896) ruling of separate but equal in U.S. public education. Many perceived Brown vs. Board of Education (1954) to be a signifier of progression and possibility for Black students in schools. However, Black students' experiences with anti-Black racism in schools are often compounded by the perpetuation of anti-Blackness within their school counseling experiences.

Anti-Black History of the School Counseling Profession

Historically, the school counseling profession has been permeated by White school counselor educators, practicing school counselors, trainees, theories and theorists, textbook authors, research methodologies, and evidence-based practices, that often reify Whiteness and White Supremacy within the field (Arredondo et al., 2020; Baggerly et al., 2017; CACREP, 2017). Scholars have also called attention to the pervasive Whiteness among counseling leadership and credentialing bodies, such as CACREP site team members and ACA, ACES, and ASCA executive board members (Arredondo et al., 2020). The ASCA (2019c) School Counselor Professional Standards and Competencies speak to the mindsets and behaviors that school counselors and school counselor trainees need in order to implement adequate school counseling practices. However, the standards and competencies are inadequate in addressing the ways that school counselors can and should engage in anti-racist counseling practices, particularly as it relates to combating anti-Blackness in schools (ASCA, 2019c). As such, the standards and competencies are deficient in holding school counseling programs and school counselor trainees accountable for engaging in anti-racist counseling in schools.

For example, the ASCA competencies call for school counselors to "act as a systems change agent to create an environment promoting and supporting student success" (ASCA, 2019c). However, the competencies fail to specifically mention race, racism, or anti-racism, which each dynamically shape the educational and learning environment for Black students. Failing to explicitly name race, racism, and anti-racism, contributes to the misguided belief that school counselor preparation programs are meeting the social, cultural, emotional, and academic needs of all students.

Similarly, ACA (2020) released an anti-racism statement, saying "Our stance is Black Lives Matter. We have a moral and professional obligation to deconstruct institutions which have historically been designed to benefit white America". What was missing from this statement, and many others, was the explicit naming of the ways that the counseling profession has historically upheld anti-Black racism and White supremacy. One of the many institutions that we must abolish includes the historical and current practices of school counseling that are rooted in anti-Blackness.

Further, school counselor education scholars have called attention to the lack of systemic training that school counselor trainees have received in terms of engaging anti-racist school counseling practices to address anti-Blackness in schools (Goodman et al. 2019; Steele, 2008). To adequately educate, supervise, and train the next generation of school counselors on how to challenge anti-Black racism, school counselor educators must demonstrate a commitment to answering the call to foster anti-racist school counselor identities among trainees, in addition to committing to engaging in anti-racist school counseling practices. This call is timely, given the historical and current state of the U.S., where Black students are pervasively viewed as disposable and culturally deficient in our educational environments.

Overview of the ASCA Ethical Standards

The counseling profession as a whole is governed by the American Counseling Association Code of Ethics (2014). School counseling has its own ethical standards set forth by the American School Counseling Association (2016a). While there is significant overlap, the ASCA Ethical Standards speak to the specificity that is the school counseling profession. Every school counseling professional (counselors, district supervisors, and school counselor educators) have an ethical obligation to provide every child with equitable access to school counseling services. In this age of emboldened racism, White supremacist views, and right-wing extremism, it is imperative now more than ever that school counselors adhere to ASCA's ethical directives.

"Ethics is knowing the difference between what we have a right to do and what is right to do (Desmarais-Morse et al., 2020)." Dr. Carolyn Stone's words during an ASCA Town Hall on racism in schools got right to the heart of the school counselor's duty to confront systemic barriers within the education system in order to ensure the success of every student. In order to confront systemic racism within schools, counselors are ethically required to increase their own cultural competence and face their own prejudices (ASCA, 2016a). The following codes of the ASCA Ethical Standards (2016a) give explicit directions:

A.1.f. Respect students' and families' values, beliefs, sexual orientation, gender identification/expression and cultural background and exercise great care to avoid imposing personal beliefs or values rooted in one's religion, culture, or ethnicity.

A.3.c. Review school and student data to assess needs including, but not limited to, data on disparities that may exist related to gender, race, ethnicity, socio-economic status and/or other relevant classifications.

A.3.d. Use data to determine needed interventions, which are then delivered to help close the information, attainment, achievement, and opportunity gaps.

A.4.c. Identify gaps in college and career access and the implications of such data for addressing both intentional and unintentional biases related to college and career counseling.

A.6.e. Refrain from referring students based solely on the school counselor's personal beliefs or values rooted in one's religion, culture, ethnicity, or personal worldview. School counselors maintain the highest respect for student diversity. School counselors should pursue additional training and supervision in areas where they are at risk of imposing their values on students, especially when the school counselor's values are discriminatory in nature. School counselors do not impose their values on students and/or families when making referrals to outside resources for student and/or family support.

A.10.a. Strive to contribute to a safe, respectful, nondiscriminatory school environment in which all members of the school community demonstrate respect and civility.

B.3.i Monitor and expand personal multicultural and social-justice advocacy awareness, knowledge, and skills to be an effective culturally competent school counselor. Understand how prejudice, privilege and various forms of oppression based on ethnicity, racial identity, age, economic status, abilities/disabilities, language, immigration status, sexual orientation, gender, gender identity expression, family type, religious/spiritual identity, appearance and living situations (e.g., foster care, homelessness, incarceration) affect students and stakeholders.

B.3.j. Refrain from refusing services to students based solely on the school counselor's personally held beliefs or values rooted in one's religion, culture, or ethnicity. School counselors respect the diversity of students and seek training and supervision when prejudice or biases interfere with providing comprehensive services to all students.

B.3.k. Work toward a school climate that embraces diversity and promotes academic, career and social/emotional development for all students.

Despite these ethical instructions, counselors are reluctant to perform anti-racism work. This explains the persistence of the disparities Black and Brown students face in the following areas: gifted education, special education, discipline, the achievement gap, and student-athletes. Some counselors may be concerned they will receive resistance from White administrators, teachers, parents, and perhaps students (Desmarais-Morse et al., 2020). The ASCA Ethical Standards (2016a) provide counselors with the cover necessary to make such bold moves.

ASCA National Model

The ASCA National Model (2019a, b) is a framework for school counselors to create comprehensive school counseling programs that meet every child's need. Programs using the ASCA National Model will have a positive impact on student discipline, close achievement gaps, and will advocate for every student (ASCA, 2019a). The ASCA National Model regulates the roles, responsibilities, and activities of school counselors as well as shifts the focus of the school counseling profession from being responsive to some students to systemically delivering academic, career, and personal/social services to all students to ensure their academic success (ASCA, 2019b). The ASCA National Model incorporates four themes: (a) leadership—taking the charge and using inimitable skills in working with several stakeholders within the school system; (b) advocacy—promoting the educational needs and opportunities of all students; (c) collaboration—working with students, teachers, administrators, parents, and community organizations; and (d) systematic change—working to remove obstacles that may impede academic opportunity and achievement (ASCA, 2019b). School counselors can use the four themes to organize and apply practical interventions.

The ASCA National Model is structurally divided into four components: foundation, management, delivery, and accountability (ASCA, 2019a). Development of each of the components will allow school counselors to be leaders and advocates while collaborating with other stakeholders as well as address systematic change (Butler-Byrd et al., 2006; Mitcham et al., 2009). The foundation component is the comprehensive school counseling program's base. It ensures that the mission and vision statements and the program goals explicitly tackle the specific needs of all students— including Black students and students of color. The management component addresses the implementation of the school counseling program. It includes a program assessment, school data utilization, an annual agreement defining the program's scope and structure and the school counselor's role, and the creation of an advisory council. School counselors should disaggregate the school's academic and behavioral data to specifically examine the issues related to all students of color (ASCA, 2019a). Moreover, school counselors must ensure the advisory council is racially/culturally diverse and includes teachers, students, parents, and community members. The delivery component focuses on how students receive direct and indirect services. Direct services to Black students must integrate culturally relevant counseling techniques and address academic, career, and personal/social issues specific to this population. Indirect services (consultation, collaboration, and referrals) can incorporate social justice, effectively working with others to develop a suitable plan of action. Finally, the accountability component employs disaggregated data analysis to assess the school counseling program's efficiency in meeting the academic, career, and personal/social needs of all students.

Gifted Education

Gifted education is inherently racist and anti-Black. Dreilinger (2020) notes that Lewis Terman, the psychologist who promoted the idea of the intelligence quotient that later paved the way for gifted testing, believed in eugenics. Intelligence testing creates barriers for identifying gifted Black American students, as scores are sometimes lower for racially and culturally diverse students (Luckey Goudelock, 2019). Despite recent efforts by the profession to provide equitable access to every student, advanced courses are still overwhelmingly White (ASCA, 2019a). White students make up 60% of gifted courses compared to 9% by Black students (Dreilinger, 2020). The Office of Civil Rights (OCR)'s data collection revealed overrepresentation of Asian and White students in gifted education programs, and American Indian, Latinx and Black students have been underrepresented in gifted education programs since 1978 (US OCR, 2004). Gifted and talented education programs are more accessible to White students than they are to Black and Brown students; these students are immensely underrepresented even when they have access to honors or advanced placement courses, with only 29% of these students enrolled in at least one AP course (UNCF, 2021). Gifted education's inequities are due to the under-referral of mostly White female teachers. Grissom and Redding (2016) discovered White teachers under-referred Black students for gifted education even though their attributes were similar to White students. Giftedness may manifest itself differently in Black American students, showing a need for differentiated means of identification (Luckey Goudelock, 2019). The current system causes gifted marginalized students to fall through the cracks by failing to identify them (Gentry, 2020). Gifted programs admissions are partial toward students with wealthy, educated parents, who are more likely to be White (Thornhill, 2019; Dreilinger, 2020). While there is a plethora of research on gifted students of color, Goings and Ford (2018) found there is little discussion about how race and poverty impact recruitment and retention of these students in gifted programs. ASCA (2019e) maintains it is the role of the school counselor to maximize access to gifted programs and advanced courses for marginalized students, students of color, English-language learners, and first-generation students.

Research also suggests that marginalized students fear the label of gifted and talented due to constant exposure to microaggressions, being seen as the representative for their entire race during certain discussions, or being taunted for "acting white" (Luckey Goudelock, 2019; Staumbaugh & Ford, 2015). Students who are twice exceptional (identified as both gifted and having a disability) often struggle with self-esteem and social interactions (Mayes et al., 2014). It is the school counselor's duty to be cognizant of the unique needs of these students and help create a school climate in which all students are comfortable embracing their intelligence, abilities, and authentic selves. The ASCA National Model provides the means to ensure the comprehensive school counseling program rises to these particular challenges.

Special Education

Over-referred by mainly White female teachers, Black and Brown children compose the majority of special education classrooms (Abidin & Robinson, 2002; Artiles et al., 2002; Harris-Murri et al., 2006). In some instances, however, Black and Brown students are less likely than their White peers to be correctly identified and to receive high quality special education services despite demonstrating similar levels of academic performance and behavior (Elder et al., 2021; Shifrer, 2018; Shifrer et al., 2011). Black students may be placed in special education at a higher rate than their peers but there is evidence that they are more likely to be identified as intellectually disabled or behaviorally disordered rather than having a learning disability such as dyslexia or other conditions such as speech or language impairment or ADHD (Artiles et al., 2002; LDAA, 2020). Students in Mayes, Hines, and Harris' (2014) study said their teachers did not follow their IEPs, were rude and hostile towards them, and had low expectations. The anti-Black nature of the special education system enables it to be weaponized against Black and Brown students to keep them from participation in general education (Shell, 2020).

School counselors provide direct and indirect services to all students in the least restrictive and inclusive settings (as determined by the student's IEP) (Tarver-Behring et al., 1998). ASCA (2016c) lists the following as appropriate school counselor responsibilities pertaining to special education:

- providing school counseling curriculum lessons, individual and/or group counseling to students with special needs within the scope of the school counseling program
- providing short-term, goal-focused counseling in instances where it is appropriate to include these strategies as a part of the IEP or 504 plan
- encouraging family involvement in the educational process
- consulting and collaborating with staff and families to understand the special needs of a student and understanding the adaptations and modifications needed to assist the student
- advocating for students with special needs in the school and in the community
- contributing to the school's multidisciplinary team within the scope and practice of the school counseling program to identify students who may need to be assessed to determine special education or 504 plan eligibility
- collaborating with other related student support professionals (e.g., school psychologists, physical therapists, occupational therapists, special education staff, speech and language pathologists) in the delivery of services
- assisting with developing academic, transition and postsecondary plans for students with IEP's and 504 plans as appropriate

School counselors are integral to special education (ASCA, 2016c; Adkison-Bradley et al., 2006; Moore et al., 2008; Shell, 2020). However, many school counseling programs do not adequately prepare their graduates for the challenges of special education (Shell, 2020). Feather and Carlson's (2019) study of CACREP-accredited counseling programs reported that roughly half of counselor educators surveyed believed they received ineffective or moderately effective preparation to handle the needs of children with disabilities. Approximately 51% of the participants believed their programs did not spend enough time on disability-related practices and policies, and 35% did not think counselors-in-training were prepared to work with students with disabilities (Feather & Carlson, 2019). Shell's (2020) phenomenological study found that high school counselors felt ill equipped to work with Black students with disabilities. They also felt sidelined because the special education teachers handle the majority of decisions regarding classes and interventions (Shell, 2020). School counselors must take their place at the table in order to advocate for Black students in special education (Owens et al., 2016).

Discipline

Discipline rates among students are disproportionately high for students of color, particularly Black students. Black students spend less time in the classroom because of discipline, which keeps them from accessing a quality education. Black students are nearly twice as likely to be suspended without educational services as White students, and Black students are also 3.8 times as likely to receive at least one out-of-school suspension as White students (UNCF, 2021). Black children represent 47% of preschoolers receiving at least one out-of-school suspension despite only comprising 19% of the nation's pre-school population, while White students represent 41% of pre-school enrollment but only 28% of those receiving out-of-school suspensions (UNCF, 2021). Boysen (2009) notes counselors see Black students as more hostile than White students despite displaying the same behaviors, thereby contributing to the discipline inequities. Black girls are seen as more mature and less innocent than their White peers, causing them to receive harsher punishments for similar behavior (Wun, 2016). Disturbingly, Black students are 2.3 times as likely to be referred to law enforcement or be arrested for a school-related incident as White students, thus fueling the school-to-prison pipeline (Hines & Wilmot, 2018; Hollinger & Hansel, 2020; Parker, 2017; UNCF, 2021).

At times, the school counselor's role regarding discipline varies from advocate to enforcer depending on the school. ASCA (2019d) states school counselors should not be disciplinarians, instead serving as collaborators for developing discipline procedures. Multi-Tiered Systems of Support (MTSS) provide a framework for which school counselors can employ the ASCA National Model to meet the needs of students requiring interventions such as individual and group counseling, classroom guidance lessons, mentorship, and peer support (Goodman-Scott et al., 2019). Counselors can provide professional development for school personnel regarding classroom management, restorative practices, and emotional regulation in order to decrease the number of discipline referrals. Counselors must interrupt the school-to-prison pipeline by any means necessary.

Opportunity Gap

Black children make up 15% of students in K-12 public schools across the United States (National Center for Educational Statistics, 2020). Yet schools seem to have challenges when it comes to creating opportunities for Black students to achieve. First-generation, lower income, Black students are underrepresented in college enrollment, 17% of Black eighth grade students read at grade level, and students at urban high schools have less information and less access to information regarding higher education (ASCA, 2016a; Kamenetz, 2018; Lynch, 2016; Paolini, 2019; Robinson & Roksa, 2016; Shamsuddin, 2016). School counselors play a significant role in predicting student college applications/enrollments, especially for underrepresented minoritized students (Cholewa et al., 2016). Rust (2019) states that addressing the academic opportunity gap related to Black students is a matter of social justice, and school counselors are central figures to work with stakeholders in addressing it.

ASCA's (2018) stance on equity for students addresses the opportunity gap between White and Black students, and mandates school counselors take systemic action to address this issue (Clemons & Johnson, 2019). The ASCA National Model includes a component called the Closing the Gap Action Plan, which enables school counselors to use data to create interventions for students in target groups (ASCA, 2019a, b). Moon and Singh's (2015) study highlights the need for school counselors to implement interventions that will target Black students and show a commitment to their success, while Rust (2019) describes ways in which school counselors can accomplish this via the ASCA National Model.

School-family-community partnerships increase the academic, career, and social/emotional development of all students and assist in the school counselor's effort to close the opportunity gap (ASCA, 2016b). Black Americans' sense of community is very strong; 80% believe community involvement is extremely important (Agboola, 2018). Community is defined as "a feeling of fellowship with others as a result of sharing common attitudes, interests, and goals (Oxford)." While the Black community is not a monolith, shared experiences prove to be the tie that binds. Black Americans have relied on each other out of necessity and survival, and most feel a strong connection to the broader Black community (Barroso, 2020). Black communities were established prior to the transatlantic slave trade and were strengthened via the intergenerational trauma of Jim Crow, the Civil Rights era, and today's Black Lives Matter era. Therefore, tapping into the invaluable resources of Black communities will prove to be the key to closing the opportunity gap for Black students.

Student-Athletes

Student-athletes are the pride of any school with a robust athletics program. Many of these athletes expect to attend college, requiring the school counselor's assistance in achieving this goal. While student-athletes generally tend to do well academically, the same cannot be said for Black student-athletes (Sabo et al., 1993). School counselors must promote college and career readiness for every student (ASCA, 2016a), yet Black male student-athletes lag behind their counterparts of all genders when it comes to receiving undergraduate degrees (Harris, 2015). Furthermore, White student-athletes are more likely to attend four-year institutions than Black student-athletes (Sabo et al., 1993). If school counseling programs were indeed comprehensive and anti-racist, these gaps would be nonexistent. Since approximately 39% of student-athletes are students of color (NCAA, 2021), school counselors must recognize the ways race impacts the quality of education they receive.

School counselors must become familiar with the eligibility rules of the NCAA, as well as state graduation requirements. Sproull (2018) highlights the necessity for counselors to be familiar with Division I, Division II, and Division III in order to effectively guide student-athletes. Counselors should incorporate academic transcript interpretation into classroom guidance lessons so all students, including student-athletes, understand their academic standing and how it impacts postsecondary opportunities. Counselors must also take care to see the Black student-athlete holistically, not just as a workhorse whose purpose is to bring the school athletic glory (Harris et al., 2020).

Case Study

Amanda is a 13-year-old Black American cisgender girl who is in the 8th grade. She comes from a single parent home and has two siblings including a twin sister. Amanda has an auditory processing disorder and a speech impediment. Amanda has a 504 for both issues, which mandates speech therapy and quiet rooms. Because of her need for quiet rooms, Amanda has been placed in a special education classroom. Amanda's self-esteem has been impacted by her experience and her behavior has sent her to the principal's office multiple times. Her grades have plummeted in all subjects except for one. Amanda has an A+ in Language Arts. She wrote and performed two original poems: one for her church's Black History Month program and one for her mother's sorority celebration of the arts. Her mother believes Amanda is linguistically gifted and wants her tested. She contacted both the gifted education coordinator and Amanda's special education case manager, but they are reluctant to call a child study meeting to explore the possibility that Amanda may be gifted.

Alarmed by her numerous trips to the office, Amanda's school counselor calls her in for a chat. Though the counselor is a White cisgender man, he and Amanda have a good rapport. Amanda shares her ongoing concerns and mentions something about her mother wanting her to be tested for giftedness. After their conversation, the counselor calls Amanda's mother and requests a conference to listen to her concerns. The counselor is upset after learning Amanda's mother requested a child study meeting and was repeatedly rebuffed. Realizing he has the power to call such a meeting, the counselor sets a meeting on behalf of Amanda and her mother. The school counselor took control of the meeting and used his privilege to advocate for Amanda and her mother. Learning of her incredible linguistic abilities and creativity, the counselor asks Amanda to write and perform an original poem during the spring honor roll assembly. This request boosts Amanda's confidence, and her grades and behavior begin to quickly improve. The child study team honored Amanda's mother's request for giftedness testing, and the results proved what she knew of her daughter all along: Amanda is exceptionally gifted.

Implications

As seen by the case study and through U.S. history, Black students have received disproportionate rates of disciplinary action and referrals for special education, while also being systematically excluded from accelerated learner spaces (e.g., AP/Honors/IB) (Morris, 2016; Evans-Winters, 2016). Instead of fighting to eradicate racist policies and holding administrators accountable, school counselors have perpetuated the educational violence inflicted upon Black students. School counselors must be on the front lines of these battles as anti-racists, ensuring that all students have fair and equitable opportunities to succeed (Foxx et al., 2020). Therefore, there are several implications for engaging with anti-racist school counseling. Implications include: (1) acknowledging the anti-Black history of the U.S.; (2) acknowledging the anti-Black history of school counseling; (3) centering anti-racist counseling theories as foundational; (4) moving beyond critical self-reflection; (5) listening to Black students, families, and communities; (6) advocating for anti-racist curricula in schools; (7) deciding what you are willing to risk; and (8) holding yourself and others accountable.

Acknowledging the Anti-Black History of the U.S.

The first truth that we must reckon with as anti-racist school counselors, is that the U.S. was founded on anti-Indigenous genocide, the free labor of enslaved African people, and inherent anti-Blackness. In the same regard, schools in the U.S. were designed with anti-Blackness in mind. They were not created to be spaces of *freedom dreaming* for Black students; instead, educational systems in the U.S. were created to spirit murder Black children (Love, 2016). We cannot simply ask school counselors to disrupt the school to prison pipeline without first naming that the school system itself functions as a system of oppression. We must first acknowledge the pervasiveness of Whiteness and White supremacy in the U.S., which has permeated U.S. systems of education and school counseling (Bell, 1995).

Acknowledging the Anti-Black History of School Counseling

Within a western context, the history of school counseling and its practices are inherently anti-Black. In many schools, school counselors are positioned as disciplinarians, which serves as a function of policing within the school system (Parker, 2017). Moreover, school counselor trainees are often taught to perceive Black students as threatening, incapable, disruptive, and culturally inept (Ford & Whiting, 2007). The majority of school counselors are White (Data USA, 2019). A review of the research exposes White school counselors' lack of racial sensitivity (Moss & Singh, 2015). Johnson and Carrico (2020) highlight the power differential between White school counselors and students of color that could impede equitable access to support and cause students of color to receive less advocacy than their White counterparts. This racist socialization is perpetuated via school counseling courses, practicum and internship experiences, and clinical supervision. Seeing Black students as a problem in need of fixing is inherently anti-Black and representative of the societal stereotypes that are perpetuated about Black people in the media, movies, educational research, and western counseling theories (Love, 2016).

Centering Anti-Racist Counseling Theories as a Foundational Practice

The counseling theories that are taught as foundational to the field are predominantly written and conceptualized by White, middle class men. Eurocentric theories and frameworks do not speak to the ways that Black students navigate the world, nor do they affirm Black ways of doing and being. Moreover, most counseling theories textbooks include a small statement at the end of the chapter addressing "cultural considerations", but fail to address how school counselor trainees should navigate anti-Blackness and anti-Black racism in schools. To push this further, school counselor educators should consider teaching anti-racist theories and frameworks (e.g., critical race theory; Black feminism; womanism; BlackCrit; CritNoir), at the beginning of the counseling theories course instead of at the end (Collins, 1989; Crenshaw, et al., 2015; Dumas & ross, 2016; Stewart, et al., 2019). School counselor trainees should be taught that anti-racist counseling is not an afterthought; rather, it is the foundation of our work.

Moving Beyond Critical Self-Reflection

Doing the work of an anti-racist school counselor requires moving beyond critical self-reflection. When White school counselors and trainees are first asked to question how they may have been complicit in perpetuating anti-Blackness in schools and their personal lives, many respond with, "there isn't a racist bone in my body!". This is part of the discomfort that comes with engaging in critical self-interrogation processes around anti-Blackness and White supremacy. Interrogating your personal biases, stereotypes, and perpetuations of anti-Blackness is only one step in the lifelong process of becoming an anti-racist school counselor. Possible assignments to facilitate this long-term learning process might include: maintaining a privilege journal; creating a digital autobiography; and cultivating anti-racist book lists for individualized learning. School counseling students should also be taught about developing an anti-racist school counselor identity and orientation, which requires school counselors to move beyond self-reflection and towards intentional anti-racist action. Ratts and Greenleaf (2017)'s work provides a leadership framework to address issues of oppression and inequality within schools using the Multicultural and Social Justice Counseling Competencies, and this framework should be integral to every school counseling course curriculum. This action might include: engaging peers and friends about anti-Black racism; acknowledging the history and current manifestations of anti-Blackness in schools and school counseling; calling attention to perpetuations of anti-Blackness within the counseling curricula; and holding their peers and future colleagues accountable for becoming anti-racist school counselors.

Listening to Black Students, Families, and Communities

One of the greatest disservices that we do as school counselor educators, practicum instructors, and clinical supervisors is not ensuring that counselor trainees have a presence within the communities that they seek to serve prior to being placed in schools. What are the implications of White school counselor trainees entering historically Black schools without any experiential knowledge of Black communities? What kind of harm do we perpetuate by failing to train school counselors to address anti-Blackness in schools? What kind of harm do we cause to Black students by neglecting to assess school counselor trainees for complicity in anti-Blackness and anti-Black racism? We must be intentional about fostering this learning and community engagement process, to ensure that Black students, families, and communities are not being exploited or harmed.

Two entities within Black communities that are often overlooked by schools and school counselors regarding community partnerships are the Black Church and Black Greek Letter Organizations (BGLOs). Research shows creating partnerships with local Black churches enhances Black student achievement, helps to provide resources (e.g. school supplies, monetary donations, food/clothing drives, etc.) to struggling families, and can offer community input for school counseling programs (Clemons & Johnson, 2019; McIntosh & Curry, 2020). BGLOs, or the Divine

Nine, offer youth programs, scholarship opportunities, and mentorship for K-12 students (Clemons et al., 2022; Jones, 2012). In the case study, Amanda's confidence received a boost from her participation in these Black community staples. These untapped resources can provide untold support to African American students and invaluable collaborative support for school counselors.

Advocating for Anti-Racist Curricula in Schools

Research shows that Black students often encounter curricula that present their culture and heritage as inherently problematic (Jones & Hagopian, 2020). School counselors have the agency to advocate for a more inclusive counseling curricula as an intentional anti-racist counseling practice. Jones and Hagopian's (2020) research shows that Black students respond more positively to the learning process when they encounter affirming images and messages about themselves in the classroom. Black Lives Matter at School is an anti-racist initiative that school counselors and school counselor educators can engage with to learn strategies for advocating for ethnic studies courses within their schools (Jones & Hagopian, 2020).

Deciding What You Are Willing to Risk

When we engage in conversations around anti-racist school counseling, it is often presented as an aspirational goal that we *hope to achieve* someday. However, the health, wellness, love, and safety of Black students is not an aspirational task on a to-do list. It is a matter of survival for Black students, their communities, and their families. Despite the popularization of anti-racist counseling conversations, book clubs, and webinars, actually doing the work of anti-racism requires sacrifice. This sacrifice might be personal, professional, or social, as the people in your life might react negatively to your desire to mitigate anti-Black racism in schools and society (Richey, 2018). What does your demonstrated commitment to anti-racist school counseling look like? What do you need to make it a reality? Are you willing and prepared to disrupt the disproportionate discipline rates of Black students in your schools? Are you willing to challenge your neighbor for perpetuating anti-Black racism by calling the police on Black children at the neighborhood pool? Are you willing to question why your school or department has not hired a Black school counselor or school counselor educator? Decide what you are willing to risk and commit to that, unapologetically. The well-being of your Black students depends on it.

Holding Yourself and Others Accountable

As anti-racist school counselor educators, each of us has a responsibility to hold ourselves accountable for doing our own work (Gonzalez & Cokley, 2021). We also have an ethical and personal responsibility to ensure that our friends, family members, students, supervisees, and colleagues also do their own work. We cannot depend on Black school counselors and our co-conspirators who believe in anti-racism to carry this burden alone. White school counselor educators in particular should take up the mantle of anti-racism, using their racial privilege to cause *good trouble*. Words are not enough; it is time for action. School counselor educators should advocate for the addition of explicit anti-racist language to the ASCA Ethical Standards. Language matters (Galloway et al., 2019), and while the standards provide direction, they do not explicitly describe the ethics of anti-racism. Leibowitz-Nelson et al. (2020) list seven ways in which school counseling professionals can implement institutional interventions: (1) explore privilege and marginalization with students; (2) connect privileged and marginalized clients with supportive individuals within social institutions; (3) collaborate with social institutions; (4) engage in social advocacy; (5) remove systemic barriers; (6) address individual and systemic inequities; and (7) collect and share data that highlight inequities.

Several options to practice self-accountability include: participating in professional development opportunities; attending continuing education workshops and presentations for strategies to mitigate anti-Blackness;

and consuming research from Black school counselor educators who are actively engaged in anti-racist school counseling practices.

Conclusion

Being a silent observer or bystander of anti-Black racism in schools, is just as harmful for Black students as actively engaging in the process of perpetuating anti-Black rhetoric and policies. Disrupting these patterns as anti-racist school counselors requires us to risk something, and to hold ourselves and others accountable for doing our work. As school counselor educators, we have a personal and professional responsibility to ensure that school counselor trainees are adequately trained to become anti-racist counselors and advocates. Additionally, other helping professionals have a responsibility to ensure the safety, support, and celebration of Black children.

Guiding Questions

1. How has anti-Blackness and anti-racism shown up in your school policies?
2. Think of the marginalized students who are labeled as having behavior challenges. How and why are they falling through the cracks?
3. Name concrete ways in which anti-Blackness and anti-racism can be eradicated from the comprehensive school counseling program using the ASCA National Model.

Quiz Questions

1. The _____ enables school counselors' use of data to create interventions for target groups.
   (a) Accountability Plan
   (b) Closing the Gap Action Plan
   (c) Foundation Plan
   (d) Management Agreement

2. _____ of Black eighth grade students read on grade level.
   a. 22%
   b. 8%
   c. 17%
   d. 11%

3. White students comprise _____ of gifted courses, while Black students make up _____.
   a. 60%; 9%
   b. 54%; 8%
   c. 68%; 13%
   d. 70%; 10%

4. Which of these is not included in the ASCA National Model themes?
   (a) Leadership
   (b) Accountability
   (c) Advocacy
   (d) Systemic change

5. Black students are more likely to be identified as intellectually disabled or behaviorally disordered rather than having a learning disability.
   1. True
   2. False

References

Abidin, R. R., & Robinson, L. R. (2002). Stress, biases, or professionalism: What drives teachers' referral judgments of students with challenging behaviors? *Journal of Emotional and Behavioral Disorders, 10*(4), 204–212.

Adkison-Bradley, C., Johnson, P. D., Rawls, G., & Plunkett, D. (2006). Overrepresentation of African American males in special education programs: Implications and advocacy strategies for school counselors. *Journal of School Counseling, 4*(16), n16.

Agboola, A. (2018). Study shows Black people support family, friends more than other groups. Black Enterprise. https://www.blackenterprise.com/

blacks-support-family-friends-more/?utm_content=buffer9bb09&utm_medium=social&utm_source=twitter.com&utm_campaign=buffer

American Counseling Association. (2014). *ACA code of ethics*. https://www.counseling.org/resources/aca-code-of-ethics.pdf

American Counseling Association. (2020, November 18). *Anti-racism statement*. https://www.counseling.org/news/updates/2020/06/22/aca-anti-racism-statement

American School Counselor Association. (2016a). *ASCA ethical standards for school Counselors*. https://www.schoolcounselor.org/getmedia/f041cbd0-7004-47a5-ba01-3a5d657c6743/Ethical-Standards.pdf

American School Counselor Association. (2016b). *The school counselor and school-family – Community partnerships*. Author.

American School Counselor Association. (2016c). *The school counselor and students with disabilities*. Author.

American School Counselor Association. (2018). *The school counselor and equity for all students*. Author.

American School Counselor Association. (2019a). *ASCA National Model Executive Summary*. https://www.schoolcounselor.org/getmedia/bd376246-0b4f-413f-b3e0-1b9938f36e68/ANM-executive-summary-4th-ed.pdf

American School Counselor Association. (2019b). *ASCA national model: A framework for school counseling programs* (4th ed.). Author.

American School Counselor Association. (2019c). *ASCA school counselor professional standards and competencies*. Author.

American School Counselor Association. (2019d). *The school counselor and discipline*. Author.

American School Counselor Association. (2019e). *The school counselor and gifted and talented student programs*. Author.

Arredondo, P., D'Andrea, M., & Lee, C. (2020). Unmasking white supremacy and racism in the counseling profession. *Counseling Today*. https://ct.counseling.org/2020/09/unmasking-white-supremacy-and-racism-in-the-counseling-profession/

Artiles, A. J., Harry, B., Reschly, D. J., & Chinn, P. C. (2002). Over-identification of students of color in special education: A critical overview. *Multicultural Perspectives, 4*(1), 3–10.

Baggerly, J., Tan, T. X., Pichotta, D., & Warner, A. (2017). Race, ethnicity, and gender of faculty members in APA- and CACREP-accredited programs: Changes over five decades. *Journal of Multicultural Counseling and Development, 45*(4), 292–303. https://doi.org/10.1002/jmcd.12079

Barroso, A. (2020). Most black adults say race is central to their identity and feel connected to a broader black community. Pew Research Center. https://www.pewresearch.org/fact-tank/2020/02/05/most-black-adults-say-race-is-central-to-their-identity-and-feel-connected-to-a-broader-black-community/

Bell, D. (1995). Who's afraid of critical race theory? *University of Illinois Law Review, 4*, 893–910.

Boysen, G. A. (2009). A review of experimental studies of explicit and implicit bias among counselors. *Journal of Multicultural Counseling and Development, 37*, 240–249.

Brown v. Board of Education, 347 U.S. 483. (1954).

Butler-Byrd, N., Nieto, J., & Senour, M. N. (2006). Working Successfully with Diverse Students and Communities: The Community-Based Block Counselor Preparation Program. *Urban Education, 41*(4), 376–401.

Campbell, S. (2012). For colored girls? Factors that influence teacher recommendations into advanced courses for black girls. *Review of Black Political Economy, 39*(4), 389–402.

Clemons, K. L., & Johnson, K. F. (2019). African American pastors and their perceptions of professional school Counseling. *The Journal of Negro Education, 88*(4), 467–478.

Clemons, K., Dodson, F., & Gregory, B. (2022). Divine Nine Connections. *ASCA School Counselor Magazine, 59*(3), 24–26.

Cholewa, B., Burkhardt, C. K., & Hull, M. F. (2016). Are school counselors impacting underrepresented students' thinking about postsecondary education? A nationally representative study. *Professional School Counseling, 19*(1), 144–154.

Collins, P. H. (1989). The social construction of black feminist thought. *Signs, 14*(4), 745–773.

Council for Accreditation of Counseling and Related Educational Programs. (2017). *CACREP vital statistics 2017: Results from a national survey of accredited programs.* http://www.cacrep.org/wp-content/uploads/2019/05/2017-CACREP-Vital-Statistics-Report.pdf

Crenshaw, K., Ocen, P., & Nanda, J. (2015). *Black girls matter: Pushed out, overpoliced, and underprotected.* African American Policy Forum and Center for Intersectionality and Social Policy Studies. https://www.atlanticphilanthropies.org/wp-content/uploads/2015/09/BlackGirlsMatter_Report.pdf

Data USA. (2019, October). *Counselors.* https://datausa.io/profile/soc/211010/

Desmarais-Morse, J., Francis, D., Parker, T., Rutledge, M., Stone, C., & Susko, J. (2020, June 12). *ASCA virtual town hall: Racism in schools*. American School Counselor Association. https://videos.schoolcounselor.org/asca-town-hall-racism-in-schools

Dreilinger, D. (2020). *Why decades of trying to end racial segregation in gifted education haven't worked*. The Hechinger Report. https://hechingerreport.org/gifted-educations-race-problem/

Dumas, M. J., & Ross, K. M. (2016). "Be real black for me" imagining BlackCrit in education. *Urban Education, 51*(4), 415–442.

Elder, T. E., Figlio, D. N., Imberman, S. A., & Persico, C. L. (2021). School segregation and racial gaps in special education identification. *Journal of Labor Economics, 39*(S1), S151–S197.

Evans-Winters, V. (2016). Schooling at the liminal: Black girls and special education. *The Wisconsin English Journal, 58*(2), 154.

Feather, K. A., & Carlson, R. G. (2019). An initial investigation of individual instructors' self-perceived competence and incorporation of disability content into CACREP-accredited programs: Rethinking training in counselor education. *Journal of Multicultural Counseling and Development, 47*(1), 19–36.

Ford, D. Y., & Whiting, G. W. (2007). A mind is a terrible thing to erase: Black students' underrepresentation in gifted education. *Multiple Voices for Ethnically Diverse Exceptional Learners, 10*(1–2), 28–44.

Foxx, S. P., Saunders, R., & Lewis, C. W. (2020). Race, gender, class, and achievement: A culturally responsive approach to urban school counseling. *Professional School Counseling, 23*(1_part_2), 2156759X19899184.

Galloway, M. K., Callin, P., James, S., Vimegnon, H., & McCall, L. (2019). Culturally responsive, antiracist, or anti-oppressive? How language matters for school change efforts. *Equity & Excellence in Education, 52*(4), 485–501. https://doi-org.ezproxy.liberty.edu/10.1080/10665684.2019.1691959

Gentry, M. (2020). *Schools often fail to identify gifted and talented students – Especially if they are black, Latino or Native American*. The Conversation. https://theconversation.com/schools-often-fail-to-identify-gifted-and-talented-students-especially-if-they-are-black-latino-or-native-american-130506

Goings, R. B., & Ford, D. Y. (2018). Investigating the intersection of poverty and race in gifted education journals: A 15-year analysis. *Gifted Child Quarterly, 62*(1), 25–36. https://doi.org/10.1177/2F0016986217737618

Gonzalez, I. A., & Cokley, R. K. (2021). The case for a core anti-racist course for counselors in training. *Teaching and Supervision in Counseling, 3*(2), 26–37.

Goodman-Scott, E., Betters-Bubon, J., & Donohue, P. (Eds.). (2019). The School Counselor's Guide to Multi-Tiered Systems of Support. Routledge.

Grissom, J. A., & Redding, C. (2016). Discretion and disproportionality: Explaining the underrepresentation of high-achieving students of color in gifted programs. *AERA Online, 2*(1), 1–15.

Harris-Murri, N., King, K., & Rostenberg, D. (2006). Reducing disproportionate minority representation in special education programs for students with emotional disturbances: Toward a culturally responsive response to intervention model. Education and Treatment of Children, 779–799.

Harris, P. C. (2015). Counseling and advising black male high school student-athletes. In *Black males and intercollegiate athletics: An exploration of problems and solutions*. Emerald Group Publishing Limited.

Harris, P. C., Mayes, R. D., Freeman, C., Eberly, B., Tatby, N., & Wiener, S. (2020). Men passionately pursuing purpose (MP3): A group counseling intervention for black male student athletes. *The Journal for Specialists in Group Work, 45*(2), 146–164.

Helmore, E. (2020, September 8). Colorado suspends black boy for playing with a toy gun during virtual class. *The Guardian*. https://www.theguardian.com/us-news/2020/sep/08/colorado-springs-boy-suspended-toy-gun-virtual-class-police

Hines, D. E., & Wilmot, J. M. (2018). From spirit-murdering to spirit-healing: Addressing anti-black aggressions and the inhumane discipline of black children. *Multicultural Perspectives, 20*(2), 62–69.

Hollinger, G. W., & Hansel, T. C. (2020). *Revisiting zero tolerance policy in public schools: The case for wraparound services, community partnerships, and anti-racist policies in alternative schooling*. Urban Social Work.

Johnson, G. S., & Carrico, J. C. (2020). School Counselors applying the ASCA 2016 ethical standards. *Journal of Counseling Research and Practice, 6*(1), 1.

Jones, K. (2012). Black Greek-letter organizations: A legacy of African American adult education, Doctoral Dissertation. https://etda.libraries.psu.edu/files/final_submissions/8025

Jones, D., & Hagopian, J. (2020). Black Lives Matter at school. Illinois: Haymaker Books.

Kamenetz, A. (2018). Suspensions are down in U.S. Schools but large racial gaps remain. Retrieved from https://www.npr.org/2018/12/17/677508707/suspensions-are-down-in-u-s-schools-but-large-racial-gaps-remain

Learning Disabilities Association of America. (2020). *Disproportionate identification of students of color in special education*. https://ldaamerica.org/lda_today/disproportionate-identification-of-students-of-color-in-special-education/

Leibowitz-Nelson, S. B., Baker, S. B., & Nassar, S. C. (2020). Multicultural and social justice counseling competencies: Institutional interventions for professional school counselors. *Journal of Counselor Leadership and Advocacy, 7*(1), 42–54.

Love, B. L. (2016). Anti-black state violence, classroom edition: The spirit murdering of black children. *Journal of Curriculum and Pedagogy, 13*(1), 22–25. https://doi.org/10.1080/15505170.2016.1138258

Luckey Goudelock, J. L. (2019). *Nurturing gifted African American children*. National Association for Gifted Children. https://www.nagc.org/sites/default/files/Parent%20CK/NAGC-TIP%20Sheet-Nurturing%20Gifted%20African%20American%20Children.pdf

Lynch, M. (2016). Black boys in crisis: They aren't reading? Retrieved from https://www.theedadvocate.org/black-boys-crisis-arent-reading/

Mayes, R. D., Hines, E. M., & Harris, P. C. (2014). Working with twice-exceptional African American students: Information for school counselors. *Interdisciplinary Journal of Teaching and Learning, 4*(2), 125–139.

McIntosh, R., & Curry, K. (2020). The Role of a Black Church-School Partnership in Supporting the Educational Achievement of African American Students. *School Community Journal, 30*(1), 161–189.

Mitcham, M., Agahe Portman, T. A., & Afi Dean, A. (2009). Role of school counselors in creating equitable—Educational opportunities for students with disabilities in urban settings. *Urban Education, 44*(4), 465–482.

Moon, N. S., & Singh, A. A. (2015). In their own voices: Adolescent African American Males' experiences of the achievement gap. *Journal of School Counseling, 13*(16), n16.

Moore, J. L., III, Henfield, M. S., & Owens, D. (2008). African American males in special education: Their attitudes and perceptions toward high school counselors and school counseling services. *American Behavioral Scientist, 51*(7), 907–927.

Morris, J. E. (2001). African American students and gifted education: The politics of race and culture. *Roeper Review, 24*, 59–62.

Morris, M. W. (2016). *Pushout: The criminalization of black girls in schools*. The New Press.

Mosley, D. V., Hargons, C. N., Meiller, C., Angyal, B., Wheeler, P., Davis, C., & Stevens-Watkins, D. (2020). Critical consciousness of anti-black racism: A practical model to prevent and resist racial trauma. *Journal of Counseling Psychology, 68*(1), 1–16.

Moss, L. G., & Singh, A. A. (2015). White school counselors becoming racial justice allies to students of color: A call to the field of school counseling. *Journal of School Counseling, 13*(5), 1–36.

Munroe, T. (2017). Enriching relational practices with critical anti-black racism advocacy and perspectives in schools. *Relational Child and Youth Care Practice, 30*(3), 32–45.

National Center for Educational Statistics. (2020). Racial/Ethnic Enrollment in Public Schools. https://nces.ed.gov/programs/coe/pdf/coe_cge.pdf

National Collegiate Athletic Association. (2021). *Diversity research: NCAA race/ethnicity and gender demographics database*. https://www.ncaa.org/about/resources/research/diversity-research

Nuamah, S. A. (2019). *How girls achieve*. Harvard University Press.

Owens, C. M., Ford, D. Y., Lisbon, A. J., & Owens, M. T. (2016). Shifting paradigms to better serve twice-exceptional African American learners. *Behavioral Disorders, 41*(4), 196–208. https://doi.org/10.17988/2Fbedi-41-04-196-208.1

Paolini, A. C. (2019). School counselors promoting college and career readiness for high school students. *Journal of School Counseling, 17*(2), n2.

Parker, L. (2017). Schools and the no-prison phenomenon: Anti-blackness and secondary policing in the black lives matter era. *Journal of Educational Controversy, 12*(1), 11. https://cedar.wwu.edu/jec/vol12/iss1/11

Plessy v. Ferguson, 163 U.S. 537 (1896).

Ratts, M. J., & Greenleaf, A. T. (2017). Multicultural and social justice counseling competencies: A leadership framework for professional school counselors. *Professional School Counseling, 21*(1b), 2156759X18773582.

Richey, K. M. G. (2018). Race in predominantly white schools: Implications for school counselors. *Electronic Theses and Dissertations. Paper, 3037*, 10.18297/etd/3037.

Robinson, K. J., & Roksa, J. (2016). Counselors, information, and high school college-going culture: Inequalities in the college application process. *Research in Higher Education, 57*(7), 845–868.

Rust, J. P. (2019). Addressing the sociocultural determinants of African American students' academic achievement: The four themes of the American school counselor association's national model and the role of school counselors. *Urban Education, 54*(8), 1149–1175.

Sabo, D., Vanfossen, B. E., & Melnick, M. J. (1993). High school athletic participation and postsecondary educational and occupational mobility: A focus on race and gender. *Sociology of Sport Journal, 10*, 44–56.

Shamsuddin, S. (2016). Taken out of context: Piecing together college guidance information in urban high schools. *The Urban Review, 48*(1), 101–122.

Shell, E. M. (2020). Exploring school counselors' preparation to address disproportionality of African American students in special education. *Teaching and Supervision in Counseling, 2*(1), 84–94. https://doi.org/10.7290/tsc020108

Shifrer, D. (2018). Clarifying the social roots of the disproportionate classification of racial minorities and males with learning disabilities. *The Sociological Quarterly, 59*(3), 384–406.

Shifrer, D., Muller, C., & Callahan, R. (2011). Disproportionality and learning disabilities: Parsing apart race, socioeconomic status, and language. *Journal of Learning Disabilities, 44*(3), 246–257.

Sproull, N. (2018, November 13). *NCAA eligibility center: Overview and updates*. ASCA Webinar Series. https://videos.schoolcounselor.org/ncaa-eligibility-center-overview-and-updates

Stambaugh, T., & Ford, D. Y. (2015). Microaggressions, multiculturalism, and gifted individuals who are black, Hispanic, or low income. *Journal of Counseling & Development, 93*(2), 192–201. Retrieved from https://doi.org/10.1002/j.1556-6676.2015.00195.x

Steele, J. M. (2008). Preparing counselors to advocate for social justice: A liberation model. *Counselor Education and Supervision, 48*(2), 74–85. https://doi.org/10.1002/j.1556-6978.2008.tb00064.x

Tarver-Behring, S., Spagna, M. E., & Sullivan, J. (1998). School counselors and full inclusion for children with special needs. *Professional School Counseling, 1*(3), 51–56.

Thornhill, T. (2019). We want black students, just not you: How white admissions counselors screen black prospective students. *Sociology of Race and Ethnicity, 5*(4), 456–470.

United Negro College Fund (2021). K-12 Disparity Facts and Statistics. Retrieved from https://uncf.org/pages/K-12-Disparity-Facts-and-Stats?gclid=CjwKCAjwy7CKBhBMEiwA0Eb7akFCwAXJ0a77KHUoq2aBCAhOxOM25IuJJWO/C1mcEPoeNGeARdJelBoCoUAQAvD_BwE

U.S. Office for Civil Rights. (2004). *Office for civil rights elementary and secondary school survey projections and documentation*. U.S. Department of Education, Author.

Watson, T. N., & Baxley, G. S. (2021). Centering grace: Challenging anti-blackness in schooling through Motherwork. *Journal of School Leadership, 31*(1–2), 142–157.

Wun, C. (2016). Unaccounted foundations: Black girls, anti-black racism, and punishment in schools. *Critical Sociology, 42*(4–5), 737–750.

Yancy, C. W. (2020). *COVID-19 and African Americans*. https://jamanetwork.com/journals/jama/fullarticle/2764789

17

Antisemitism and Islamophobia: Old and Dynamic Racisms

Waleed Y. Sami and Aliza H. Lambert

On October 27th, 2018, a gunman named Robert Bowers stormed the Tree of Life Synagogue located in Pittsburgh, Pennsylvania and opened fire with assault rifles and multiple handguns on the worshipers during Shabbat morning services. The horror that unfolded was all- consuming, and resulted in the murder of 11 congregants, with several others wounded. To date this was the largest massacre of Jews in US history, though synagogue shootings and bombings are commonplace. This particular massacre shook the American Jewish community, as Bowers's words reverberated: "All Jews must die" (Gessen, 2018, para 1). A short while before the shooting, investigations revealed that Bowers had posted on a social media website named *Gab*, several hateful and antisemitic statements, along with a call to attack the HIAS organization (Hebrew Immigrant Aid Society). HIAS is a Jewish run non-profit refugee resettlement agency that has operated for over a hundred years within the United

W. Y. Sami • A. H. Lambert (✉)
Virginia Commonwealth University, Richmond, VA, USA
e-mail: samiwy@vcu.edu; ahweiss@vcu.edu

© The Author(s), under exclusive license to Springer Nature Switzerland AG 2022

K. Johnson et al. (eds.), *Developing Anti-Racist Practices in the Helping Professions: Inclusive Theory, Pedagogy, and Application*,
https://doi.org/10.1007/978-3-030-95451-2_17

States. One of Bower's social media posts revealed a startling but old connection, when he said: "Open you Eyes! It's the filthy evil jews Bringing the Filthy evil Muslims into the Country!!" (Gessen, 2018, para 1).

Within Bower's white supremacist worldview, there exists an alliance between Jews and Muslims, bent on dominating a White and Christian civilizational identity. Many forms of white supremacist literature are marked with apocalyptic calls for defense of White Race. This collection of hate, calls for fighting back against Jewish plans to change the demographic nature of American society. Specifically, this attack was motivated by Bower's understanding of how HIAS was aiding Muslim immigrants and refugees resettle from war-torn lands. Thus, the most violent antisemitic attack in American history carried the intersection of Islamophobia and anti- immigrant hysteria as well. This is not an accidental connection. Indeed, the history of antisemitism and Islamophobia within Western society is old but dynamic, and predates the founding of the United States. This latent force was active during the beginning of this nation, as potential citizenship for Jews and Muslims (and Catholics) caused quite a political controversy in the late 1700s (Spellberg, 2014). It should also be noted that many of the African slaves in America and the Western hemisphere were Muslim as well, during several phases of the trans- Atlantic slave trade (Spellberg, 2014). Thus, Jews and Muslims have firm roots in the beginnings of the United States, and both forms of racism are intertwined and a part of our historical landscape. The authors will advance a theoretical basis for including Islamophobia and antisemitism concurrently within this chapter, dedicated to helping professionals and their antiracist practice. Understanding both racisms is critical for anti-racist work, and forms an integral piece for social justice praxis.

When assessing the historical and contemporary impact, it is notable that both forms of systemic discrimination represent old manifestations of the religious Other. Renton and Gidley (2017) argue that antisemitism and Islamophobia share a "relationship in this sense of simultaneous epistemological connectedness and political divergence," (p. 6). Despite different political antecedents, both Jews and Muslims have been targeted historically as threats to a Christian identity and heresy in traditional Europe (Renton & Gidley, 2017); however, this xenophobia and discrimination was not limited to religious ideology alone. As the transformation to secular nation states began post-Enlightenment, justifications evolved to racial and national fears (Renton & Gidley, 2017). This demonstrates the evolutionary nature of historical antisemitism and Islamophobia, and recognizes it as not contingent on a specific theology or politics; but rather its own dynamic, that accommodates many different politicized manifestations.

The definitional features and structures of antisemitism and Islamophobia are conceptually challenging, but also share important features (e.g., both groups seen as subversive, radical, alien). We will explore these features in detail later in the chapter. The history of exclusion has been theorized to serve different purposes. Within old European nation-states, Jews were a minority to single out, ostracize, and murder in order to defend an ethnically pure nation-state (Bunzl, 2007). However, as the importance of the nation-state has declined in recent years from the emergence of globalization, Islamophobia now seeks to defend a pan-European and Western civilizational identity under siege (Bunzl, 2007).

Additionally, while the underlying premise of these exclusions may theoretically differ over time, the practical implications of this xenophobia are similar. In fact, Jews and Muslims are the mutual target of far-right political groups across a variety of nations. Historically speaking, Jews and Muslims share the dubious distinction of being racialized as cultural and racial Others (Green, 2015). As noted in the opening description of the Tree of Life massacre, Jews and Muslims occupy mutual reinforcing genealogy within ever-growing white supremacist literature (Jansen & Meer, 2020; Meer & Noorani, 2008). Edward Said, the famous scholar of Orientalism and post-colonial studies, noted the deep similarity between antisemitism and anti- Muslim prejudice within popular imagination, arguing that they were practically interchangeable in contemporary society (Rubin, 2015). These same prejudices are deeply manifested within the recent refugee crises of our generation as well. For example, the banning of Syrian refugees and the larger Muslim Ban enacted by the US government, mirrors the discourse over the exclusion of Jewish refugees fleeing the Holocaust in WW2 (Klein, 2015; Wyman, 1985). For instance, *Das Kleine Blatt* (1939), an Austrian newspaper in the 1930s, depicted the flood of Jewish refugees as a threat to the European heartland. In contemporary times, *The Daily Mail* (2015), a British

Newspaper, depicted the Syrian refugees as rats, threatening Europe almost a hundred years later. Both images are still online and are noted in our reference section. Indeed, it is not a coincidence that the largest ethnic cleansing in Europe, post Holocaust, directly targeted Bosnian Muslims in the 1990s. Thus, the dehumanizing discourse from the past and present carries a remarkable and troubling similarity.

As antiracist helping professionals, we must be aware of the historical, structural, and present, challenges of bigotry and prejudice towards Jews and Muslims in our society today. Creating intentional conversations around religious diversity in training programs and familiarizing yourself with some of the basic themes of both racisms, are concrete steps to undertake in order to help develop your anti-racist pedagogy. This chapter will aid with your understanding of both of these discriminations. Additionally, it will equip you with knowledge and insight into the historical and present features of religious bigotry. Lastly, it will promote self-reflection of internalized biases, and allow the reader to critically examine politicized discourses around Jews and Muslims in America.

The Current Problem

Background on Antisemitism

There has been a steady increase in antisemitic hate crimes in the United States (ADL, 2020). In 2011, there were 771 FBI reported antisemitic hate crimes. While a slight dip in hate crimes towards Jews was noted in 2014, the numbers rose again to their highest mark between 2017 and 2019. These numbers were reported at around 953 hate crimes in 2019. It is noteworthy that the number of Americans that believe Jews face discrimination has increased by 20% from 2016 and was reported at 64% (Pew Research Center, 2019). The number of Americans that believe Jews face "a lot" of discrimination has gone from 13% to 24% (Pew Research Center, 2019). What has antisemitism specifically looked like in the United States, and where did it come from? America has had a consistent history of antisemitism. However, there are critical moments in US history, particularly beginning in the 1900s, that typify such prejudice.

Many may be unfamiliar with the Leo Frank case that took place in Atlanta Georgia, when Frank (a Jewish man) was wrongfully convicted and sentenced to the rape and murder of a Mary Phagan, a young Christian girl (Michael, 2005, p.102). Though Frank's sentence was reduced, he was dragged by a group of well-known and established southern gentlemen (a minister, two judges, and a sheriff) and lynched in 1915. Paranoia and conspiracies surrounding Jews historically as sexual predators, and killers of Christians (particularly Christian children), was exacerbated through the wrongful conviction and later lynching of Frank (Goldstein, 2006). The murderers were never convicted and supported publicly, which helped them band together to become the Knights of Mary Phagan.

Conspiracy theories and disease run rampant with Jewish scapegoating, and are an essential feature of antisemitism. One of the most egregious examples being the contemporary pandemic of COVID-19 linked to Jews, in order to corrupt the economy to make money, biological weaponry, and blood libel (Gerstenfeld, 2020). Jews have been targeted by neo-Nazis and white supremacists deliberately spitting on Jews to encourage the spread of COVID-19 through the Jewish community (Margolin, 2020). Jews have also been blamed for the spread of COVID-19, as a manifestation of long-standing disease conspiracies accusing Jews of spreading such diseases, and personifying poison (Antisemitic Conspiracy Myths, 2020). Blood libel is a conspiracy theory that dates back to the Middle Ages in Europe, when the Jews were blamed for numerous plagues (Gerstenfeld, 2020). A modern example of blood libel in America is QAnon believers that "falsely claim the cabal is abducting children to kill them and harvest their blood for a chemical known as adrenochrome, which is used to extend their lives"(Southern Poverty Law Center, 2020). QAnon has emerged in many ways, most noticeably in the political sphere, where about 90 candidates that ran for office in 2020 had shared QAnon messaging or openly stated their belief in this conspiracy theory (Southern Poverty Law Center, 2020). Conspiracy theories can be politicized in democratic societies, as we saw in Germany with the rise of Nazism that thrived on Jewish conspiracy theories. These false beliefs about the Jewish people's connection to plague and COVID-19, have led to accusations and strengthened fear of Jews within society. These features, combined with the historic racialization of Jews as an Other, have cemented antisemitism in the taxonomy of racism (Elukin, 2020).

Racializing Jews was a Nazi strategy during World War II, and was used as an ideological pretext to marginalize and eventually eliminate them (United States Holocaust Memorial Museum, 2021). Comics, cartoons, and booklets circulated depicting the very physical traits that made Jews not traditionally Aryan looking, with a lack of pureness. Jews were known as a cultural and racial Other, and this corroborated the very fear people had of personality traits and motives believed to be possessed by all Jews. In contemporary America, Jews have now become racialized as white (Gordon, 2016; Goldstein, 2006) and can be seen as both white and as an ethnic and religious minority. It is important to note the basis of pathologizing for Jews is measured on the scale of whiteness, which is used to determine one's humanity depending on where they fall on the scale. Being a religious minority, yet identifying with contemporary American whiteness, creates a space for both privilege and discrimination to cohabitate.

Racialization of the Jews in America, however, has been most noticeable in our history through the trope of creating a white nation, free of racial and ethnic minorities. The most notorious embodiment being the Ku Klux Klan, which is antisemitic and anti-black, and has carried on centuries of domestic terrorism. However, more subtle forms of racialization still manifest. A longstanding effort to racialize Jews was apparent when photographs of about a dozen Jewish Brandeis students, graduates, faculty, and staff were shared on a white supremacist forum. The slander spewed by these white supremacists included calling these Jews, and thousands of others in this thread, "greasy," and "pure evil" (Gould & Schaffel, 2019). Jews were profiled in 21 pages of "evidence" within the forum, spanning across many Jewish sects. One forum member called Jews the children of Satan and another referred to the international Hillel organization "a group of Jewish supremacist thugs" (Gould & Schaffel, 2019). This online thread that began in 2018, snowballed from an article in The Jewish Chronicle from 2012 of a woman, being told by a doctor she could have rhinoplasty to make her less Jewish and more beautiful (Gould & Schaffel, 2019). This tension between distinguishing racial traits of Jews, as distinct from "purer" racial phenotypes, provides the grounds to legitimize bigotry, and perpetrates conspiracy theories and fears throughout the general population.

The history of antisemitism runs deep and intersects with the history of Islamophobia. One of the most prominent points of intersections is the racialization of both religious communities. In studying *Jews of Color in North America* (Gordon, 2016) stated that: "The prototypical term *raza* from which the word "race" emerged was, after all, a Medieval Spanish word to refer to breeds of dogs, horses, Jews and Moors (Afro-Muslims)" (p.105). This follows the legacy of the *Reconquista* and Inquisition, which saw the Iberian Peninsula come under complete domination of King Ferdinand and Queen Isabella, leading the forcible conversion and ethnic cleansing of Jews and Muslims. As noted earlier, both groups inhabited shared spaces of exclusion which often intersected. We will review the background of Islamophobia and note the congruent similarities.

Background on Islamophobia

Islamophobia is a modern term, developed to describe bigotry, discrimination, and innate fear of Muslims (Green, 2015). Islamophobia is the discrimination and the prejudice against Muslims, or simply: anti-Muslim racism (Green, 2015). The term Islamophobia was coined by a British anti-racist non-profit organization called Runnymede Trust in 1997 (Conway, 1997). The nonprofit organization was commissioned by the British government to investigate and come up with solutions to help inform policy in creating a more inclusive and safer British society. The Runnymede Trust first introduced the concept of Islamophobia to the public, and noted that a theoretical conceptualization needed to be created in order to combat rising discrimination against Muslims in England. The Runnymede Trust also attempted to conceptualize modern antisemitism in England as well. While initially created for the British Public, these features of Islamophobia, and the word itself, has become the contemporary way of describing racism against Muslims throughout the West, and the rest of the world (Green, 2015).

Islamophobia and its history present an alarming challenge in contemporary America, and in many parts of the world. Hate crimes, assaults, and other forms of intimidation against Muslim-Americans have increased since 9/11, after an escalation and a plateau (Kishi, 2017). Hate crimes (as collected by the FBI), are often a poor way to grasp the enormity of discrimination, as they are routinely underreported and undercounted (Kishi, 2017). Other measures can help us understand this dynamic. The Pew Research Center, an internationally recognized expert on polling, demographics, and social insight, released a feelings thermometer in 2014, measuring how Americans feel towards all major religious groups in the nation. The results showed Americans report the "coldest" feelings towards Muslims, compared to every other major religion within the United States (though the feelings have gotten slightly warmer since) (Greenwood, 2017b). Indeed, a Gallup poll found that 4 out of 10 Americans feel some sort of prejudice towards Muslims, higher than any other major religious group within the United States (The Gallup Center for Muslim Studies, 2010). Furthermore, 4 in 10 Americans also believe that Islam promotes violence, though that position is distinctly impacted by a respondents age, education, and political partisanship (Pew Research Center, 2019). Large numbers of Americans continue to hold negative views believing that some, to most Muslims are Anti-American, along with recent polls demonstrating that 50% of Americans believe Islam is fundamentally incompatible with democracy (Greenwood, 2017b). Even when holding no personal prejudices against Muslims, one third of Americans still hold unfavorable opinions about Islam, or believe that Islam is inherently intolerant of other religions (Gallup Inc., 2020). This dynamic is incredibly alarming as it demonstrates that many Americans can withhold personal prejudice towards individuals, but still have ideologically derived unfavorable opinions about the religion at large. This can make them passive supporters of systemic discrimination against Muslims. Indeed, this sentiment is found in Europe too, with a recent survey ranking Muslims just below drug addicts, as the least desired neighbors throughout several European nations (Gallup Inc., 2020).

Not coincidentally, this hostility is reflected within the lives of Muslim-Americans. Out of all major religious groups, Muslims self-report the highest level of personal experiences of discrimination and prejudice, on par with rates self-reported by Black and Latino Americans (Gallup Inc., 2020). Furthermore, 42% of Muslim-American students report being bullied for their faith, four times greater than the general public, and greater than peers of other faiths and/or identities (Moghaed & Chouhoud, 2017). This is likely due to adult and staff participation in bullying, which pushes the threshold of bullying to such a high degree (Moghaed & Chouhoud, 2017).

Muslim-Americans find themselves at the nexus of the security, surveillance, and carceral state within the United States. A stunning example was revealed in 2012, when a team of reporters from the Associated Press (AP), won a Pulitzer award for uncovering the systemic spying, infiltration, and coercion of informants by the NYPD on the Muslim-American population (The Pulitzer Prizes, 2012). This sprawling, domestic spying operation encompassed several states, and spied on the daily lives and interactions of Muslim-Americans in their homes, restaurants, mosques, colleges, and political events (The Pulitzer Prizes, 2012). This operation was overseen by the Demographics Unit of the NYPD, and hundreds of millions of dollars were devoted to this domestic spying operation, which involved violations of constitutional rights and invasive surveillance. Furthermore, the program involved deep infiltration into friend groups, with undercover agents pretending to convert in order to secretly record conversations, and mass surveillance of over 250 mosques and student groups across the northeast (The Pulitzer Prizes, 2012). Despite millions of dollars, violations of constitutional rights, and CIA influence, the program yielded very little intelligence "successes' 'to justify its existence. It was finally disbanded after pressure from various civil rights groups and Muslim advocacy organizations.

This domestic surveillance and coercion are not atypical in the lives of Muslims within the United States. Indeed, the American Civil Liberties Union (ACLU) noted in a letter to President Obama in 2014, that: "the government's domestic counterterrorism policies treat entire minority communities as suspect, and American Muslims have borne the brunt of government suspicion, stigma and abuse," (American Civil Liberties

Union, 2014, p. 1). These deep links with the security state are also demonstrated with domestic mass incarceration. For example, despite Muslims being close to or under, one percent of the American population, they make up about nine percent of state prisoners (Muslim Advocates, 2019). Within the carceral system, Muslims face large hurdles are further policed for their faith, and often denied constitutionally protected religious rights (Muslim Advocates, 2019).

Within the "History of Islamophobia", we will discuss some of the historical and modern currents that have led to contemporary society viewing Muslims through a War on Terror security lenses, justifying state and social discrimination against them. As helping professionals, it is important to have insight into the dynamics of discrimination against Muslims and Jews in our society today. These insights are a necessary first step in developing practical and concrete interventions within the classroom, clinical practice, and the larger political sphere to combat these systemic prejudices. Your clients and students will have to navigate multiple layers of state and social discrimination, potentially impacting the therapeutic relationship and how they perceive professional help and support.

History and Features of Antisemitism

Difficulty in Defining Antisemitism

Defining antisemitism is quite complex for a multitude of reasons. Firstly, "antisemitism, is an idea that is profoundly anachronistic; it is unbounded by time or context" (Elukin, 2020, p. 20). Antisemitism infects perceptions that morph through time to meet the needs of people to scapegoat entire communities for social problems. Secondly, antisemitism is unique and quite different from other types of prejudice. Antisemitism feeds on social paranoia and links Jews with false explanations of very complex economic, social, and political problems in society. These false ideas have formed surrounding Jewish communities span across eras, cultures, and geographic locations, to justify the violence and discrimination faced by

Jews. Thus, Jewish minority communities in society are often unique intersections of social identity. However, this uniqueness has made them a target in many European nations historically, with the Holocaust being the most dramatic example. Lastly, Jews increasingly own multiple ethnic identities (Magid, 2012, p. 102). Jews have immigrated to America from all over the world, particularly during pogroms and the events leading up to the Holocaust (Goldscheider, 2009). Jewish communities are historically diverse, with many such as the Sephardic and Mizrahi communities that are interwoven with historic Muslim and Christian populations throughout the Middle-East and North Africa. Jewish communities have also been present in Ethiopia for several thousand years, and Ashkenzai Jews are a part of larger European diasporas. As generations continue to grow, Jews continue to diversify, thus further complicating the narrative and manifestation of antisemitism in everyday lives of Jews.

Antisemitism as a term has epistemological origins in the nineteenth century in Austria, but originated as an ideal, centuries prior (Elukin, 2020). The term antisemitism came out of necessity to conceptualize a form of political discrimination, as politicians used pseudo-science and racialized language to distinguish between Aryans and Semites, in order to inhibit Jews from receiving civil rights across central Europe (Elukin, 2020). Antisemitism fed into depictions of Jews that became formulaic and scientifically racist, reflecting racial concerns of that time (McGeever & Virdee, 2017). As noted by Linda Martín Alcoff, when a racialized identity is invisible, fear is created and an existential enemy can be erected (1999).

This social fear parallels that of Islam, and is apparent in the similar tactics of Othering both Jews and Muslims. It is noticeable that there are racial and social traits considered "Jewish" and exhibiting these traits is unacceptable and reprehensible. For example, money management has been linked to Jewish racial character historically as a stereotype, but is related to how Jews were marginalized from other forms of career and job opportunities in Europe. Along with social marginalization, Jews were also falsely accused of spreading plagues through poisoning wells during 1348–1349 (Elukin, 2020). Associating Jews with money and disease is a historic, European trope that can re-emerge in contemporary moments.

The rise of antisemitism in literature is often categorized as ethnic prejudice, which includes concepts such as scapegoating and ethnic competition. Jews have been feared for their religious beliefs, racial characteristics, their economic behavior, and their leading roles in subversive European political movements, such as socialism (Brustein & King, 2004, p. 38). Thus, antisemitism is a form of xenophobia that is complex and widespread through a spectrum of mediums, such as religion, politics, and economics (Brustein & King, 2004). This difficulty in defining antisemitism acts as another accelerant of antisemitism; being that it is so amorphous and can be applied with flexibility to suit scapegoating needs.

The Holocaust for American Jews and Identity Development

The Holocaust for American Jews cannot be separated from American Jewish identity. Identity development for American Jews is complex, much like for other Americans (Magid, 2012). Jewish Americans often reflect on America's role during the Holocaust. In the alarming antisemitism leading up to the Holocaust, America and other countries stood idly by, as pogroms mounted in Europe. A notable instance was the call for help that was unanswered during the Evian Conference in 1938 (Brustein & King, 2004). During the conference, countries sent condolences and pledges of support to the Jewish refugees, yet many countries still denied accepting them. Not only were borders closing to let Jews in, but they were also diverting more refugees (Brustein & King, 2004). Notably, the Dominican Republic and Costa Rica increased their refugee quotas, but the message was already sent, as the world cast away German and Austrian Jewish refugees.

America further perpetuated negligence by failing to pass the Wagner-Rogers Child Refugee Bill, a bill that would have opened America's borders to 20,000 Jewish refugee children, and by denying entry to the 936 Jewish refugees aboard the St. Louis (Brustein & King, 2004). There has been much debate about the presence and role of America during WWII. Wyman (2019), argues that Roosevelt's indifference to Jewish refugees and their annihilation is one of the black marks on American history (p. 219). Though America had resources and feasible plans, the very fear of hindering war efforts was strong enough to drown out the desire to save Jewish refugees (Wyman, 2019).

Antisemitism Meaning

Antisemitism is an ideology; it is a framework for how one can see the world. When we look at antisemitism as an ideology, one can describe its contours succinctly. These contours involve an irrational inclination to defend groundless beliefs about Jews (Marcus, 2015). This ideology can be synonymous with illusion, giving people the grounds to victimize Jews. It is also conveniently generalizable, as America grapples simultaneously with its illusive fear of Muslims. For both Jews and Muslims, the ideology of antisemitism and Islamophobia is coercive, paving a way for united fear and subjection to spread.

What happens out of this fear is a true, almost metaphysical vision. This antisemitism gives way to, as Marcus (2015) notes a: "double illusion in which first the Jew disappears behind 'the Jew,' and then the underlying trauma that caused this distortion is forgotten" (p.27). This trauma results in seeing the Jewish person as truly the very object of fear itself, and not always the human features behind the fear. Dehumanization is a necessary process to engage in antisemitism, and thus is congruent with how we understand racism. This ideology is also systemic, in the sense that for it to be cyclical, people must have a lack of awareness and interest in how impactful and historical this discrimination is on our society. Thus, despite the progress Jewish citizens in America have made since WW2, the tropes of antisemitism can be re-deployed to suit national crises (e.g., COVID-19), in order to serve this consistent need to scapegoat. Now that we have discussed some of the features and histories of antisemitism, we will explore Islamophobia. As an antiracist professional, you will be able to quickly notice and point out the similarities that emerge and make them intertwined, yet distinct phenomena.

History and Features of Islamophobia

Similar to antisemitism, Islamophobia's definitional structure can be complex, and creates further questions about the nature of the word. Indeed, bigotry against Muslims has a long and dynamic history. Initially, Islam was viewed as a demonic heresy, and as a punishment for sins committed by Christians (Green, 2015). This morphed into a cultural and civilizational anxiety, as wars erupted over resources and territory, culminating in the tragic Crusades, which lasted for several hundred years (Green, 2015). These Crusades also included Jews as their target. However, it is important to note that there were harmonious inter-faith communities and intellectual exchanges through the medieval ages, and one shouldn't view the entirety of Muslim-Christian relations through simple, geo-political conflict. With the dawn of the Enlightenment, there was some progress in engaging with Islamic thought. Many diverse Western intellectuals and leaders, such as Goethe, Nietzsche, Carlyle, Gibbon, Napoleon, and Benjamin Franklin, spoke highly of some of the features of the faith (Tolan, 2019). However, with the advent of European colonization and the latter twentieth and twenty-first century, bigotry of Muslims shifted from Christian ideological justifications, to political, secular, and militaristic ones, in order to justify colonization and resource extraction (Tolan, 2019). This captures the dynamism of the contemporary forms of Islamophobia, which re-hashes and surfaces old tropes in deployment of new ideologies. It is important to note that theological or secular justifications have been historically utilized to support Islamophobia, and aren't inherent to either ideology. This mirrors the history of antisemitism as well.

Islamophobia has several features, and we will list them before going into detail. (1). Islam as monolithic and static, (2). Islam as separate and other), (3). Islam as inferior, (4). Islam as the enemy, (5). Muslims are manipulative, (6). Discrimination is justified, (7). Muslim criticisms of the West are invalid, (8). Anti-Muslim discourse is natural (Conway, 1997). As seen above, these features echo antisemitism closely.

Islam as Monolithic and Static

This feature refers to a conception of Islam as being essentialized, or made up of fundamental, uncomplicated essences that define and predict the behavior of its adherents. This neglects the diversity, plurality, and history of the faith, and removes any complicated engagement with it (Conway, 1997). Perhaps the easiest way to understand this feature, is the constant linkage Islam has with terrorism and extremism in our consciousness (Green, 2015). Violent acts committed by Muslims are somehow indicative of the fundamental nature of Islam, as encouraging violence. When Muslims don't commit violence, however, or are the victims of violence (by Muslims or non-Muslims), then this is considered in light of other circumstances, and not influenced by their faith. Thus, when Muslims commit violence, it is due to their faith. When they engage in social justice or are victims of violence, that can't possibly be associated with their faith, making the connection to Islam as monolithic and static entity complete (Conway, 1997). Thus, Islam's intellectual and cultural diversity is eliminated in favor of promoting a black-and-white worldview.

Islam as Separate and Other

Islam as Other, refers to labeling Islam as an alien belief system, that shares nothing in common with other belief systems, values, and normative ethics found in any other society (Conway, 1997). A brief look at history easily refutes this point, as various Islamic civilizations have enriched and been enriched by various other cultures, belief systems, and values across much of the world (Conway, 1997). Indeed, one of the deep ironies is that Islam is often held up as a paradigmatic Other to Western Enlightenment values, when various Muslim philosophers, scientists, and thinkers helped contribute to the Enlightenment (Tolan, 2019). Green (2015, p. 14), demonstrates this modern attitude by discussing Switzerland's 2009 mosque minaret ban, by quoting a member of the Swiss People's Party who backed the ban, as describing Christian Churches as representing diversity and tolerance, and Islamic Mosques as representing the opposite of tolerance. The Islamic Tradition is as diverse and pluralistic as any other, and can't be easily summarized in a generalizable way. This Other-ing reflects a false binary, and is integral to Islamophobia.

Islam as Inferior

Islam as inherently inferior closely aligns with it being a complete Other (Conway, 1997). If a religion, ethnic group, country, or a community is a cultural Other and a permanent outsider, it likely means that the faith will also be inferior in values. For example, Islam is often accused of being barbaric, inherently sexist, and more totalitarian, in comparison to enlightened, gender-equal, and rational Westerners (Green, 2015). Indeed, this formulation has gripped the minds of many policy makers, government agencies, and security networks with Western nations for many years, influencing policy (Esposito, 1999). This is best articulated in the infamous "Clash of Civilizations" thesis advocated by academic Samuel Huntington, who argued that population growth amongst Muslim-majority nations would lead to inevitable war. This was due to the inherent incompatibility with universal liberal, Western values (Huntington, 2011). Originally published in the early 90s, this thesis has become the underlying ideology that guides much of the policy choices by the political elite of today (Kumar, 2015). This inherent, civilizational inferiority sets the stage for policies and political agendas that create systematic marginalization.

Islam as the Enemy

The features of discrimination are intertwined and linked with each other. If one chooses to believe that another religious group is an alien Other and inferior, it is not surprising that they will represent an existential enemy. Islam is viewed as an enemy, precisely because inherent essences of violence, conquest, and subjugation are ascribed to Islam's fundamental qualities, not political choices made by Muslim groups in response to contingent events (Green, 2015). An excellent example was the rise of ISIS (The Islamic State of Iraq and Syria), an extremist group that was able to seize control over a large swath of land in the Levant area of the Middle East for a few years. ISIS was an outgrowth of the insurgency against the American occupation in Iraq, starting in 2003. Accompanying their rise were gruesome acts of atrocity and conquest over their opponents (whether they were Muslims or non-Muslim), and a string of high-profile terrorist incidents around many parts of the world. Many commentators simply argued that ISIS was not an extreme group of Muslims radicalized through perpetual war and trauma, rather just the realization of Islam itself, as naturally violent and blood-thirsty. This is despite the reams of evidence to the contrary, and the fact that most of the victims of ISIS were Muslims themselves (Sandberg & Colvin, 2020). Contrary evidence didn't matter to this formulation, as Islam's inherent quality of aggression was confirmed in the eyes of many due to ISIS's behavior. Indeed, empirical analysis of the media overwhelmingly focuses on the violent behavior of Muslims, contributing to the underlying feature of Islamophobia (Green, 2015). Thus, Muslims can be characterized as permanent and existential enemies, due to Islam's inherent aggressive pathologies.

Islam as Manipulative

Muslims as manipulative refers to how they may appear as normal citizens and neighbors, interested in the same things you are (e.g. family, health, education, jobs), but that are stealthily attempting to undermine our democratic values (Conway, 1997). In this conceptualization, Muslims are represented as a 5th column of duplicitous people within a society, ready to undermine and destroy it secretly from within. An example of this is the idea that Muslims will secretly hide their faith or their devotion from scrutiny through a practice called *Taqiyya* (note the historical similarities with Jews being seen as subversive). *Taqiyya* was a practice undertaken by medieval *Shia* Muslims to escape oppression and discrimination at the hands of authorities. In modern times, this has become a standard Islamophobic talking point, as individuals point to this historical practice as evidence that Muslims can manipulate and hide their true intentions. Ben Carson, a 2016 Republican nominee for president, and the Secretary of Housing and Urban Development under President Trump's administration, told the *Hill* newspaper that: "Taqiyya is a component of Sharia that allows, and even encourages you to lie to achieve your goals" (Kessler, 2015). Another example is the concept of "Love Jihad" in India. Islamophobic Indian authorities have long sought to enact a law to "protect" Hindu women from marrying Muslim men (Rao, 2011). Their claim is that Muslim men seduce and Hindu women into falling in love and converting, leaving their families and faith, despite there being no evidence of this practice (Rao, 2011). Claims of romantic seduction and demographic anxiety are found in England (The Guardian, 2017) and Israel as well (Frenkel, 2009).

Racism Against Muslims Is Justified

As the features of Islamophobia (built on fear and Othering) are maintained, it is natural to arrive at the conclusion that racism against Muslims must be justified for social safety (Conway, 1997). Indeed, some of the critiques offered by individuals critical of the world Islamophobia, point to marked differences between racism and prejudice, and being critical of a religion's underlying philosophy, thought, and practices. The former they deem to be unacceptable, the latter they believe is a part of intellectual freedom. Thus, many Islamophobic individuals couch their bigotry in freedom of speech, and thought. This is easily refuted by pointing out that Muslims are racialized individuals within the social sphere (Gotonda, 2011). This racialization is inscribed in law and practice, as profiling and surveillance are justified on racialized grounds. Sam Harris, the famous neuroscientist and atheist thinker, argued that profiling Muslims in an airport line is an acceptable security practice (Green, 2015). One can't profile without salient physical evidence, as religious thought and association are internal and should in theory, carry no racial features. However, Muslims are racialized as brown-skinned, turbaned, scarf-wearing, bearded, and menacing within the popular imagination (Gotonda, 2011). Non-Muslims, such as Sikhs, Hindus, and Catholic Latinos have also been racially harassed as Muslims, due to these features. This racialization is similar to the Jewish experience as well. Thus, when Muslims are profiled, they are automatically racialized. This is contrary to the actual demographic make-up of the Muslim-American community, which is deeply diverse and has no ethnic or racial majority within it (Greenwood, 2017a).

Racialization of Muslims as non-White, and denying citizenship to them has also contributed to the racialization of Islam in America. For example, Christian immigrants from Lebanon have been able to justify citizenship cases in the early 1900s due to their association with Christianity, which is racialized as White within American legal tradition (Beydoun, 2014). The same immigrants from Lebanon, who happened to be Muslim, were denied citizenship on the basis that their Islamic association made them non-White (Beydoun, 2014). Thus, the racialization of Islam in America has a deep history with systemic features. Islamophobia follows the well-worn path of racism, and is not congruent with the political values of free- speech.

Muslim Critiques of the West Are Invalid

This feature functions as a "one-way street", according to Green (2015, p.17). The "West" can critique the features of Islam that are deemed incompatible with liberal civilization, but any response by Muslims that complicates the binary is rejected outright. For example, whenever violence or dysfunction is perpetrated by Muslims, Islam is often used as the explanatory variable to understand the phenom, as opposed to contingent geopolitics and historical dynamics. However, whenever Muslims critique Western imperialism, intervention, global capitalism, or point to the natural divides within many Western nations among race, language, and social class that can lead to violence, these are considered out of the pale and not serious. Muslim clients and students often find their explanations, defenses, or critiques invalidated or stymied within popular discourse, leading them to lose trust with institutions and professionals. As noted above, empirical analysis of media content featuring Muslims skews overwhelmingly towards Islamophobic tropes, in order to profit off of alarm and fear.

Anti-Muslim Discourse Is Normal

Indeed, one of the striking features of Islamophobia today is the deep consensus between different political classes, whether liberal or conservative, on the threat of Muslims. This normalizes Islamophobic discourse, and challenges any ability to hold individuals and institutions accountable. For example, noted public liberal comedian Bill Maher, has openly expressed contempt over demographic births of Muslims in Western nations, and argued that ISIS is too similar to the "Muslim world" (Jalabi, 2014). Aforementioned Sam Harris, argues that: "Islam contains specific notions of martyrdom and jihad that fully explain the character of Muslim violence" (Harris, 2011). Furthermore, many political parties on the right throughout Europe and America, are characterized by nationalist politics and anti-immigration policies, that feature Islamophobic discourse and policy (Hafez, 2014). This is despite them adopting certain liberal, domestic positions on marriage and sexuality. Thus, anti-Muslim discourse does not easily fall into left or right ideological camps, and is normalized across a broad spectrum of political thought.

None of these features eliminate intellectual critique of the Islamic faith, or adherence to any of its core beliefs and practices. One can for example, not believe that the Qur'an is the divinely revealed word of God (a baseline Muslim belief), without utilizing Islamophobic features. Indeed, there exists a myriad of different literature examining, debating, and pursuing deeper questions around the religion in various Islamic Studies fields around the world, without defaulting to discourse that treats the faith as monolithic, an alien Other, or Muslims as manipulative enemies (Green, 2015). Mastering the understanding of Islamophobia, allows helping professionals to engage in social justice concerns around the status of Muslims and to be critical of discourse around Islam that is politicized in our society against your Muslim clients and co-workers.

Conclusion

As noted in the introduction, Islamophobia and antisemitism carry congruent similarities of exclusion, discrimination, and racial Other-ing within the West. Suffice to say that the problem of both discriminations is not wholly a Western phenomenon anymore, and within international politics, both are likely to be found in any society and nation today. This chapter provides broad features of both discriminations, along with current knowledge of contemporary events within the United States that carry antisemitic and Islamophobic features. Knowledge of the features of both discriminations will help the professional in understanding the role they will play in your clients, patients, and colleague's lives. Additionally, both phenomena can serve as a place for advocacy and social justice. Lastly, they will equip the practitioners with critical and historical perspectives to place these discriminations in context whenever they resurface within society.

Various helping professionals of diverse disciplines will benefit from incorporating the knowledge provided in the preceding sections. As systemic and historic forms of racism and religious bigotry, antisemitism and Islamophobia have complicated overt and latent expressions that can be found in a variety of contexts in society. As noted above, they continue to manifest in dangerous ways through our contemporary moment. Thus, there is a strong likelihood that your students, clients, and patients from these backgrounds orient themselves in ways to protect from these racisms. Understanding their history and how they appear socially through politics, media, and educational systems, will allow you to become an ally of these communities, while not essentializing them into fundamental characteristics that are not dynamic and diverse.

Antisemitism and Islamophobia are acute and dangerous forms of racism and discrimination. Antiracism practice cannot be complete without a comprehensive and thorough understanding of them. This understanding gives way to necessary self-reflection. Our hope is that the practitioner engages with the text and critically assesses their own interactions with antisemitism and Islamophobia. While this chapter focused on features of discrimination against Jews and Muslims, it is not exhaustive of all forms of discrimination and bigotry towards individuals who practice a faith. Indeed, Sikhs, Hindus, Catholics, Mormons, and indigenous religions have faced forms of exclusion, discrimination, and bigotry as well. This chapter cannot document the unique dynamic behind all of these discriminations. However, we invite professionals to develop and incorporate antiracist frameworks to help educate and advocate for all of those who face persecution, due to their faith.

The following are concrete steps that any helping professional can take to commit to the safety of Muslim and Jewish clients and students:

- As a provider you can add the religious holiday Google calendar to your personal calendar. To do this, go into your Google calendar and select the plus sign next to the "other calendars" section. Then you can search different religious holidays to add (e.g. Muslim Holidays and Jewish Holidays). Though holiday start times and dates vary throughout the world for the Muslim and Jewish communities, due to the adherence to the lunar calendar, having a general awareness of when holidays fall is important. This can help guide when you have social events, meetings, and due dates for assignments, and generally make your coworkers and students feel welcome by acknowledging their diversity.
- Professionals and educators can collaborate with reputable national organizations that focus on civil rights and advocate for anti-discrimination laws and regulations to be upheld. Specifically, the Anti-Defamation League (ADL), and the Council of American-Islamic Relations (CAIR), provide national support, training, and legal advocacy for Jews and Muslims. This collaboration could entail training and resources directed at students and other professionals, so they have a baseline awareness of both racisms and their structural solutions.
- Safe spaces for Muslim and Jewish students don't naturally exist, so creating these spaces is even more necessary. To do this you can set aside time and space for conversations with your students and colleagues about religious diversity and discrimination they may face. Be intentional by setting a topic of discussion and parameters to again ensure safety. You can create a suggested agenda and get feedback from members of the community.

  Having group discussions creates a community of people, who can open the door to meaningful conversations. Creating intentional discussion and meeting groups in early training programs that are focused on religious pluralism can expose students and future professionals to deeper relationships and decrease potential alienation. In order to prevent alienation, making clear statements about religious pluralism can help promote feelings of safety amongst a diverse array of students.

- Educators can make intentional connections with various Jewish and Muslim communities around their area, and invite them to speak about their unique faith and traditions. This early exposure can be very powerful for setting the tone of inclusion and diversity. If connections are challenging to make, educators can reach out to various Muslim and Jewish colleagues within the helping professions to help fill this critical gap.
- Students and professionals must be critical consumers of popular media, news, and government policy. Especially if these policies include security-based measures that target entire communities. As mentioned in the chapter, the history of Islamophobia and antisemitism is deep and infects depictions, perspectives, and popular narratives/framing of stories. Questioning how conflicts and narratives are framed through popular media and mainstream news is important, as Jews and Muslims are often impacted by national and international critical incidents that place their respective communities under the crosshairs. Both communities are often deeply connected with their international co- religionists, and feel kinship within the diaspora. Thus, critical incidents happening outside of the United States can potentially impact the functioning of your students/colleagues. For example, noting how the War on Terror marginalizes Muslims domestically and creates chaos for them abroad is an important context for how Muslim- Americans navigate their experiences with the media and official policy-making institutions.

We are hopeful that the next generation of Americans transitioning into the helping professions, are able to become aware of both racisms, and help promote concrete steps within their practice to alleviate some of the challenges posed within the text.

Guiding Questions

1. Antisemitism is at an all-time low

    - True
    - False

2. 42% of Muslim-American students report being bullied for their faith, four times greater than the general public, and greater than peers of other faiths and/or identities (Moghaed & Chouhoud, 2017). This is largely due to:

   A. Students and their misunderstandings of Islam
   B. The school curriculum failing to address religion due to the division of church and state
   C. Adult and staff participation in bullying
   D. Political allegiance and geographic location

3. CAIR and ADL are________?

   A. Government programs
   B. Intelligence services
   C. Different religious doctrines
   D. Muslim and Jewish civil rights agencies

4. Jewish refugees during World War 2 were accepted in this country, as it increased its quota for refugees:

   A. Dominican Republic
   B. United States
   C. Finland
   D. Canada

5. Jews and Muslims have both become racialized, meaning they are considered races of people instead of religious people.

   A. True
   B. False

6. All of the following are concrete steps to create safe spaces for Muslim and Jewish students except:

   A. Add the religious holiday Google calendar to your personal calendar.
   B. Set aside time and space for conversations with your students and colleagues.
   C. Ask your students to give lectures about their religion
   D. Be critical consumers of popular media and news.

7. Which of following is not a feature of Islamophobia:
   A. Islam as the dominate world religion
   B. Islam as Separate and Other
   C. Islam as Inferior
   D. Islam as the Enemy
8. All of the following are conspiracy theories about Jews except:
   A. Jews drink blood of Christian children
   B. COVID-19 is linked to Jews, in order to corrupt the economy
   C. Jews spread the plague through poisoning wells during the plague in 1348–1349
   D. America is the most Jewish populated country in the world.

1. What are the similarities that you note with the other chapters on antiracism? How does racism against religious minorities differ? How is it similar?
2. Discuss the differences and similarities between Islamophobia and antisemitism. Were you surprised?
3. Process the congruencies between various refugee crises in our contemporary moment and the past. What is it about refugees that provokes polarized reactions throughout history?
4. Discuss the concrete steps outlined at the end of the chapter. Will they be easy or hard to implement? What are the potential barriers?

References

Alcoff, L. M. (1999). Toward a phenomenology of racial embodiment. *Radical Philosophy*, (95), 15–26.

American Civil Liberties Union. (2014). *Civil rights groups ask administration to explain NSA surveillance of American Muslims*. https://www.aclu.org/press-releases/civil-rights-groups-ask-administration-explain-nsa-surveillance-american-muslims

Antisemitic conspiracy theories, Qanon movement on the rise with spread of covid-19. *World Jewish Congress*. (2020, November 30). https://www.worldjewishcongress.org/en/news/antisemitic-conspiracy-theories-qanon-movement-on-the-rise-with-spread-of-covid-19-11-1-2020

Anti-Defamation League. (2020). Audit of antisemitic incidents 2019. Retrieved from https://www.adl.org/audit2019

Beydoun, K. A. (2014, November 22). *Between Muslim and white: The legal construction of Arab American identity*. SSRN. https://papers.ssrn.com/sol3/papers.cfm?abstract_id=2529506

Brustein, W. I., & King, R. D. (2004). Anti-Semitism in Europe before the holocaust. *International Political Science Review, 25*(1), 35–53. https://doi.org/10.1177/0192512104038166

Bunzl, M. (2007). *Anti-Semitism and islamophobia: Hatreds old and new in Europe*. Prickly Paradigm Press.

Conway, G. (1997). *Islamophobia*. Runnymede Trust. Commission on British Muslims and Islamophobia. https://www.runnymedetrust.org/companies/17/74/Islamophobia-A-Challenge-for-Us-All.html

Das Kleine Blatt. (1939, February 2). *Enormous profits* [Cartoon]. The New Humanitarian. https://www.thenewhumanitarian.org/photo/201511191600190569/cartoon-depicting-jewish-refugees-rats-thrown-out-germany-and-nazi-occupied

Elukin, J. (2020). Antisemitism: Understanding its meaning, context, and history when teaching the holocaust. In L. J. Hilton & A. J. Patt (Eds.), *Understanding and teaching the holocaust* (pp. 19–31). The University of Wisconsin Press.

Esposito, J. L. (1999). *The islamic threat: Myth or reality?* (3rd ed.). Oxford University Press.

Frenkel, S. (2009, October 12). Vigilantes patrol for Jewish women dating Arab men. *National Public Radio*. https://www.npr.org/templates/story/story.php?storyId=113724468

Gallup, Inc. (2020, June 8). *Islamophobia: Understanding anti-Muslimism sentiment in the west*. Gallup.Com. https://news.gallup.com/poll/157082/islamophobia-understanding-anti-muslim-sentiment-west.aspx

Gerstenfeld, M. (2020). *The COVID-19 crisis: Impact and implications* (pp. 41–45, Rep.), E. Karsh (Ed.). Begin-Sadat Center for Strategic Studies. https://doi.org/10.2307/resrep26356.12.

Gessen, M. (2018, October 28). Why the tree of life shooter was fixated on the Hebrew immigrant aid society. *The New Yorker*. https://www.newyorker.com/news/our-columnists/why-the-tree-of-life-shooter-was-fixated-on-the-hebrew-immigrant-aid-society

Goldscheider, C. (2009). Immigration and the transformation of American Jews. In R. D. Alba (Ed.), *Immigration and religion in America: Comparative and historical perspectives* (pp. 198–214). New York University Press.

Goldstein, E. L. (2006). *The price of whiteness: Jews, race, and American identity*. Princeton University Press.

Gordon, L. R. (2016). Rarely kosher: Studying jews of color in north America. *American Jewish History, 100*(1), 105–116. https://doi.org/10.1353/ajh.2016.0006

Gotonda, N. (2011). The racialization of Islam in American law. *The Annals of the American Academy of Political and Social Science, 637*, 184–195. https://doi.org/10.2307/41328573

Gould, J., & Schaffel, C. (2019, August 29). Photos of Brandeis students, staff found on white nationalist forum. *The Justice*. https://www.thejustice.org/article/2019/08/photos-of-brandeis-students-staff-found-on-white-nationalist-forum

Green, T. H. (2015). *The fear of Islam: An introduction to Islamophobia in the West*. Fortress Press.

Greenwood, S. (2017a, July 26). *1. Demographic portrait of Muslim Americans*. Pew Research Center's Religion & Public Life Project. https://www.pewforum.org/2017/07/26/demographic-portrait-of-muslim-americans/

Greenwood, S. (2017b, July 26). *7. How the U.S. general public views Muslims and Islam*. Pew Research Center's Religion & Public Life Project. https://www.pewforum.org/2017/07/26/how-the-u-s-general-public-views-muslims-and-islam/

Hafez, F. (2014). Shifting borders: Islamophobia as common ground for building pan-European right-wing unity. *Patterns of Prejudice, 48*(5), 479–499. https://doi.org/10.1080/0031322x.2014.965877

Harris, S. (2011, May 25). Bombing our illusions. *HuffPost*. Retrieved March 15, 2022, from https://www.huffpost.com/entry/bombing-our-illusions_b_8615

Huntington, S. P. (2011). *The clash of civilizations and the remaking of world order* (A ed.). Simon & Schuster.

Jalabi, R. (2019, February 17). A history of the bill maher's "not bigoted" remarks on islam. *The Guardian*. Retrieved March 15, 2022, from https://www.theguardian.com/tv-and-radio/tvandradioblog/2014/oct/06/bill-maherislam-ben-affleck

Jansen, Y., & Meer, N. (2020). Genealogies of 'Jews' and 'Muslims': Social imaginaries in the race–religion nexus. *Patterns of Prejudice, 54*(1–2), 1–14. https://doi.org/10.1080/0031322x.2019.1696046

Kessler, G. (2015, September 22). Ben Carson's claim that 'Taqiyya' encourages Muslims 'To lie to achieve your goals'. *Washington Post.* https://www.washingtonpost.com/news/fact-checker/wp/2015/09/22/ben-carsons-claim-that-taqiyya-encourages-muslims-to-lie-to-achieve-your-goals/

Kishi, K. (2017, November 15). *Assaults against Muslims in U.S. surpass 2001 level.* Pew Research Center. https://www.pewresearch.org/fact-tank/2017/11/15/assaults-against-muslims-in-u-s-surpass-2001-level/

Klein, J. (2015, November 16). What's next after Isis's Paris massacre. *Front Page Magazine.* https://archives.frontpagemag.com/fpm/whats-next-after-isiss-paris-massacre-joseph-klein/

Kumar H. M. (2015). Responding to western critiques of the muslim world: Deconstructing the cliché of islamophobia and the genealogies of islamic extremism. *British Journal of Middle Eastern Studies, 42*(4), 579–598. https://doi.org/10.1080/13530194.2015.1037247

Magid, S. (2012). The Holocaust and Jewish identity in America: Memory, the unique, and the universal. *Jewish Social Studies: History, Culture, Society, 18*(2), 100–135. https://doi-org.proxy.library.vcu.edu/10.2979/jewisocistud.18.2.100

Marcus, K. (2015). The Ideology of the new antisemitism. In A. H. Rosenfeld (Ed.), Deciphering the new antisemitism (pp. 21–41). Indiana University Press. Retrieved November 08, 2020, from https://www.jstor.org/stable/j.ctt18crxz7

Margolin, J. (2020). White supremacists encourage their members to spread coronavirus to cops, and Jews, FBI says. *ABC News.* https://abcnews.go.com/US/white-supremacists-encouraging-members-spread-coronavirus-cops-jews/story?id=69737522

McGeever, B., & Virdee, S. (2017). Antisemitism and socialist strategy in Europe, 1880–1917*: An introduction. Patterns of Prejudice, 51*(3–4), 221–234. https://doi.org/10.1080/0031322X.2017.1349606

Meer, N., & Noorani, T. (2008). A sociological comparison of Anti-Semitism and Anti-Muslim sentiment in britain. *The Sociological Review, 56*(2), 195–219. https://doi.org/10.1111/j.1467-954x.2008.00784.x

Michael, R. (2005). World War I and the Leo frank case. In *A concise history of American antisemitism* (pp. 101–126). Rowman & Littlefield.

Mogahed, D., & Chouhoud, Y. (2017, March). American muslim poll 2017: Muslims at the crossroads. *Institute for Social Policy and Understanding*. https://www.ispu.org/american-muslim-poll-2017/

Muslim Advocates. (2019, July). *Fulfilling the promise of free exercise for all: Muslim prisoner accommodation in state prisons*. https://muslimadvocates.org/wp-content/uploads/2019/07/FULFILLING-THE-PROMISE-OF-FREE-EXERCISE-FOR-ALL-Muslim-Prisoner-Accommodation-In-State-Prisons-for-distribution-7_23.pdf

Pew Research Center. (2019, April 15). *Sharp Rise in the Share of Americans Saying Jews Face Discrimination*. Pew Research Center — Discrimination & Prejudice. https://www.pewresearch.org/politics/2019/04/15/sharp-rise-in-the-share-of-americans-saying-jews-facediscrimination/

Rao, M. (2011). Love jihad and demographic fears. *Indian Journal of Gender Studies, 18*(3), 425–430. https://doi.org/10.1177/097152151101800307

Renton, J., & Gidley, B. (2017). *Antisemitism and islamophobia in Europe: A shared story?* (1st ed.). Palgrave Macmillan.

Rubin, A. N. (2015). Orientalism and the history of western anti-Semitism: The coming end of an American taboo. *History of the Present, 5*(1), 95–108. https://doi.org/10.5406/historypresent.5.1.0095

Sandberg, S., & Colvin, S. (2020). 'ISIS is not Islam': Epistemic injustice, everyday religion, and young Muslims' narrative resistance. *The British Journal of Criminology, 60*(6), 1585–1605. https://doi.org/10.1093/bjc/azaa035

Southern Poverty Law Center. (2020, October 27). What you need to know about Qanon. Retrieved from https://www.splcenter.org/hatewatch/2020/10/27/what-you-need-know-about-qanon

Spellberg, D. (2014). *Thomas jefferson's qur'an: Islam and the founders* (Illustrated ed.). Vintage.

The Daily Mail. (2015, November 16). *MAC ON... Europe's open borders* [Cartoon]. *Daily Mail.Com*. https://www.dailymail.co.uk/news/article-3321431/MAC-Europe-s-open-borders.html

The Gallup Center for Muslim Studies. (2010, January 5). *In U.S., religious prejudice stronger against Muslims*. Gallup.Com. https://news.gallup.com/poll/125312/Religious-Prejudice-Stronger-Against-Muslims.asp

The Guardian, G. S. (2017, May 8). BNP leader "warned of multiracial hell hole." *The Guardian*. https://www.theguardian.com/uk/2006/jan/17/thefar-right.politics

The Pulitzer Prizes. (2012). Matt apuzzo, adam goldman, eileen sullivan and chris hawley of the associated press. *The 2012 Pulitzer Prize Winner in*

Investigative Reporting. Retrieved March 15, 2022, from https://www.pulitzer.org/winners/matt-apuzzo-adam-goldman-eileen-sullivan-and-chris-hawley

Tolan, J. (2019). *Faces of Muhammad: Western perceptions of the prophet of Islam from the middle ages to today*. Princeton University Press.

United States Holocaust Memorial Museum. Antisemitism in History: Racial Antisemitism, 1875–1945. *Holocaust Encyclopedia*. https://encyclopedia.ushmm.org/content/en/article/introduction-to-the-holocaust. Accessed on 22 Jan 2021.

Wyman, D. S. (1985). *Paper walls: America and the refugee crisis 1938–1941* (Rev. ed.). Pantheon.

Wyman, D. S. (2019). *The abandonment of the Jews: America and the Holocaust, 1941–1945*. Plunkett Lake Press. Retrieved from: http://holocaust.umd.umich.edu/news/uploads/PEC_Niewyk_rescue_1993.pdf

18

Diversity, Equity & Inclusion Training in a New Key: Adapting a Race-Class Lens for the Helping Professions

Daniel José Gaztambide, Dashawn Ealey, and Bora Meraj

Diversity, Equity, and Inclusion (DEI) training has become more visible in the public consciousness alongside backlash by right-wing commentators deriding DEI and critical race theory as divisive anti-White discourses that discourage the pursuit of the American Dream (Butcher & Gonzalez, 2020). Given legitimate questions of DEI's effectiveness (Dobbin & Kalev, 2018), a rigorous re-evaluation is in order. Within clinical psychology, the American Psychological Association's *Multicultural Guidelines* stress an ecological and intersectional approach to DEI in practice, research, and training (Clauss-Ehlers et al., 2019). Despite calls for weaving DEI throughout training, questions remain as to how to do so effectively (Benuto et al., 2018), a concern shared by other helping professions (see this volume). DEI training, defined as "cultural competence" in clinical psychology, is heterogeneous, ranging from didactics on

D. J. Gaztambide (✉) • D. Ealey • B. Meraj
The New School for Social Research, New York, NY, USA
e-mail: gaztambd@newschool.edu; ealeyd@newschool.edu; merab625@newschool.edu

© The Author(s), under exclusive license to Springer Nature Switzerland AG 2022

K. Johnson et al. (eds.), *Developing Anti-Racist Practices in the Helping Professions: Inclusive Theory, Pedagogy, and Application*,
https://doi.org/10.1007/978-3-030-95451-2_18

specific groups to implicit bias in the therapeutic relationship (Benuto et al., 2018). While DEI training increases knowledge about specific groups, change in attitudes and skills is mixed (Benuto et al., 2018). The emphasis on knowledge of specific cultural groups can foment "neutral stereotyping," the belief that once the client's identities are "known," one "understands" the client without exploring whether they find their identities relevant to their presenting problem in psychotherapy (cf. Leslie et al., 2020). Scholars proposed "cultural humility" as a complement to cultural competence, underscoring a *not-* knowing stance and openness to how the patient identifies in their own terms (Hook et al., 2017). Though an important client-centered framework, cultural humility has been scrutinized as lacking attention to issues of power and social justice (Abe, 2020).

Reflecting these theoretical evolutions, while student perceptions of DEI in clinical training have improved over time, Black and other underrepresented students rate multicultural training more negatively and their programs as less receptive to diversity, with better outcomes for programs with a diversity committee (Gregus et al., 2020). Relatedly, DEI training often presents a "zero-sum" (cf. McGhee, 2021) perspective on privilege that evokes resistance to reflecting on one's social position. Too neat a division between "being a (perfect) White ally" and "being racist" in current conceptualizations of "White psychology" can trigger avoidance and resistance among White trainees oriented around protection from the "racist = bad person = *me*" association (Nnawulezi et al., 2020; cf. Shepherd, 2019). Without minimizing the importance of reflecting on privilege, it is nonetheless important to meditate on what kinds of approaches *facilitate* such reflection, for both non-White and White trainees.

Although less commented in the literature, DEI training in mental health fields maintain a bifurcation between "general skills" and "culturally competent skills," suggesting that clinicians must learn two separate bodies of knowledge: "general psychotherapy" applicable to "everyone," and then later in training something called "culturally competent psychotherapy" applicable to the "alien other" (Brown, 2008). The former may involve addressing early attachment trauma, distorted cognitions, or skill deficits, whereas the latter addresses the effects of racism, cisheterosexism, and classism (among other isms). As commented by some of my (DG) students of color, this creates a "two-tier" system of human suffering (something I also experienced as a graduate student). Our training is structured in such a way that when sitting with a White cis- heterosexual male client, for example, we are biased to think about "universal" processes such as early childhood trauma in a manner devoid of culture, power, and context, whereas for BIPOC, LGBTQ+ and cis-women clients the import of social determinants may be over emphasized and overlook other features of clinical care. This concern brings discussions of DEI face to face with fundamental questions of human suffering.

Approach of This Chapter: The Race Class Lens

Without asserting a facile universalism or a stereotyping relativism that marginalizes oppressed communities, we approach this question of human suffering from an intersectional (Crenshaw, 1990; Taylor, 2016), Liberation Psychology (Freire, 1972; Martín-Baró, 1994), and critical race theory approach as informed by the Race-Class Lens (López, 2019). The Race-Class Lens is a product of the Race-Class Narrative Project (López, 2019; McGhee, 2021), a mixed-methods research study led by progressive think tank Demos. Field research informed by this framework highlights the need for a paradigm shift in our thinking of social justice. Instead of framing racism as *primarily* a conflict between White people and people of color, the Race-Class Lens sheds light on how racism is a weapon of class warfare waged by the wealthy against all of us. In addition, we will note how the Race-Class Lens can help us understand intersections with other aspects of identity which may also serve as axes of division to maintain inequality. We will position ourselves in relation to this project before engaging in a critique of current DEI thinking, practice, and evidence-base. We will also review cross-disciplinary research on race and inequality to frame our understanding of human suffering, and show how the Race-Class Lens recontextualizes many of the assumptions of DEI in the helping professions. We end with preliminary recommendations on how training programs can structure DEI training "in a new key" through adoption of this lens. In sum, if we grasp the interconnectedness of suffering for both oppressor and oppressed, support intrinsic motivation for social justice, and center the systemic context, we can develop a curriculum in which social justice is a matter of course as opposed to an ancillary component of training for all trainees—Black, White, or Brown.

Using the Race-Class Lens, we will develop a mode of thinking about suffering that recognizes privilege while accounting for its *costs* to both oppressor and oppressed. We offer an invitation that includes White people (and other privileged identities) as part of the process of social change—a process that requires the "sum of us" to succeed (McGhee, 2021). The idea that the privileged also suffer costs from conditions of inequality is grounded in some of our most radical traditions. Latin American Liberation Psychology (Freire, 1972; Martín-Baró, 1994) and the Black Radical Tradition (see Ahad, 2010) orient us to how oppressor and oppressed are dehumanized by inequality though in distinct ways. This idea can sometimes have an abstract quality where it is not altogether clear *how* the privileged "suffer" from the systems that benefit them. The task of this chapter will be to make the case for the material and psychological basis for this oft-forgotten assertion in our radical traditions, rendering a more integrative vision for social justice training within the helping professions and clinical psychology in particular. That way, we can move beyond bifurcated notions of suffering and toward understanding how the suffering of both oppressor and oppressed are *critically different though intimately related.*

Positionality Statement

DG: I am a White Puerto Rican cisgender man born and raised on the island, now living in New York City during the COVID-19 pandemic. I name my Whiteness in recognition of how colorism and anti-Blackness privilege me even as my Puerto Ricanness led me to experience discrimination and precarity. I grew up in a context in which *familismo*—the centrality of the family—was weaponized as a tool of racial, gender, and sexual control. Homosexuality was explicitly positioned as a threat to the sanctity of *la gran familia Puertorriqueña* ("the great Puerto Rican family"), even as having darker skin was tacitly emplaced as a greater threat. One should not—stated out loud and a whisper—be "unequally yoked" with a partner who was *darker* skinned, for one had to *mejorar la raza*, "improve the race." The reality of my Black, Brown, and LGBTQ friends and family put me on a collision course *with familismo*, yet paradoxically on its behalf at the same time. I can to realize that it was queer negativity, not queerness, that was a threat to my friends, family, and community—my understanding of family had to be transformed. I see the process of transforming our values in the interest of justice similarly as an intricate part of social change. I not only seek methods to engage privileged people, but also members of my community who internalized an identification with oppressive systems.

BM: I am an Albanian-Canadian, cisgender "Eastern European White" woman born in Albania and displaced as a child to the island of Crete. At age seven, my parents paid a smuggler to help us cross the border to Greece during a precarious political period. Four years later we arrived in Toronto, crossing another border but this time "legally," then becoming a Canadian citizen. My awareness of anti-Black racism took full shape in Toronto. As an "illegal immigrant" in Greece, I experienced first-hand those intangible boundaries delineating who can be part of the nation and who cannot, making immigrants feel out of place no matter how hard they try to assimilate. Whereas my "Eastern European" identity led to xenophobia in Crete, my Whiteness protected me from more severe backlash. Both my whiteness and my Canadian identity afford me the privilege of walking down the street without suspicion or fear. Having experienced discrimination side by side with the freedoms afforded by my Whiteness, I came to realize that just as I have the right to inhabit the world without fear, so do others in my community—people of color, LGBTQ+ people, and other marginalized peoples. I joined DG in this chapter because I deeply value critical self-reflection on intersecting identities and articulating a narrative that frames anti-racism as work that benefits all of us. I see this approach as the only way forward.

DE: I am a Black cisgender queer man and psychology graduate student, born and raised in a women-led, multigeneration household in Brooklyn, New York. Although my community devoted itself to the African proverb, "It takes a village to raise a child," I quickly understood the messy intersections of my queer and racial identities as byproducts of inflexible gendered and racialized interactions I experienced as a child. Attending a predominantly White liberal arts college as a first-generation student triggered the sudden moment my personal life, colored by childhood experiences, became political. The cold reality was that my hopes and dreams were gendered, racially segregated, sexually oppressive, and interrupted by multiple oppressive systems. At the same time, I understood the systems that rendered me sub-human also afforded me privileges as a cisgendered man, a cisgendered Black man, and a cisgendered Black man with privileged abilities. As you'll read in this chapter, privilege is dynamic, and the maintenance of systems that engender privilege, regardless of the personal benefits, ultimately disadvantages us all. For this reason, I tailor my personal and academic pursuits to dismantling oppressive systems and healing those traumatized by their insidious influence.

Our process (DG, DE, BM) writing this chapter included heartfelt debate, dialogue, and self-exploration of our relationships to privilege and marginalization. The "paradigm shift" that switching from a racial justice to a Race-Class Lens involved—and its implications for gender and sexuality—evoked strong reactions and the temptation to "dig in" to discourses in our broader culture that commodify suffering and set people up to compete against each other for "who suffers more" (Sue et al., 2019). Such conversations were difficult and painful, but led to the realization that the only way forward is for us to reach across—often through—our vulnerabilities.

A Critical Examination of DEI: Theoretical and Empirical Reviews

DEI training proliferated across the helping professions and human resources industry in the wake of public outcries against racist incidents. For instance, on May 29th, 2018 Starbucks encouraged nearly 175,000 employees to undergo a mandatory four-hour racial bias training after a barista called the police on two Black men waiting at a table in one of its

Philadelphia stores. While the move was lauded as representing the "mainstreaming" of DEI, there is a notable lack of agreed-upon metrics for evaluating its effectiveness (Eberhardt, 2018; Noon, 2018). While DEI training is the go-to practice for addressing bias in organizations, the underlying philosophies and pedagogical practices make certain assumptions about power, privilege, and bias that undercut stated goals of DEI training. These assumptions include:

1. Short-term, one-size-fits-all *didactic* training that is generic, superficial in nature, and promotes conformity (as opposed to dynamic, context sensitive, and dialogical);
2. Social injustice should be framed primarily in terms of "oppressor versus oppressed" (as opposed to ideological weapons wielded by the rich against all of us);
3. The locus of change is individual psychology and interpersonally prejudiced behavior (as opposed to building relationships to change the larger politico-institutional context);
4. Implicit bias and behavior is primarily internal, intractable, and resistant to change (as opposed to communal, malleable, and responsive to change);
5. DEI training values such as racial justice are transparently valuable, and resistance to these values is evidence of bias (as opposed to requiring persuasion and engagement).

We will critique and present alternatives for each of these assumptions over the course of this chapter drawing on contemporary DEI scholars and researchers.

Limitations of "Cookie Cutter" Knowledge, "Zero-Sum" Framing, and the Focus on the Individual

When short-term and without follow-up, DEI training risks promoting stereotypes through a "museum-tour" approach to diversity, biasing practitioners to apply a cultural lens when it may not be relevant or experienced as stereotyping by clients (Shepherd, 2019). Relatedly, the "business argument for diversity" (Kidder et al., 2004) appeals to the profit motive of corporations, disciplining workers while providing legal protection against litigation (Newkirk, 2019). More attention should be given to the motivations of *people*, not the legal, political, and economic interests of institutions. DEI training can introduce shallow understandings of power and privilege that diluting the importance of structural racism, defining it in individual-interpersonal terms that increase the likelihood of division and conflict while leaving institutions "off the hook" from systemic change (Carter et al., 2020).

Focusing squarely on disciplining individuals can trigger a "shame and blame" cycle that *backfires* by increasing prejudiced behavior adversely impacting minority individuals, and reducing support for diversity policies (Devine et al., 2002; Dobbin & Kalev, 2018; Legault et al., 2011; Leslie et al., 2014; Shepherd, 2019). Framing interracial interactions primarily through the lens of a "culture clash" between "White and non-White" produces exactly that—racial antagonists trapped in a zero-sum game (McGhee, 2021). When DEI is framed as a strategy that facilitates *one's own* goals and values, it provides intrinsic motivation to reduce bias (Devine et al., 2002; Legault et al., 2011; Forscher et al., 2019), and makes it easier to tolerate the fear of losing status (Kidder et al., 2004, p. 82).

Limitations of Psychologistic Bias and Rigid Conceptions of the Self as Intractable to Change

Noon (2018) summarizes the underlying theory behind popular conceptions of unconscious bias: it is learned in childhood and reinforced through family, peers, and the surrounding culture, influences behavior, is deeply ingrained, and is rigid and intractable toward change. Following an almost Freudian topography of the unconscious, individuals are "repressed racists" (e.g. unconscious) who need to bring their biases "to the surface" (e.g. insight) to change racist behavior. Even White liberals, "once they have recovered from the shock of finding out they are really a racist deep down, they might change, but equally they might decide this is beyond their control and not alter their behaviour" (Noon, 2018,

p. 202). They might conclude that "nothing can be done," aside from the purification ritual of "confessing" their racism and privilege, relieving their personal anguish without changing racist structures. Whites who commit to anti-racist action may do so out of a moral sense of "it's the right thing to do." Although appreciative of our White allies, we contend that this is a dangerous proposition placing people of color at the behest of White people's benevolence. We advocate for an approach that stresses social justice not as charity (which can be given and taken away), but an act of survival against systems that threaten the well-being of all of us. This requires a shift in perspective from a) the individual to an unambiguously structural lens, and b) rigid notions of the self to a more fluid one. In this view, bias is not locked in a Freudian basement but derives "from social context… It requires looking within and beyond the individual" (Noon, 2018, p. 205).

When implicit bias is examined at the individual level it is inconsistently related to outcomes, but at the aggregate level of counties or states they are associated with discrimination (Payne et al., 2017). Instead of conceptualizing implicit bias as intractable *individual* attitudes, it is better seen as a constitutionally "*social* phenomenon that *passes through* individual minds, rather than residing in them," (p. 236, emphasis added; cf. Payne et al., 2019). What is measured in studies of implicit bias is the "wisdom of crowds"—the *availability* of stereotypes in our socio-political surroundings, rendered *accessible* by social and political discourse (Payne et al., 2017). Media depictions, culture, political messages and systems "trickle down" to everyday experiences, including daily and tacit observations of who is high or low status (cf. Ayala-Lopez & Beeghly, 2020). Implicit bias, then, is a psychological *symptom* of systemic structures, widespread due to discourses that "repeatedly raise the accessibility of stereotypic concepts" (Payne et al., 2017, p. 242). This points to *malleability* and *fluidity* in the accessibility of bias, suggesting individuals *oscillate* in their beliefs depending on their availability and accessibility at a given time and place. For example, structural variables—such as faculty and student diversity, diversity policies, robust financial aid—predict implicit bias in universities even as individual bias oscillates, often returning to the institutional "mean" after DEI interventions (Vuletich & Payne, 2019). If so, changes to the context (structures, policies, messaging) can reduce the availability bias, and its accessibility to individual minds.

Empirical Support for DEI: Yes and No, Caveats and Concerns

The effects of DEI training on attitudes and behavior are meager (e.g. may not last past a few days), but more robust when complemented by other initiatives focused on awareness and skills over time (Bezrukova et al., 2016). In line with our critiques above, recent DEI scholarship calls for prioritizing structural programs over individual consciousness raising (Carter et al., 2020; Onyeador et al., 2021). Recommendations include (a) a core message centering diversity in organizational values and mission, (b) opportunities for positive intergroup contact (without burdening marginalized groups), and (c) affinity groups for underrepresented members that provide social support, mentoring, and skills in how to cope with discrimination (Bernstein et al., 2020; Dobbin & Kalev, 2018; Onyeador et al., 2021). DEI training should also provide education about bias and tools to manage emotional reactions, reflect on bias, and change behavior (Carter et al., 2020; Onyeador et al., 2021). Carter, Onyeador, & Lewis Jr. (2020) argue a moderate amount of discomfort can be "a critical catalyst" for self-reflection, "Persuasion is often most successful when people are presented with a moderately disturbing outcome and strategies they can use to avoid that outcome" (p. 64).

However, the framing that being confronted with one's racist beliefs induces a "moderately disturbing outcome," (e.g. realizing one is a racist) which can then be "escaped" by reducing implicit bias (e.g. changing racist beliefs) sidesteps the question of *why* a White participant would be *intrinsically* motivated to change in the first place aside from a moral injunction or to avoid punishment. We will review a promising approach to DEI addressing this, Intergroup Dialogue (Gurin et al., 2013), and note its strengths and limitations.

Dialogical Approaches to DEI: The Case of Intergroup Dialogue

When DEI is framed as *inclusive* of majority groups this lowers reactance, emphasizing a perspective centering marginalized communities while stressing "that the majority culture is an important part of that multiculturalism" (Dobbin & Kalev, 2018, p. 51). When individuals perceive themselves as standing to gain from a common ingroup identity that both transcends *and* recognizes differences they are more likely to tolerate conflict and value diversity more (Bernstein et al., 2020). Contact increases intercultural competence (Meleady et al., 2020), and confers additional benefits conducive to psychological flexibility, the ability to situations that involve cognitive dissonance, multiple perspectives, and creative problem solving (Meleady et al., 2019). Being a member of a labor union, for example, and collaborating across race on economic interests reduces White racial resentment while increasing support for universal redistributive policies and policies that specifically benefit African-Americans (Frymer & Grumbach, 2021). Drawing on the intergroup contact literature, Intergroup Dialogue (IGD) brings together groups comprised of communities experiencing asymmetrical conflict (e.g. White and Black people/people of color, men and women). Across randomized controlled trials and process-outcome studies (Frantell et al., 2019; Rodríguez et al., 2018), IGD has been shown to facilitate ally-ship, exploration of privilege, perspective taking, bias reduction, improved interpersonal skills, and preparedness for social action. Core processes include active listening, addressing conflict in session, emotional expression, and developing a politicized identity connected to systems of power and privilege (Frantell et al., 2019).

Inspired by Paulo Freire's (1972) work, IGD takes a critical-dialogic approach emphasizing dialogue, empathy and relationship. Rather than beginning with didactics, IGD groups focus on building relationships and trust alongside training in communication and conflict resolution skills *prior* to conversations on power and privilege. This includes active listening skills to weather moments of conflict and facilitate reflection (Gurin et al., 2013, p. 61–62). Once that groundwork is set, IGD groups begin exploring differences and commonalities around identity and inequality, controversial issues (e.g. criminal justice reform, immigration, etc), processing power dynamics that emerge in group, engaging in exercises focused on the value of solidarity, and organizing to plan and take social justice action.

Underlying this process, Gurin, Nagda, and Zuniga (2013, p. 34–35) stress the importance of exploring differences in power *and* articulating common values to move beyond diversity and toward action on systems of inequality. IGD draws on established trust and values to "survive" moments of tension—arguably, an "optimal" amount of conflict. However, we question the extent to which IGD fully articulates a rationale for privileged group members to even engage in such dialogues. If the goal is for privileged group members, in solidarity with marginalized group members, to engage in action on behalf of the latter (and presumably, not themselves) we encounter the problem of motivation anew. Again, to the extent social justice projects require solidarity with other marginalized groups and privileged allies, this cannot depend on the "good will," guilt, or shame of privileged groups. In what follows we show that it is in White people's (and other privileged group's) *best material and psychological interest* to be allies, and center solidarity as the goal of any meaningful DEI project in the helping professions. To articulate this view, we situate our theory of suffering and privilege in the context of our unequal world.

Racial Fear Ideology, Inequality, and Public Goods

U.S. elite ideologies evolved in the 1950s and 60s to mystify inequality by arguing that the cause of racial inequality was either a Black "culture of poverty" *or* White cultural racism. Hence, social justice was *not* to be found in political economic change but hygiene programs to either rehabilitate Black people's cultural stagnation or individual White people's ontological racism—setting the stage for both racial fear politics and the "management" of individual bias by DEI initiatives (Reed, 2020). These historical trends have implications for our struggles today. Despite the rise of inequality during COVID-19, this has not increased U.S. public support for redistribution despite declared opposition to inequality—higher inequality prompts support for government intervention, but this is moderated by trust in government itself (MacDonald, 2020). Trust in government as a vehicle for redistribution is dampened by racial fear messages and meritocratic ideologies (López, 2019; Macdonald, 2021). As income inequality rises so does relative deprivation and the threat of losing one's status in the hierarchy—the *perception* of scarcity leads to higher support for the right's racist rhetoric, restriction of civil rights and anti-redistribution policy (Engler & Weisstanner, 2020). Even among "the 1%" there exists a hierarchy where status anxiety and competition abounds as elites compete for material and symbolic position (Mechanic, 2021)—even bragging rights on who makes it into space *first*.

When inequality is rendered invisible through meritocracy and social mobility, this leads to policies rewarding the rich while "draining the pool" for the rest of us (McGhee, 2021). But when people engage in social comparisons with the wealthy, support for redistribution increases (Condon & Wichowsky, 2020). Hence Condon and Wichowsky (2020) write, "All of these factors—class segregation, perceptions of risk and economic anxiety, race, and gender—govern whether people look up, look down, or avoid comparisons altogether" (p. 158).

A Crown of Thorns: A Dynamic Theory of Privilege and Suffering

Part of the power of racism comes from neutralizing multiracial solidarity and deepening racial and economic inequality. Our perspective on this dynamic is informed by W.E.B. Dubois' (1935) meditations on the "wages of Whiteness." While White people may be exploited under capitalism through lower wages, they are "compensated [by] a sort of *public and psychological wage*" (p. 700), material and symbolic privileges operating as a psychic salve for their pain. Afropessimists like Wilderson (2020), commenting on non-Black people of color, similarly define anti-Blackness as "a healing balm for the human mind" (p. 200). Non-Black people of color may suffer due to exploitation, racism and anti-immigrant sentiment, and *yet*, because they are not Black, be granted higher status on a racial hierarchy that soothes their pain. As James Baldwin once said, "You knew *you* were not on the bottom, because the Negro was there."

Borrowing Marx's (1844) critique of religion, we might say that anti-Blackness is "the opium of the masses." We posit that privilege advantages that are relative in nature, resulting in what Marx called an "illusory happiness." Hence, we must upend the illusory happiness that privilege affords, and the system those privileges make us attached to. Borrowing from Marx again, to "call on [White and non-Black people] to give up their illusions about their condition is to call on them to *give up a condition that requires illusions*." We critique privilege *as* an illusion not in the sense that it is not real, but that its promises are transient. We do so to shed light on "*that vale of tears* of which [privilege] is the *halo*," strapped to our heads like a crown of thorns. This image evokes the privilege of royalty, along with the damage that comes with thorns drawing your blood. The privilege this crown of thorns confers is an opiate that numbs our pain, yet like any drug, has benefits and costs. With continued use, the drug begins to damage your body. You take more of the drug to manage its symptoms until it becomes fatal.

Wilkinson and Pickett (2020) review an interdisciplinary literature on the effects of income inequality on societal well-being. As income inequality rises, psychosocial outcomes worsen— worse life expectancy, infant and adult mortality, child well-being, medical well-being, educational attainment, social mobility, mental illness, substance use, child maltreatment, homicides, and population in prison. The inequality-outcome relationship is mediated by social capital (e.g. trust and social bonds). With lower trust and support, people are more likely to focus on where they stand on a hierarchy (status anxiety), resulting in exaggerated domination and submission behaviors to either achieve higher status or protect the self. Ideologies and behaviors to preserve status have a soothing, emotion regulation effect for *both* high and low-status ethnic groups—both can rationalize their position in the hierarchy (Sengupta et al., 2017; cf. Cameron et al., 2016). For low status groups, meritocracy promises that if they "work hard" and dissociate from "the undeserving" they too can "climb to the top."

Although income inequality results from anti-redistributive, pro-wealth austerity policies (Bor et al., 2017), we must grasp the *fusion* of race and capitalism. Racial fear ideologies *drive* White status anxieties and politicians who enact policies restricting civil rights, increase inequality, and deploy rhetoric that fuels racial violence—"draining the pool" of resources so *the other* cannot have them, and depriving oneself in the process (McGhee, 2021). Attempts by Whites to hurt Black and other people of color, and the privileges that result from such efforts, *have a cost* measured in suicide deaths (often from guns purchased to protect against "the other"), worse health and restricted healthcare for all, and decaying schools leading to lower life expectancy *for White people and in particular White men* (Metzl, 2019). It is not that the suffering of White people is on the same plane as that of people of color. Rather, White privilege is a system that confers material and symbolic advantages *even* as it extracts a cost.

An analogy with gender, gender identity, and sexuality is illustrative. Cisheteropatriarchy confers privilege to cisgender (especially but not only White) heterosexual men while threatening the bodily, cultural and economic life of cisgender women, LGBTQ people and in particular Transgender women. At the same time, the demands of hegemonic masculinity posit toxic ideals most cisgender men cannot achieve, leading to adverse mental and medical outcomes including substance use, depression, and higher rates of suicide (Barber et al., 2019). Rising income inequality threatens job security and men's ability to *fulfill* hegemonic masculine ideals (e.g. being a "provider," "top dog," etc), allowing right-wing rhetoric to *blame* women and LGBTQ people for the "crisis in masculinity," fueling homicides, sexual violence, and support for anti-egalitarian policies (cf. Krems & Varnum, 2017; Kosakowska-Berezecka et al., 2020). Gender and income inequality intersect to impact mental health—gender inequality disproportionately affects women's mental health, income inequality is more likely to be associated with men's mental health, while a country's wealth *worsens* gender disparities (Yu, 2018), leading to a cycle of intersecting and additional impact for women further complicated by class, race, gender identity and sexuality

(Crenshaw, 1990). Patriarchy as a weapon of capital combines ideology, culture, and structural forces to wound men, then *weaponize* those wounds against women and LGBTQ people, with male privilege functioning as a crown of thorns.

The privilege afforded to men, like Whites, include performing violence on the other deemed to be the source of their suffering. However, hegemonic masculinity, like Whiteness, is a preposition in constant state of disrepair, requiring continued maintenance. This dialectic between performance and failure produces a constant malaise—why do I suffer? That suffering is directed where the powerful need us to look—who is up? Who is down? And where am *I*? Ideology's answer is that because of *them* you lost your rightful place, and we *will make you great again*. An example at the nexus of Whiteness and hegemonic masculinity comes to mind— a gun manufacturer's promotion, "Consider your man card reissued" (Metzl, 2019, p. 61).

One final note before turning to the Race-Class Lens. Given the negative relationship between income inequality and social trust (Wilkinson & Pickett, 2020), one would imagine that racial division would worsen trust in tandem. The opposite seems to be true—economic inequality *positively* moderates the impact of racial diversity on social trust (Kim et al., 2020). "Ironically," Kim, Kim, & Altema (2020) write, "given the dominance of racial divisions in American politics, the rise of income inequality seems to open a new horizon through which *more people are motivated to bond together and invest in collective activities*" (p. 25, emphasis added). Hence, racial and economic inequality may interact in ways that create an aperture for building solidarity for social change.

The Race-Class Lens

Given the dynamic nature of privilege and inequality, we can better understand the limitations of many DEI interventions. To the extent DEI conceptualizes race, racism, and privilege as a zero-sum game—as fundamentally a conflict between White people versus people of color—it becomes fairly obvious why this generates resistance among White people. Our call is not to silence race talk, but to engage in more effective and mutative race talk with the Race- Class Lens as a guide. The Race-Class Narrative Project (findings summarized in López, 2019), found that aside from Americans who consistently endorse progressive or reactionary racist beliefs (23% and 18%, respectively), most Americans (59%) form part of the "persuadables" in between. Rather than a reasoned political "middle," persuadables *toggle* fluidly and ambivalently between progressive and reactionary views. Conversant with a recent study of White ambivalence among practitioner graduate students (Nnawulezi et al., 2020), "making room for complex moving away and moving toward may open new avenues for facilitating the development of racially-conscious and critical practitioners" (p. 371). Depending on how available and accessible these beliefs are, persuadables might believe that talking about race is necessary to move toward equity *and* that talking about race will make things worse.

López (2019) shows how the right and center-left deploy narratives of racial fear in which people of color—in particular, Black people—are dangerous and undeserving, government should not be trusted as it coddles the undeserving, and one should trust the market as the solution to our problems. This message was endorsed highly among Whites *and also among communities of color*. Not surprisingly, when participants were exposed to traditional racial justice messaging—racism by White people harms people of color, we must come together to end racism, etc—they saw those messages as divisive and "racist." Participants of color *also* resisted discussion of racism as White-over-non-White as itself racist, stressing personal responsibility and minimizing structural oppression. Those who acknowledged structural racism were nonetheless pessimistic about the possibility of change, *defaulting* to personal responsibility as a matter of survival.

Given the racial fear message divides and conquers while empowering the wealthy, López (2019) and his collaborators developed the Race-Class message "urging people to join together across racial lines, to distrust greedy elites sowing division, and to demand that government work for everyone" (p. 174). The Race-Class message (1) calls out racism as a weapon of class division deployed by greedy economic elites, (2) calls for multiracial solidarity, and (3) connects working together with building a "government for all." One example of a Race- Class message would be the following:

> No matter our color or where we come from, we all want a future for our children. But greedy politicians hurt everyone by cutting taxes to the rich and defunding social services. Then they point the finger for hard times at Black people, immigrants, and the poor. We must come together with people from all walks of life to fight for our future, just like we won better wages, safer workplaces, and civil rights in our past. That way, we can build a government that works for all of us whether we're Black, White, or Brown.

The Race-Class message is not new, but stems from the Black and Queer Black Feminist radical tradition from Dubois to the Combahee River Collective (Taylor, 2016). In wrestling with racial capitalism, these traditions "[posit] that Black salvation requires cross-racial solidarity and likewise that white salvation requires precisely the same" (López, 2019, p. 181).

The Race-Class message was more convincing than racial fear, colorblind-economic, and racial justice messages across progressives and persuadables (López, 2019). Focus groups with participants found that although White people and people of color were resistant to seeing racist intentions in everyday people, they were more willing to see racism as something weaponized by elites (p. 185). Echoing the review above, participants could "readily grasp purposeful division, as they see it in their families, their workplaces, in community groups, and very much in politics. And they know that coming together is the clear solution" (p. 185–186). Participants were *more* enthusiastic when (a) race was explicit in messaging (not color-blind) and (b) stated that all racial groups *including Whites* are hurt by racism and would benefit from social change.

The idea that Whites would benefit from multiracial solidarity short-circuits two core elements of the ring-wing's narrative—(1) talking about racism means blaming Whites, and (2) addressing racism means a net loss for Whites (López, 2019, p. 188). These are two stories that mainstream racial justice discourse, including much DEI training, unfortunately *reinforce* time and again. If racial fear messages hurt us *because* they trigger status anxiety among White people and people of color who desire a higher place in the hierarchy, and then weaponize those fears against all of us, it behooves us to not do our opponents' work for them. Further, participants of color responded positively to the Race-Class message when benefits to Whites in addition to themselves were emphasized, instilling greater confidence in solidarity when they perceive that Whites have a stake in working together (López, 2019, p. 190). A Race-Class Lens recognizes White privilege, but instead of individual condemnation opens an invitation that includes White people as part of the solution. It answers the question "why do I suffer?" by turning social comparison away from one another and "upward" toward the powerful, centering social justice work as something that requires the "sum of us" to succeed (McGhee, 2021).

Lopez draws on critical race theorist Derrick Bell's theory of interest convergence— racial progress is more likely when Whites recognize it can benefit them as well. This is more than mere self-interest, as it taps into intrinsic and self-motivated morals and values. López (2019) writes,

> [it] involves providing for one's family and especially one's children; receiving what you merit measured against what others receive and deserve; and self-respect as well as status in the community. In other words, most people do not sharply distinguish between morality and self-interest. Rather, they blend them together, typically in terms heavily influenced by cultural norms. This means people tend to reject moral claims that run counter to their sense of what helps them and their family. (p. 192)

When people understand how a given task or perspective will advance their goals, they become *more open* to being pushed morally. To give another analogy, when I (DG) realized my beliefs around family, race and sexuality were fueled by colonial patriarchal mores that hurt me as a cisman (e.g. no room for vulnerability, getting into fights), empowered politicians whose policies hurt my Black and Brown LGBTQ family and friends, and emboldened violence in the community, I could no longer hold those views.

The cognitive dissonance I wrestled with through adolescence—homosexuality threatens family, members of my family are gay, cut them off to protect family, but cut off my family to protect family?—demanded a *reformulation* of my values that extended the frame of what family and *familismo* is. This dissonance was not something instilled from outside (which would have likely evoked resistance), but something that developed *inside* in the context of my evolving environment and experiences. This experience transferred to all LGBTQ and Black people whether they were Puerto Rican or not. Hence, the survival of my loved ones depends on a multiracial coalition of LGBTQ and cisheterosexual people.

Conclusion and Training Implications

In the context of COVID-19, race talk is no less fraught. Critical perspectives on DEI training, especially within clinical psychology and other helping professions, are needed now more than ever. We recognize that among DEI trainers and scholars we have approached the issue backwards by leading with the moral demand to be anti-racist without first articulating the concrete benefits to both White people and people of color. Narratives specific to our helping professions must center how anti-racism fulfills our deepest values and material needs—whether White, Black, or Brown. Once that groundwork is laid, more traditional DEI work such as reflecting on privilege can then follow. Not as external demand but as a task that is *internally valued* as necessary for the survival of those we value most. "Once people understand" Lopez (2019) writes, "that the greater threats in their lives come from economic titans rather than from other working families, that new understanding quickly finds expression in moral terms" (p. 193).

This chapter labored to dig deep into the underlying premises of DEI training, criticizing them "from within" with the goal of developing a more coherent and effective vision. We summarize some of the more robust and evidence-based DEI components in our review below, framed from the perspective of the Race-Class Lens. Although this is not a "how to" chapter, we offer the following for clinical psychology programs, while acknowledging they may be applicable to other helping professions as well. We organize them around *content and structural* recommendations, and *process and pedagogical* recommendations:

Content and Structural Recommendations

- Center social justice and cultural humility within a scientist-practitioner-advocate training model (Nadal, 2017; Mallinckrodt et al., 2014) *infused* with the Race-Class Lens. Training programs should retain an emphasis on the needs of oppressed communities along with an analysis of suffering that accounts for (a) *why* marginalized and dominant groups suffer and (b) *how* that suffering is connected. This should be infused throughout the curriculum so teaching, supervision, and research connects back to a social justice vision and the value of solidarity. Further, connect this vision to trainees' values and training goals to foment intrinsic motivation for social justice work.
- Recruit more diverse faculty, students, and staff as an ongoing goal. In training programs and cohorts that are predominantly White, stress across curriculum how White people are still affected by the "structural fallout" of Whiteness and White supremacy. Put bluntly, race *still* matters, perhaps more so, whether the helping professional and client are both White, or an institution is predominantly White.
- Frame discussions of bias as predominantly contextual and fluid rather than individual and fixed, consider what contextual changes can reduce the availability and accessibility of implicit bias. For example, creating opportunities for intergroup contact around shared goals, lowering the value (and thus, accessibility) of zero-sum racial fears.
- Alongside a diversity, inclusion, and social justice committee, create spaces that are not necessarily DEI-specific providing opportunities for diverse students to collaborate on a shared task. For example, a student union where trainees brainstorm and advocate for curricular changes that benefit their learning goals to faculty and staff. Encouraging participation from students across identities will promote positive contact around shared goals. Adding a Race-Class Lens may highlight for students how race, labor, and economics intersect in the political economy of the helping professions, further incentivizing how reforming training programs carry benefits for all.

Process and Pedagogical Recommendations

- Infuse a dynamic theory of suffering across the curriculum to connect training, research, and practice back to social justice values. Do not limit such conversations to a "diversity course," or to the issues of marginalized communities—as if race is not relevant in work with White clients, or gender in work with cis-male clients. Articulate how the suffering of privileged and underprivileged groups are *qualitatively different though related*.
- Provide communication and conflict resolution skills training as part of exploring issues of identity. In addition, provide coping skills for students of color dealing with racism in the helping professions, and for White students to cope with anxieties when discussing race. Reinforce how dialogue across difference results in a "solidarity dividend" (McGhee, 2021) benefitting White and BIPOC students alike. Frame an optimal amount of conflict as a healthy part of building solidarity and connection.
- When addressing conflict that emerges in training programs, center a systemic as opposed to individual analysis inspired by the Race-Class Lens. What real and imagined scarcities in the context are underlying this conflict? How can the relational and institutional context be changed in a way that thaws resistance and promotes dialogue?
- When engaging in discussions of privilege, acknowledge intersectionality while addressing the avoidant use of marginalized identity to prevent reflection on a privileged identity (Nnawulezi et al., 2020). For example, a White male student from a working class background may assert that he cannot be privileged because of the deprivation he experienced as a child. A Race-Class approach would validate the reality of their suffering, while also connecting that suffering to how racism has led *precisely* to worse conditions for working class—including White—people. Active listening and empathy can help thaw resistance to discussing privilege by validating underlying vulnerability. By connecting their vulnerability to the different-but-related vulnerability of people of color, this can open another path to reflecting on how, alongside

their pain, there is *privilege* that they hold, which is itself a contributor to their pain.

- Alongside didactic courses on intervention and cultural competency, offer skills and process-oriented IGD groups to foment reflection on privilege, identity, and social action. Reframe IGD groups from the perspective of the Race-Class Lens—instead of framing dialogue on racism with the goal of getting White students to change for people of color, center discussions on how racism *disproportionately* impacts people of color while also exerting a cost for Whites. Again, the goal is not to "even the playing field" so that Whites are "also oppressed" by racism. The goal is to make clear that social justice is not the sole purview of trainees of color, and that White trainees should not participate in social justice out of charity, but shared vulnerability.

Coda: To Liberate Ourselves and Our Oppressors

Helms (1990) outlined a process for developing a "healthy White identity" defined by the "abandonment of racism and the development of a non-racist White identity" (p. 49). This includes a search for redefinition, "Who am I racially?" and "Who do I want to be?" (p.62). At the end of that journey, White people no longer feel the need to either "oppress or idealize" people of color, as race is no longer a source of threat or sanctuary (p. 66). This chapter was motivated by suffering, and the urgent necessity to change the conditions that produce that "vale of tears" of which Whiteness is the halo, even if this means challenging deeply held assumptions in our values. We have undertaken this project in the spirit of a deeper calling, what Freire (1972) called the "humanistic and historical task of the oppressed: to liberate themselves and their oppressors as well" (p. 21). This task requires a particular kind of vulnerability and the willingness to open ourselves up to being challenged by our colleagues committed to racial justice work. For only from vulnerability can we find the strength to free the other as well as ourselves. Because that is our true calling—to be free.

Guiding Questions

- When delivering services within your specific helping profession, what kind of theories or frameworks do you draw on when helping clients of color? What kind of theories or frameworks do you draw on when helping White clients? In what ways are they similar, in what ways are they different?
- What would it mean to consider that White people both benefit and are harmed by Whiteness? What would it mean to consider this if you are a helping professional of color? A White helping professional?
- Coming together across racial lines could provide an opportunity for solidarity or collaboration, but also pain and harm. Thinking about your own identity, what would make you hesitant about a multiracial coalition? What would you need to feel safe in a cross-racial space?
- Given the review of the more effective DEI initiatives above, which findings surprised you? Which confirmed your pre-existing beliefs about DEI?
- As a trainee or educator in the helping professions, which of the more effective components of DEI reviewed above are already implemented in your program? Which ones are missing? What would need to change in your training setting to be a more inclusive and space for educators and trainees?

Quiz Questions

1. The Race-Class Lens argues that White people suffer the same as people of color.

   True_____ False_____

2. DEI research shows that the effects of multicultural training can be meager, unless it is supported by longer-term institutional policy, opportunities for positive intergroup contact, and core values that make diversity and equity central to an institution's mission.

   True_____ False_____

3. Economic inequality leads to racism. Therefore, addressing economic issues will alleviate racism.

True_____ False_____

References

Abe, J. (2020). Beyond cultural competence, toward social transformation: Liberation psychologies and the practice of cultural humility. *Journal of Social Work Education, 56*(4), 696–707.
Ahad, B. S. (2010). *Freud upside down: African American literature and psychoanalytic culture*. University of Illinois Press.
Ayala-Lopez, S., & Beeghly, E. (2020). Explaining injustice: Structural analysis, bias, and individuals. In *An introduction to implicit bias* (pp. 211–232). Routledge.
Barber, K., Bridges, T., & Nelson, J. D. (2019). Mitigating the harms of masculinity: A symposium on the APA guidelines for psychological practice with boys and men. *Men and Masculinities, 22*(5), 905–908.
Benuto, L. T., Casas, J., & O'Donohue, W. T. (2018). Training culturally competent psychologists: A systematic review of the training outcome literature. *Training and Education in Professional Psychology, 12*(3), 125–134.
Bernstein, R. S., Bulger, M., Salipante, P., & Weisinger, J. Y. (2020). From diversity to inclusion to equity: A theory of generative interactions. *Journal of Business Ethics, 167*(3), 395–410.
Bezrukova, K., Spell, C. S., Perry, J. L., & Jehn, K. A. (2016). A meta-analytical integration of over 40 years of research on diversity training evaluation. *Psychological Bulletin, 142*(11), 1227.
Bor, J., Cohen, G. H., & Galea, S. (2017). Population health in an era of rising income inequality: USA, 1980–2015. *The Lancet, 389*(10077), 1475–1490.
Brown, L. S. (2008). *Cultural competence in trauma therapy: Beyond the flashback*. American Psychological Association.
Butcher, J., & Gonzalez, M. (2020). Critical race theory, the new intolerance, and its grip on America. *Heritage Foundation Backgrounder, 3567*, 1–42.
Cameron, C. D., Harris, L. T., & Payne, B. K. (2016). The emotional cost of humanity: Anticipated exhaustion motivates dehumanization of stigmatized targets. *Social Psychological and Personality Science, 7*(2), 105–112.

Carter, E. R., Onyeador, I. N., & Lewis, N. A., Jr. (2020). Developing & delivering effective anti- bias training: Challenges & recommendations. *Behavioral Science & Policy, 6*(1), 57–70.

Clauss-Ehlers, C. S., Chiriboga, D. A., Hunter, S. J., Roysircar, G., & Tummala-Narra, P. (2019). APA multicultural guidelines executive summary: Ecological approach to context, identity, and intersectionality. *American Psychologist, 74*(2), 232.

Condon, M., & Wichowsky, A. (2020). Inequality in the social mind: Social comparison and support for redistribution. *The Journal of Politics, 82*(1), 149–161.

Crenshaw, K. (1990). Mapping the margins: Intersectionality, identity politics, and violence against women of color. *Stanford Law Review, 43*, 1241–1299.

Devine, P. G., Plant, E. A., Amodio, D. M., Harmon-Jones, E., & Vance, S. L. (2002). The regulation of explicit and implicit race bias: The role of motivations to respond without prejudice. *Journal of Personality and Social Psychology, 82*(5), 835.

Dobbin, F., & Kalev, A. (2018). Why doesn't diversity training work? The challenge for industry and academia. *Anthropology Now, 10*(2), 48–55.

Dubois, W. E. B. (1935) 1973. *Black reconstruction in America, 1860–1880*. Atheneum.

Engler, S., & Weisstanner, D. (2020). The threat of social decline: Income inequality and radical right support. *Journal of European Public Policy*, 1–21.

Forscher, P. S., Lai, C. K., Axt, J. R., Ebersole, C. R., Herman, M., Devine, P. G., & Nosek, B. A. (2019). A meta-analysis of procedures to change implicit measures. *Journal of Personality and Social Psychology, 117*(3), 522–559.

Frantell, K. A., Miles, J. R., & Ruwe, A. M. (2019). Intergroup dialogue: A review of recent empirical research and its implications for research and practice. *Small Group Research, 50*(5), 654–695.

Freire, P. (1972). *Pedagogy of the oppressed*. Penguin.

Frymer, P., & Grumbach, J. M. (2021). Labor unions and White racial politics. *American Journal of Political Science, 65*(1), 225–240.

Gregus, S. J., Stevens, K. T., Seivert, N. P., Tucker, R. P., & Callahan, J. L. (2020). Student perceptions of multicultural training and program climate in clinical psychology doctoral programs. *Training and Education in Professional Psychology, 14*(4), 293–307.

Gurin, P., Nagda, B. R. A., & Zúñiga, X. (2013). *Dialogue across difference: Practice, theory, and research on intergroup dialogue*. Russell Sage Foundation.

Helms, J. E. (1990). *Black and White racial identity: Theory, research, and practice*. Greenwood Press.
Hook, J. N., Davis, D., Owen, J., & DeBlaere, C. (2017). *Cultural humility: Engaging diverse identities in therapy*. American Psychological Association.
Kidder, D. L., Lankau, M. J., Chrobot-Mason, D., Mollica, K. A., & Friedman, R. A. (2004). Backlash toward diversity initiatives: Examining the impact of diversity program justification, personal and group outcomes. *International Journal of Conflict Management, 15*, 77–102.
Kim, M. S., Kim, D., & Altema McNeely, N. (2020). Race, inequality, and social capital in the US counties. *The Social Science Journal*, 1–19.
Kosakowska-Berezecka, N., Besta, T., Bosson, J. K., Jurek, P., Vandello, J. A., Best, D. L., … Žukauskienė, R. (2020). Country-level and individual-level predictors of men's support for gender equality in 42 countries. *European Journal of Social Psychology, 50*(6), 1276–1291.
Krems, J. A., & Varnum, M. E. W. (2017). More than just climate: Income inequality and sex ratio are better predictors of cross-cultural variations in aggression. *Behavioral and Brain Sciences, 40*, 58.
Legault, L., Gutsell, J. N., & Inzlicht, M. (2011). Ironic effects of antiprejudice messages: How motivational interventions can reduce (but also increase) prejudice. *Psychological Science, 22*(12), 1472–1477.
Leslie, L. M., Bono, J. E., Kim, Y. S., & Beaver, G. R. (2020). On melting pots and salad bowls: A meta-analysis of the effects of identity-blind and identity-conscious diversity ideologies. *Journal of Applied Psychology, 105*(5), 453–471.
Leslie, L. M., Mayer, D. M., & Kravitz, D. A. (2014). The stigma of affirmative action: A stereotyping-based theory and meta-analytic test of the consequences for performance. *Academy of Management Journal, 57*(4), 964–989.
López, I. H. (2019). *Merge left: Fusing race and class, winning elections, and saving America*. The New Press.
Macdonald, D. (2020). Trust in government and the American public's responsiveness to rising inequality. *Political Research Quarterly, 73*(4), 790–804.
Macdonald, D. (2021). Immigration attitudes and White Americans' responsiveness to rising income inequality. *American Politics Research, 49*(2), 132–142.
Mallinckrodt, B., Miles, J. R., & Levy, J. J. (2014). The scientist-practitioner-advocate model: Addressing contemporary training needs for social justice advocacy. *Training and Education in Professional Psychology, 8*(4), 303–311.
Martín-Baró, I. (1994). *Writings for a liberation psychology*. Harvard University Press.

Marx, K. (1844). Contribution to the critique of Hegel's philosophy of right. *Deutsch-Französische Jahrbücher, 7*(10), 261–271.

McGhee, H. (2021). *The sum of us: What racism costs everyone and how we can prosper together*. One World/Ballantine.

Mechanic, M. (2021). *Jackpot: How the super-rich really live—And how their wealth harms us all*. Simon and Schuster.

Meleady, R., Crisp, R. J., Hodson, G., & Earle, M. (2019). On the generalization of intergroup contact: A taxonomy of transfer effects. *Current Directions in Psychological Science, 28*(5), 430–435.

Meleady, R., Seger, C., & Vermue, M. (2020). Evidence of a dynamic association between intergroup contact and intercultural competence. *Group Processes & Intergroup Relations*, 1–21.

Metzl, J. M. (2019). *Dying of whiteness: How the politics of racial resentment is killing America's heartland*. Hachette UK.

Nadal, K. L. (2017). "Let's get in formation": On becoming a psychologist–activist in the 21st century. *American Psychologist, 72*(9), 935–946.

Newkirk, P. (2019). *Diversity, Inc.: The failed promise of a billion-dollar business*. Hachette UK.

Nnawulezi, N., Case, K. A., & Settles, I. H. (2020). Ambivalent white racial consciousness: Examining intersectional reflection and complexity in practitioner graduate training. *Women & Therapy, 43*(3–4), 365–388.

Noon, M. (2018). Pointless diversity training: Unconscious bias, new racism and agency. *Work, Employment and Society, 32*(1), 198–209.

Onyeador, I. N., Hudson, S. K. T., & Lewis, N. A., Jr. (2021). Moving beyond implicit bias training: Policy insights for increasing organizational diversity. *Policy Insights From the Behavioral and Brain Sciences, 8*(1), 19–26.

Payne, B. K., Vuletich, H. A., & Brown-Iannuzzi, J. L. (2019). Historical roots of implicit bias in slavery. *Proceedings of the National Academy of Sciences, USA, 116*(24), 11693–11698.

Payne, B. K., Vuletich, H. A., & Lundberg, K. B. (2017). The bias of crowds: How implicit bias bridges personal and systemic prejudice. *Psychological Inquiry, 28*(4), 233–248.

Reed, T. (2020). *Toward freedom: The case against race reductionism*. Verso Books.

Rodríguez, J., Nagda, B. R. A., Sorensen, N., & Gurin, P. (2018). Engaging race and racism for socially just intergroup relations: The impact of intergroup dialogue on college campuses in the United States. *Multicultural Education Review, 10*(3), 224–245.

Sengupta, N. K., Greaves, L. M., Osborne, D., & Sibley, C. G. (2017). The sigh of the oppressed: The palliative effects of ideology are stronger for people living in highly unequal neighbourhoods. *British Journal of Social Psychology, 56*(3), 437–454.

Shepherd, S. M. (2019). Cultural awareness workshops: Limitations and practical consequences. *BMC Medical Education, 19*(1), 1–10.

Sue, D. W., Sue, D., Neville, H. A., & Smith, L. (2019). *Counseling the culturally diverse: Theory and practice.* John Wiley & Sons.

Taylor, K. Y. (2016). *From# BlackLivesMatter to black liberation.* Haymarket Books.

Vuletich, H. A., & Payne, B. K. (2019). Stability and change in implicit bias. *Psychological Science, 30*(6), 854–862.

Wilderson III, F. B. (2020). *Afropessimism.* New York: Liveright.

Wilkinson, R., & Pickett, K. (2020). *The inner level: How more equal societies reduce stress, restore sanity and improve everyone's well-being.* Penguin Books.

Yu, S. (2018). Uncovering the hidden impacts of inequality on mental health: A global study. *Translational Psychiatry, 8*(1), 1–10.

19

Antiracism and Health: An Action Plan for Mitigating Racism in Healthcare

Janice Hawkins, Leslie Hoglund, Jamela M. Martin, Marvin T. Chiles, and Kimberly Adams Tufts

Introduction

Racial and ethnic minorities experience a disproportionate burden of poor health outcomes. Unequal treatment and lack of patient-provider concordance in healthcare results in power differentials, lower quality of care, increased prevalence of disease, and poor health outcomes. Racism, alongside other inequitable determinants of health, is a significant contributor to negative health outcomes. Evidence of racism exists among

J. Hawkins (✉) • L. Hoglund • J. M. Martin • M. T. Chiles
Old Dominion University, Norfolk, VA, USA
e-mail: JHawkins@odu.edu; lhoglund@odu.edu; jm1marti@odu.edu; mchiles@odu.edu

K. A. Tufts
Hampton Veterans Medical Center, Hampton, VA, USA
e-mail: Kimberly.AdamsTufts@va.gov

© The Author(s), under exclusive license to Springer Nature Switzerland AG 2022

K. Johnson et al. (eds.), *Developing Anti-Racist Practices in the Helping Professions: Inclusive Theory, Pedagogy, and Application*,
https://doi.org/10.1007/978-3-030-95451-2_19

healthcare professionals at rates comparable to the general population (Hall et al., 2015; Paradies et al., 2014).

The stress of racism has been found to contribute to a phenomenon termed *weathering* (Geronimus, 1992). Weathering is described as the impact of chronic social and environmental stressors that diminish health over time. Chronic stress impacts diseases at the cellular level through repeated activation of the sympathoadrenal system, leading to cumulative hastening of aging, inflammation, and cell stress (Chae et al., 2020). Hence, it is hypothesized that persistent exposure to structural racism and social stress results in the early onset of chronic disease and increased morbidity and mortality due to premature physiologic aging (Geronimus, 1992). Confronting systemic structural racism and the subsequent social, economic and political oppression mitigates the weathering effect and positively influences health outcomes (Geronimus, 2001). This chapter examines the link between racism and the weathering effect on health. Additionally, an action plan is provided for individuals and organizations who are ready to enact change.

Background

The World Health Organization (WHO) describes the social, economic and physical "conditions in which people are born, grow, live, work and age" as the social determinants of health (WHO, 2020). Racism is specifically identified as a health determinant (Office of Disease Prevention and Health Promotion [ODPHP], 2020). The disproportionate burden of the COVID- 19 pandemic in Black and Brown communities has amplified pre-existing inequities in the healthcare system. Socioeconomic disadvantages rooted in racism have resulted in higher rates of comorbidities and societal burdens that increase vulnerability to COVID-19 (Laurencin & McClinton, 2020; van Dorn et al., 2020; Webb Hooper et al., 2020; Yancy, 2020).

Historical Influences

Healthcare inequities have been long established in the United States (US). Historians have found that the chains of slavery have not only stamped Blacks with an inferior racial classification, but also rendered them defenseless against the violence of dehumanizing healthcare practices designed to justify scientifically their 'inferiority'. During the sixteenth and seventeenth century, Europeans used the commodification of slave labor as a lens to investigate Black bodies. Methods ranging from tasting sweat to grabbing genitalia helped them conclude that the minute biological differences between Black and White bodies, mainly skin color, reflected a natural, inherent black inferiority (Hogarth, 2017). The practices and inhumanity of slavery influenced conventional medical knowledge. The current notion that Blacks have higher pain tolerance, still seen as scientific fact by some, came directly out of America's initial encounter and perfection of chattel slavery (Salvitt, 1978).

As the nation around them became more dependent on slave labor in the nineteenth century, the need to commodify slavery anchored the inequities that birthed modern American healthcare. Slave owners hired physicians to maintain the capacity of work and productivity as well as the marketability of slaves (Baptist, 2014). Their medical assessments reinforced conventional knowledge that racial difference was a biological fact that predestined Whites to be superior to Blacks. A healthy Black man was a slave who appeared to be physically able to work. Assessment of Black women's health was tied to their ability to operate as field workers and breeders (Cooper Owens, 2018; Fett, 2002).

Formal slavery ended in 1865. However, structural racism and inherent discrimination did not. The post Civil War era brought new healthcare challenges for thousands of sick and dying freed men and women whose former masters were no longer bound by profit to 'care' for them. The US government filled this void by tasking the Freedmen's Bureau with providing healthcare to former Black slaves. Their intention was to convert the formerly enslaved into autonomous, taxable free laborers. This profit-seeking agenda, combined with a mix of malice and incompetence, resulted in neglectful inadequate healthcare, turning many of the

Black sick into the Black dead. The Bureau's systematized neglect was now the governmental standard (Downs, 2012).

Structural racism linked to post Civil War Jim Crow laws favors majority populations and limits the capacity of minorities to improve their socioeconomic status. Historically, minorities have not had equal access to educational and occupational opportunities (Yearby, 2018). The segregation of neighborhoods by race, initiated in the late nineteenth century, still persists today. Residents of lower socioeconomic neighborhoods, often minorities, have limited healthcare access and lower quality care. Minorities also experience higher rates of hiring discrimination, unemployment and overrepresentation in lower paying service occupations (Solomon et al., 2019).

Limiting educational and occupational opportunities for minorities results in a racial wealth gap and negatively impacts our economy. Economists estimate the wealth of average White families at more than ten times the wealth of average Black families. The wealth gap translates to a projected loss of one to 1.5 trillion dollars to the US economy over the next several years (Noel et al., 2019). Structural racist practices such as hiring discrimination, biased standardized educational testing, and neighborhood segregation is associated with decreased utilization of preventive health care services (Henning-Smith et al., 2019) resulting in increased healthcare costs (Castro Sweet et al., 2020; Dehmer et al., 2017; Lee et al., 2018) and ultimately, lower life expectancy (O'Brien et al., 2020). Hence, race-based inequities cost billions of annual dollars in healthcare spending and lost productivity (LaVeist et al., 2011).

These inequities are also reflected in the limited racial and ethnic diversity of the healthcare workforce. By the 1940s, nearly 90% (less than 200 annually) of Black physicians received training at Black medical schools, specifically Howard and Meharry (Byrd & Clayton, 2000; JBHE Foundation, 2000; Rudwick, 1951). Historically, Blacks represented 10% to 12% of annual graduating medical professionals (Butler, 2012; JBHE Foundation, 1997). Patients expect providers like them. Yet, there are often racial, ethnic, and class differences between patients and healthcare professionals. As a whole, healthcare professionals represent privileged majority populations. Notably the largest group of healthcare professionals, nurses, are 73.3% White (Health Resources and Services

Administration, 2019) while physicians are 56.2% White (Association of American Medical Colleges, 2020) and often come from higher socioeconomic backgrounds (Youngclaus & Roskovensky, 2018). In a systematic review of 37 studies, White physicians demonstrate higher levels of implicit bias than Black physicians (Maina et al., 2018).

The lack of patient-provider concordance in healthcare is a form of institutional racism. Distrust of discordant patient-provider relationships is rooted in historical norms of discrimination, unethical harm and treatment, and inferior care. Patient-provider concordance, highest among Whites, mediates trust, adherence, disease management, and less attrition in follow-up (Poma, 2017). Notably, race concordance in healthcare is associated with greater patient satisfaction and improved health outcomes (Cooper & Powe, 2004; LaVeist & Nuru-Jeter, 2002; Poma, 2017; Street et al., 2008).

Health Inequities

The sequela of structural racism and its manifestations including the implied biological inferiority of Black and Brown populations, economic and educational disadvantages, and patient-provider discordance have been associated with healthcare inequities and poor health outcomes. Racism and discrimination have been linked to decreased life expectancy associated with higher rates of heart disease, cancer, diabetes, obesity, poor oral health, depression, maternal morbidity, infant mortality, and more. Well documented negative cardiovascular impacts linked to racism and discrimination include hypertensive disorders, myocardial ischemia, dysrhythmias, hypercholesterolemia, and hyperglycemia. Studies have demonstrated a relationship between racism and negative cancer outcomes (Beyer et al., 2017; Dawes et al., 2016; Moore et al., 2013; Sighoko et al., 2017).

Maternal stress is a known contributor to poor fetal and maternal outcomes. The stress of discrimination has been specifically linked to preterm births and low birth weights. Black women frequently enter prenatal care at later gestational stages and have fewer prenatal care visits, a trend that is at least partially attributed to experiences of racism and discrimination in healthcare (Gadson et al., 2017). Black and Indigenous American babies are twice as likely to die before their first birthday compared to White babies (Centers for Disease Control and Prevention [CDC], 2020a). Increased rates of infant mortality, preterm births and low birthweight babies have been directly linked to structural racism and associated inequities in educational, economical and occupational opportunities (Beck et al., 2020; Wallace et al., 2017).

Significantly, women with Arabic sounding names who gave birth in California within six months after 9/11 had more low birth weight and preterm babies in contrast to a comparable group of women who gave birth the previous year (Lauderdale, 2006). Similarly, Latino women had a 24% increase of low birth weight infants after a traumatic U.S. Immigration and Customs Enforcement raid in Iowa. This increase occurred in both immigrant and US born Latino women. Non-Latino White women who gave birth in the same facilities during the same time period did not have a change in birth weight outcomes (Novak et al., 2017). Maternal mortality rates are also 2–5 times higher for Black and Indigenous American women than for White women in the US (CDC, 2019). Regardless of socioeconomic status, Black and other minority women experience a system of unequal treatment and limited access to quality healthcare that results in less than optimal maternal and infant outcomes (Beck et al., 2020).

Deliberate antiracist measures are necessary to promote greater health equity for chronically oppressed or disadvantaged populations. Measures to address systemic racism in healthcare must include action framed by a social-ecological perspective, informed by data, and grounded in the context of lived experiences. Collective impact principles, including community dialogue and engaged civic leadership, must be incorporated to effectively address racism in healthcare with the goal of positively influencing health outcomes.

Call to Action

Removal of structural and systemic barriers that have consistently plagued underrepresented racial and ethnic minority groups and resultant health inequities can facilitate the achievement of optimal health outcomes (Nardi et al., 2020). A number of tools and strategies are emerging to address negative social determinants of health. Mutual goals shared across all areas of government include the application of a "health in all policies" strategy to close existing health gaps, and the use of health impact assessments to review needed, proposed, and existing social policies for their likely impact on health (ODPHP, 2020). The CDC's (2020b) 10 Essential Public Health Services (10 EPHS) framework supports an immediate call to action for addressing racism in healthcare (see Fig. 19.1) and describes action points designed to achieve equity in healthcare. The broad areas of action are assessment, policy development, and assurance as follows:

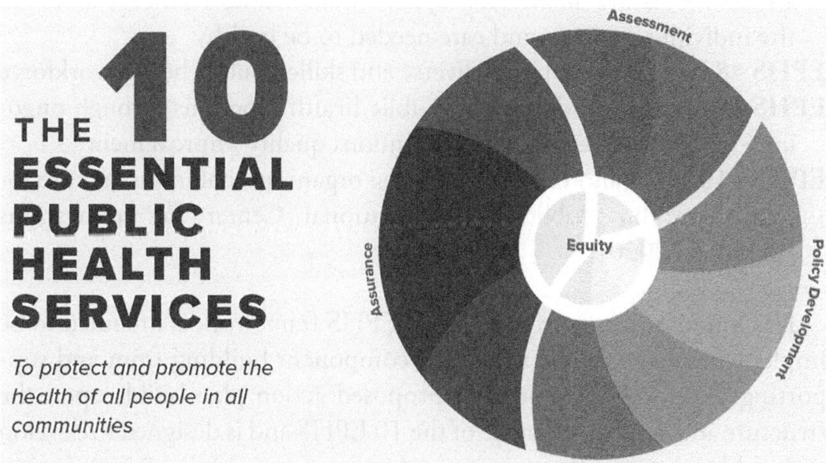

Fig. 19.1 The 10 essential public health services. (Public Health National Center for Innovations [PHNCI], 2020)

Assessment

- **EPHS #1** Assess and monitor population health
EPHS #2 Investigate, diagnose, and address health hazards and root causes

Policy Development

- **EPHS#3** Communicate effectively to inform and educate people about health
EPHS #4 Strengthen, support, and mobilize communities and partnerships to improve health
EPHS #5 Create, champion, and implement policies, plans, and laws that impact health
EPHS #6 Utilize legal and regulatory actions designed to improve and protect the public's health

Assurance

- **EPHS #7** Assure an effective system that enables equitable access to the individual services and care needed to be healthy
EPHS #8 Build and support a diverse and skilled public health workforce
EPHS #9 Improve and innovate public health functions through ongoing evaluation, research, and continuous quality improvement
EPHS #10 Build and maintain a strong organizational infrastructure for public health. (Public Health National Center for Innovations [PHNCI], 2020)

It is important to note that the 10 EPHS framework is intended to be implemented as a whole, with each component building from and supporting the next. Therefore, the proposed action plan builds upon the structure and general guidance of the 10 EPHS and is designed to develop actionable measures that can be undertaken at multiple socioecological levels to mitigate racism in healthcare.

Action Plan

Racism is a root cause of the social arrangements that ***allocate life*** *to some and* ***premature death*** *to others. (Arrianna Planey, MA, PhD).*

The striking persistence of health inequities for racial and ethnic minorities can be attributed to partial approaches in addressing root causes. It is clear that racism results in disparate health outcomes at the individual level. However, this myopic focus on implementing individual-level solutions has not brought about an equitable healthcare system but has led to limited success in addressing what are largely systemic issues. A typical approach to solving issues of racism and disparities might include raising awareness of inequities (cultural competency module trainings, diversity and inclusion-based courses, diverse conversations, implicit bias training) and improving opportunities for minorities to participate in efforts to reduce prejudice (research participation, community engaged initiatives) (Williams & Cooper, 2019). These approaches are not enough, and will never be, because they fail to account for the ecological impacts of policy and practice. Even when individuals within the systems support antiracist attitudes and behaviors, the same views are not always ingrained within the systems and structures. To be clear, these approaches are valuable and necessary, yet they only address issues at a singular ecological level.

Healthcare institutions are rooted in institutional racism, structural violence, and historical injustice and must direct efforts to confront and reverse these pervasive social constructs (King & Redwood, 2016). Historical abuses are well-known in research like the Tuskegee Syphilis Study (Sharma, 2010), and more recently, the revelation of the prolific and unfettered use of "HeLa" cells from Henrietta Lacks, a Black woman with cervical cancer who never consented to her cells being taken (Beskow, 2016). Hospitals, clinics, and public health departments are parts of a larger ecosystem that struggles to reduce Black maternal and infant mortality, decrease heart disease, diabetes, stroke, and hypertension, and improve life expectancy. This is often because health administrators and helping organizations that serve the myriad of Black communities are rarely influenced by them, especially when it comes to strategies and interventions that address poor health status (Noonan et al., 2016). Helping professionals will not be able to address complex and intersectional inequities on their own or in a silo (Cahn, 2020), however, they can seek to eliminate inequities in healthcare settings by investing in marginalized communities (King & Redwood, 2016). It will require mutually- reinforcing action at the structural and institutional levels and be guided by community influence and public policy level changes to shift course toward systems of care that create and protect equity.

To mitigate racism's impacts on health, we must actively acknowledge and seek ways to address all the contributing factors from a holistic, ecological, top-down approach. The social- ecological model (Bronfenbrenner, 2008) is a recognized systematic method for understanding health outcomes, including issues specific to underserved populations (Reno & Hyder, 2018). Social-ecology theory posits that multiple levels of influence shape individual outcomes, with factors at the highest levels influencing factors at successive levels. To sustain efforts over time, it is necessary to act across several levels of the model simultaneously (CDC, 2020b). Therefore, to address racism holistically, we must address root causes at public policy, community, organizational, and interpersonal levels and not just at the individual level. The proposed action plan considers the need for action at all levels of influence, with a goal of creating sustainable, impactful measures for imploring change via five key factors for action: (a) collective impact, (b) data-informed by real-life context, (c) community dialogue, (d) civic agency and leadership, and (e) system and structure revisions (see Fig. 19.2).

Fig. 19.2 Action plan key factors. (Original graphic: Leslie Hoglund)

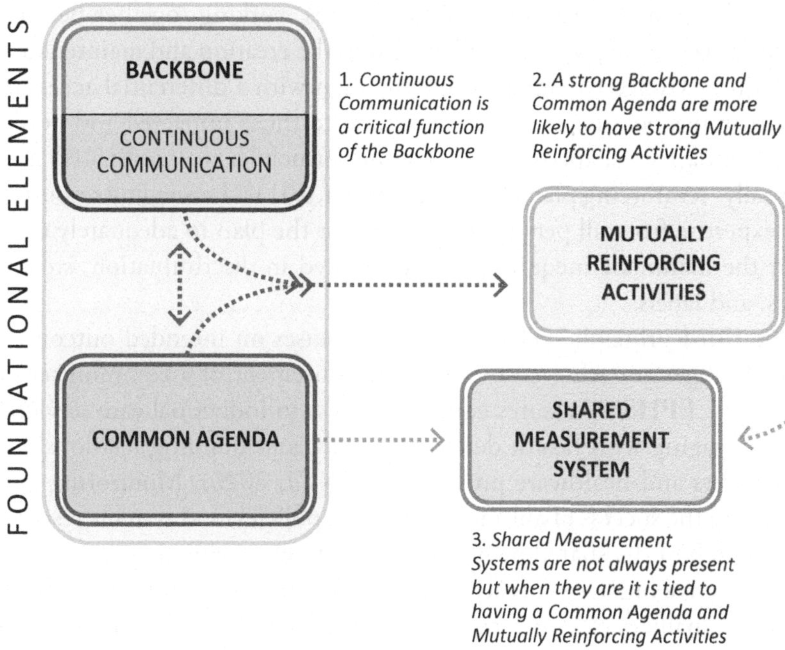

Fig. 19.3 The relationship between the collective impact conditions. (ORS Impact, 2018)

Collective Impact, a Structured Way to Achieve Antiracism

Collective impact works on social problems to bring about systemic change for population-level outcomes (see Fig. 19.3). The five collective impact principles give practitioners a framework to advocate for what works and to actively pursue social change (Kania & Kramer, 2011). Deconstructing and reshaping systems and institutions is generational work, and **first** requires a shared vision and agenda for change through strategic and intentional partnerships. In some places, there is much to discover about what works. Authentically engaging communities as partners is critical for and required to address cultural racism to bring forward antiracist impact. This aligns with **EPHS #4** as a mechanism for convening, facilitating, and contributing expertise to solutions (PHNCI, 2020).

To achieve health equity, it takes all of us working together because racism drives social policies that have led to the creation and maintenance of inequity. Collective impact does not align with a differential access to opportunities because the goal is listening to those impacted and developing initiatives shaped by the **second** principle: a coordinated and mutually- reinforcing plan (Kania & Kramer, 2011). Leveraging resources and expertise from all perspectives allows for the plan to adequately confront the manmade inequities that are rooted in discrimination, stereotypes, and labels.

The **third** principle collective impact focuses on intended outcomes. Thus, changes are achieved by shared measurement of a common set of indicators. **EPHS #7** assures equitable access to individual care services, when engaging with health delivery systems, and building relationships with payers and healthcare providers (PHNCI, 2020). Monitoring and evaluating the success of antiracist activities, policies, and systems rests on the strength of the shared ownership around measurement.

A collective impact approach requires administrators and practitioners to intentionally decide to focus on mutually derived goals and elevate a culture of collaboration that shares and releases power and authority (Stachowiak & Gase, 2018). Credit is only given to the achievement of the goals of antiracism, not to individuals. Continuous communication and backbone support – the **fourth** and **fifth** principles – guide and advance strategy, policy, system, and environmental changes for reparation, alignment, and improvement. A diverse organization of leadership, staff, and capacity to backbone or manage the work is critical to collective impact's success (Stachowiak & Gase, 2018). **EPHS #8** implores the role of building and supporting a diverse and skilled workforce that encompasses a broad spectrum of cultural competencies and humilities.

Racial justice has been described as the "proactive reinforcement of policies, practices, attitudes and actions that produce equitable power, access, opportunities, treatment, impacts and outcomes for all" (Lawrence & Keleher, 2004, p. 2). **EPHS #6** supports legal and regulatory actions to protect communities from hazardous conditions that cause health crises (PHNCI, 2020). The goal of employing a collective approach is to create antiracist systems, policies, and practices to accelerate racial justice (Ogden, 2017).

Data-Informed By Real-Life Local Context

Being data-informed means we ground and validate the data in the real-life context of lived experiences, deliberately and specifically with those who are negatively impacted and who experience poor health outcomes. The quantitative data shows disparities and inequities in health outcomes; it is well established why these exist and who they impact the most. Still, there is not enough emphasis and priority on how these data are qualitatively grounded in the community. This is a primary factor for accelerating antiracist action – by translating data into real action. **EPHS #1** and **EPHS #2** rely on the strength of multi-sector collaboration and the use of real- time data, technology, and innovation to assess, monitor, and improve population health (PHNCI, 2020). Disaggregating data to illuminate root causes of inequities must be backed by community voice.

For decades, we have been highlighting the impact of healthcare inequities and their associated less than optimal health outcomes without an understanding of how structural racism informs the social determinants of health and lived experiences of those who are impacted (Kilbourne et al., 2006). The data provides evidence that there is a reason to intervene; to change policy and practice. However, our traditional approaches to data collection and the very nature of those data, implies bias (Owens & Walker, 2020). Therefore, the data must be evaluated to determine whether it tells the whole story or the right story. We do this by collecting qualitative data that seeks to understand multilevel determinants, primary individual's beliefs and preferences, effective organization and communication of services because the goal is trust (Kilbourne et al., 2006). Once we, as antiracist practitioners, know what the data informs about how assets and resources can be expanded, enhanced or created, we can champion indicators for interventions that promote further engagement of communities, providers, and policymakers. **EPHS #9** ensures that improvement derives from utilizing data to inform decision-making processes, both quantitatively and qualitatively (PHNCI, 2020). Linking data together for monitoring of solutions assures alignment and congruence with what works for the population being served.

Listening Generously Through Community Dialogue

Community and patient population dialogue is about robust, ongoing conversation with those who are most affected by oppressive systems of disadvantage, racism, and injustice (Lowery, 2017). As antiracist helping professionals, we must listen and hear what the community is saying needs to change and act accordingly. Because we do not inherently know their truth and our implicit bias may cloud our ability to hear it. Practicing decoloniality and antiracism principles take concerted effort and is demonstrated by humility and solidarity (Watkins et al., 2018). Community dialogues offer an approach to collectively understand words and behaviors, apply them to examine our own biases and prejudices, and diminish faulty characterization or condemnation (Lowery, 2017).

Listening generously through community dialogue means giving our undivided attention to those who experience and are impacted by racism and other prejudice. We are not accustomed to doing this work, we tend not to do it or we do not do it well (Lowery, 2017). Listening generously means staying present and engaged, even when it is uncomfortable and feels daunting, and seeking to understand through care and empathy (Came & Griffith, 2018). Antiracist professionals are curious and open to influence because they strongly value what works to improve outcomes for patients, not what is easy for them as professionals. **EPHS #3** expects an asset-based approach that addresses equity through health education and communication, including cultural and linguistically appropriate methods and materials (PHNCI, 2020).

EPHS #2 is about identifying problems and hazards affecting the population and using the agency and power of the community to discuss and dialogue toward solutions (PHNCI, 2020). True community dialogue can lead to a healthier community. Creating a safe and relaxed opportunity for dialogue is based on respect, one speaker at a time, being tough on ideas and not on people, and making the success of the dialogue the responsibility of everyone present. A helping professional can facilitate dialogue with any group of patients or members of the community. They do not have to be experts but must remain neutral so the group can address quality of life improvements through systems change, building capacity and leveraging resources, and measuring progress and outcomes. Becoming antiracist is deeply rooted in community dialogue circles (Love & Muhammad, 2017; Rodríguez et al. 2018; Watkins et al., 2018). There are many emerging examples of antiracism dialogue offerings at colleges, universities, and schools and other organizations such as the Antiracism Study-Dialogue Circles (ASDIC Curriculum, 2020), AWARE-LA (2020), and the Active Voices' (2009) Closer to the Truth Project.

Elevating Civic Agency and Leadership

Engaged civic leadership means that the ownership for organization and mobilization rests in the community or population in which the change in outcomes is expected and needed. Unprecedented numbers of American citizens voted in the 2020 general election. Civic life has come alive beyond the traditional and led to galvanized social movements like Black Lives Matter, MeToo and TimesUp, among others, to root out prejudice, discrimination, and racial injustice. Hashtags and performative actions are not enough. Changing how resources and power are distributed and mobilizing allies and supporters through civic leadership will bring about antiracist policies and practices (Came & Griffith, 2018).

EPHS #5 aims to elevate policies, plans, and laws that correct historical injustices for fair and just health and well-being (PHNCI, 2020). A criticism of the collective impact principles is that it fails to elevate advocacy and empowerment for systems change as strongly as some would desire (Wolff et al., 2016). Collaborative action that incites transformative changes in power, equity, and justice is the goal. But led by who? The usual suspects of healthcare administrators, local government officials, social workers, public health directors, or by the people most disenfranchised, marginalized, and oppressed? Health in all policies assures that for any decision an organization or institution might consider, the voice of impacted people must be sought out and considered.

Community resilience is a common aspiration for many Black communities. There is recognition and appreciation that people have their own agency and power, and can explicitly address and deconstruct the policies, systems, and practices entrenched with injustice and racism.

Patients, beneficiaries, and community members rarely have equal power at determining goals and allocation of resources, but that is exactly what is needed to elevate civic agency and leadership. While collective impact principles promote antiracism from the top down, civic agency aimed at health equity is the grassroots approach built on community organization. This is when intentional engagement is attentive to power differentials that puts patients in the position as advisor to test ideas, interpret data, make decisions, and address other issues that impact their lives (Pastor et al., 2018; Wolff et al., 2016). Civic agency puts solving problems, healing, and improving quality of life ahead of partisan politics, religion and faith, income status, race and ethnicity, and meritocracy (King & Redwood, 2016). Ownership is evidenced by being involved at every step and level so that the community and the partners both hold themselves accountable for the outcomes. **EPHS #6** adds equity to the legal and regulatory functions of government, institutions, and organizations by assuring protection of communities exposed to unsafe water, lack of food, and exposure to other hazardous conditions, such as racial injustice, that promote injury, disease, or death (PHNCI, 2020).

Community organizing is one of the most effective ways to leverage the power to demand and share in decision-making and structure the building of power to prioritize leaders, specifically, those who are impacted by racism. Power is deliberately released by those who are professionally paid to work on these issues, for example, those who are in the helping professions. It is not adequate for White professionals to simply acknowledge the power and privilege associated with their whiteness. The intrinsic motivation of helping professionals is evidenced by using power and privilege to undo racism in all of its forms, especially in alliance with others. Leaders know how to mobilize resources and people, to move from talk to action, and create the right structure for long-term antiracist transformation in systems, policies, and practices (Pastor et al., 2018). Civic leadership develops the capacity for conflict and flexibility in order to manage and reshape the culture toward equity as the driving force of antiracist action (Wolff et al., 2016).

Necessary Systems and Institutional Changes

The last element of the antiracist action plan is shifting systems and institutions to center and rest on equity and justice. This work must begin now and be an intentional action as a matter of priority. Disrupting the structures that are not working, that rigidly protect status quo and perpetuated inequities, is monumental. **EPHS #10** stresses the critical elements of organizational structure and influences research, innovation, health policy, and linkages to academia (PHNCI, 2020). The expectations for this service include ethical leadership and governance, strong decision-making and communications, accountability, transparency, inclusiveness, and integration in planning capacities. It requires the most decisive leadership and vision to develop and reconstruct antiracist structures within systems and institutions.

Dismantling systems and institutions is looked at as counterculture: "If it's not broken, why fix it?" But broken for whom? If a system, structure, or institution does not work for a considerable percentage of the population served, it would be advantageous to change and adapt to make it work. Dynamics of power, money, law, and politics significantly influence the types and rate of antiracist change that any helping profession system or institution would consider implementing. Breaking the cycle of ongoing inequity can be done. It must be done. **EPHS #6** focuses on public policy and regulation that can be implemented to ensure equity and quality in health care, with the goal being to protect the community and reduce exposure to diseases that can cause health crises (PHNCI, 2020). To be a helping professional means we advocate for the upstream where healthy people stay healthy, and we focus on the improvement of the conditions and factors that impact outcomes at all levels.

EPHS #5 emphasizes community health assessment and community health improvement planning processes to legitimize antiracist policies, plans, and laws for implementation (PHNCI, 2020). The goal of antiracist systems and institutions is rooted in justice. Margaret and Came (2019) debuted guiding questions to shape new paradigms to inspire organizations' antiracist action. Asking these questions at the executive levels will challenge current settings and structures. There must be humility in asking these questions because what is learned may be uncomfortable or difficult to accept.

1. What is our strategy for understanding and addressing racism in our workplace?
2. What is our strategy for achieving equity in our institution?
3. How are minority and indigenous peoples' health aspirations being prioritized and funded?
4. Who is missing from the decision-making table?
5. Who are we accountable to and for what?
6. How do our recruitment processes reflect and value cultural and political competencies?
7. How are we equipping staff to work across differences to understand their own power and position?
8. What mechanisms do we have to encourage each other to embrace our responsibilities and the roles we can take up from within our own cultural contexts?
9. What mechanisms do we have in place to make our work transparent and open to feedback?
10. What mechanisms do we have in place to ensure new relationships can be sustained? (Margaret & Came, 2019, pp. 320–322, 324).

Centering on healing is a part of dismantling racist structures and institutions. How does this affect the spirit of our patients, our staff, our community, and world? When relationships are emboldened and initiatives led by minority and indigenous people are supported and invested in, we see improvement in ways that lead to outcomes that lessen inequity and champion justice.

Communicating agency, elevating authority, and amplifying ability allows people who have been marginalized, who are forced to fit into systems that do not work, to make their own decisions and control the outcomes (Margaret & Came, 2019).

EPHS #7 aims to strengthen the relationships between public health, healthcare delivery systems, health care providers, and payers for the purpose of equitable access to preventive health services (PHNCI, 2020). Dominant cultures carry power designed for White people, and this privilege protects systems and institutions from addressing racism and injustice (Margaret & Came, 2019). An "unlearning and relearning" allows us to integrate new knowledge and skills into systems and institutional environments. Every day is an opportunity to communicate knowledge that promotes antiracism to lead the thoughts of others toward eradicating the racism entrenched in our systems and institutions. **EPHS #3** maintains accurate, timely, and appropriate communication with emphasis on assets and equity. Health education and communication science outline cultural and linguistically appropriate materials and channels (PHNCI, 2020).

The intended outcomes of this action plan is a just and equitable system of helping, healthcare, and public health. It is no longer acceptable to believe that our present institutional and organizational structure are sufficient for everyone's needs. We know health inequities exist and now we must reverberate the call for change and antiracist action.

Conclusion

The aim of this chapter was to offer an action plan to effectively address racism in healthcare and with the goal of positively influencing health outcomes. It has been well- established that racial and ethnic minorities experience a disproportionate burden of poor health outcomes with unequal treatment and lack of patient-provider concordance resulting in power differentials, lower quality of care, and increased prevalence of chronic disease. Despite our nation's attempts to address healthcare inequities at the individual level, health disparities for racial and ethnic minorities persist. It is known that persistent exposure to structural racism and social stress results in the early onset of chronic disease due to premature physiologic aging and increased morbidity and mortality. To create real, sustainable change, it is critical that we begin to address the root causes of the inequities at systemic and organizational, as well as individual, levels. Removal of structural and systemic barriers, which have consistently plagued underrepresented racial and ethnic minority groups, is particularly time-sensitive given our nation's current state of social unrest. Systems and institutions must act now, with intent and active prioritization, to begin shifting to a model of equity and justice. The action plan presented in this chapter promotes five key factors for action which can serve as guiding principles for tangible change. For healthcare organizations and professionals, application of this type of action plan must begin with a critical self-analysis. Supportive leadership, structural support (such as amended hiring practices, review of standing policies, coordination of activities, distribution of authority, and re/allocation of resources), and inter-organizational change agents are necessary. The tenets of the aforementioned framework can be used as a guide for normalization and acculturation of antiracist change.

A shared vision and agenda for change; a coordinated and mutually-reinforcing plan; the delineation of intended outcomes; guiding and advancing strategy; and policy, system, and environmental changes for reparation, alignment, and improvement are all actions that can be tailored to the needs of any profession. Similarly, grounding data in the real-life context of lived experiences, listening generously to individual and population-based needs, and elevating civic leadership within the context of a specific field (such as engineering, the arts, education, and business management to name a few) can initially be framed by the theoretical underpinnings of that specific discipline and then be furthered molded by the broader principles of an interprofessional antiracist action plan. Notably, the information presented in this chapter is useful to other helping professions and is not specifically limited to healthcare. Institutions, organizations, and individuals from all disciplines can utilize this action plan to promote tangible change in racist practices. The action plan presented herein is framed by the 10 Essential Public Health Services (10 EPHS). This interprofessional framework supports an immediate call to action for addressing racism in *healthcare*. The embedded five collective impact principles provide interprofessional teams with a foundational framework for actively pursuing social change through a deconstruction and reshaping of systems and institutions. Hence, these principles are broad enough to support interprofessional collaborative teams who seek to dismantle anti-racist practices.

Going forward, institutions and systems who choose to be antiracist and implement an action plan highlights a prioritization for the conditions and factors that generate and create equity and justice for all. It is deliberate and intentional and must be met and achieved through cultural humility and acceptance that institutions and systems must be improved—to actualize on the salutogenic vision whereby recipients of our services actually experience better health and wellness. We can be actively antiracist and uproot the racism embedded in the helping professions and dynamically change institutions, systems, and culture for optimal health outcomes.

1. In what ways does structural racism impact health outcomes?
2. What are some of the factors beyond individual choices and health practices that impact health outcomes?
3. What are some of the factors that positively or negatively impact health in your own community?
4. What role does implicit bias play in health inequities? What strategies can you identify to address implicit bias?
5. How can you use your knowledge of the existence of racism in healthcare to influence change?

Chapter Quiz

1. The five key factors for the action plan for mitigating racism in healthcare are collective impact, data-informed by real life contact, community dialogue, civic agency and leadership and:

   a. Public policy engagement
   b. System and structure revisions
   c. Diversity and inclusiveness training
   d. Grassroots advocacy

2. The CDC's 10 Essential Public Health Services framework offers specific guidelines under three broad areas of action. Which of the following is not one of the three broad areas of action?

   a. Assessment
   b. Policy development
   c. Assurance
   d. Evaluation

3. All but which of the following is noted in this chapter as an associated benefit of patient- provider concordance?
   a. Increased levels of trust
   b. Better patient outcomes
   c. Equal access to care
   d. Greater patient satisfaction
4. The social, economic, and physical conditions in which people are born, live, work and age are known as:
   a. The social determinants of health
   b. Socioeconomic status
   c. Institutional racism
   d. Collective impact
5. Structural racism and the resulting health inequities have been linked to higher rates of:
   a. Diabetes
   b. Heart disease
   c. Infant mortality
   d. All of the above
6. Racism in American healthcare is an issue that historians have traced back to?
   a. Jim Crow
   b. Slavery
   c. Civil War
   d. The 1960s
7. Which of the following is NOT a part of the Action Plan to create equity within healthcare?
   a. Creating a shared vision and agenda between providers and communities.
   b. Contextualizing data within the lived experiences of patients.

c. Elevating and prioritizing healthcare policies that correct historical injustices.
d. Allowing trained experts to have the final say in healthcare policy and procedures.

References

Active Voice. (2009). *The closer to the truth project: Facilitation and dialogue guide*. https://www.racialequitytools.org/resourcefiles/closer.pdf

ASDIC Curriculum. (2020). *Antiracism study-dialogue circles*. https://www.asdicircle.org/

Association of American Medical Colleges. (2020). *Diversity in medicine: Facts and figures 2019 executive summary*. https://www.aamc.org/data-reports/workforce/report/diversity-medicine-facts-and-figures-2019

AWARE-LA. (2020). *What we do*. https://www.awarela.org/what-we-do

Baptist, E. (2014). *The half has never been told: Slavery and the making of American capitalism*. Basic Books.

Beck, A. F., Edwards, E. M., Horbar, J. D., Howell, E. A., McCormick, M. C., & Pursley, D. M. (2020). The color of health: How racism, segregation, and inequality affect the health and well-being of preterm infants and their families. *Pediatric Research, 87*(2), 227–234. https://doi.org/10.1038/s41390-019-0513-6

Beskow, L. M. (2016). Lessons from HeLa cells: The ethics and policy of biospecimens. *Annual Review of Genomics and Human Genetics, 17*, 395–417. https://doi.org/10.1146/annurev-genom-083115-022536

Beyer, K. M. M., Bemanian, A., McGinley, E. L., Nattinger, A., & B. (2017). Institutional racism, segregation, and breast cancer outcomes. *Journal of Clinical Oncology, 35*(5_suppl), 199.

Bronfenbrenner, U. (2008). Ecological models of human development. In M. Gauvain & M. Cole (Eds.), *Readings on the development of children* (5th ed., pp. 14–19). Worth Publishers.

Butler, B. M. (2012). Shifting patterns in the premedical education of African Americans and the role of the HBCU. *Journal of African American Studies, 15*(4), 541–556. https://doi.org/10.1007/s12111-010-9135-0

Byrd, W. M., & Clayton, L. (2000). *An American health dilemma: A medical history of African Americans and the problem of race—Beginnings to 1900*. Routledge.

Cahn, P. S. (2020). How interprofessional collaborative practice can help dismantle systemic racism. *Journal of Interprofessional Care, 34*(4), 431–434. https://doi.org/10.1080/13561820.2020.1790224

Came, H., & Griffith, D. (2018). Tackling racism as a "wicked" public health problem: Enabling allies in anti-racism praxis. *Social Science & Medicine, 199*, 181–188. https://doi.org/10.1016/j.socscimed.2017.03.028

Castro Sweet, C., Bradner Jasik, C., Diebold, A., DuPuis, A., & Jendretzke, B. (2020). Cost savings and reduced health care utilization associated with participation in a digital diabetes prevention program in an adult workforce population. *Journal of Health Economics and Outcomes Research, 7*(2), 139–147. https://doi.org/10.36469/jheor.2020.14529

Centers for Disease Control and Prevention. (2019). *Racial and ethnic disparities continue in pregnancy-related deaths.* https://www.cdc.gov/media/releases/2019/p0905-racial-ethnic-disparities-pregnancy-deaths.html

Centers for Disease Control and Prevention. (2020a). *Infant mortality*. https://www.cdc.gov/reproductivehealth/maternalinfanthealth/infantmortality.htm#mortality

Centers for Disease Control and Prevention. (2020b). *The 10 essential public health services.* https://www.cdc.gov/publichealthgateway/publichealthservices/essentialhealthservices.html

Chae, D. H., Wang, Y., Martz, C. D., Slopen, N., Yip, T., Adler, N. E., Fuller-Rowell, T. E., Lin, J., Matthews, K. A., Brody, G. H., Spears, E. C., Puterman, E., & Epel, E. S. (2020). Racial discrimination and telemore shortening among African Americans: The Coronary Artery Risk Development in Young Adults (CARDIA) study. *Health Psychology, 39*(3), 209–219. https://doi.org/10.1037/hea0000832

Cooper, L., & Powe, N. (2004). *Disparities in patient experiences, health care processes, and outcomes: The role of patient-provider racial, ethnic, and language concordance*. The Commonwealth Fund.

Cooper Owens, D. (2018). *Medical bondage: Race, gender, and the origins of American gynecology*. University of Georgia Press.

Dawes, S. M., Tsai, S., Gittleman, H., Barnholtz-Sloan, J. S., & Bordeaux, J. S. (2016). Racial disparities in melanoma survival. *Journal of the American Academy of Dermatology, 75*(5), 983–991. https://doi.org/10.1016/j.jaad.2016.06.006

Dehmer, S. P., Maciosek, M. V., LaFrance, A. B., & Flottemesch, T. J. (2017). Health benefits and cost-effectiveness of asymptomatic screening for hypertension and high cholesterol and aspirin counseling for primary prevention. *Annals of Family Medicine, 15*(1), 23–36. https://doi.org/10.1370/afm.2015

Downs, J. (2012). *Sick from freedom: African-American illness and suffering during the civil war and reconstruction*. Oxford University Press.

Fett, S. (2002). *Working cures: Healing, health, and power on southern slave plantations*. The University of North Carolina Press.

Gadson, A., Akpovi, E., & Mehta, P. K. (2017). Exploring the social determinants of racial/ethnic disparities in prenatal care utilization and maternal outcome. *Seminars in Perinatology, 41*(5), 308–317. https://doi.org/10.1053/j.semperi.2017.04.008

Geronimus, A. T. (1992). The weathering hypothesis and the health of African-American women and infants: Evidence and speculations. *Ethnicity & Disease, 2*(3), 207–221.

Geronimus, A. T. (2001). Understanding and eliminating racial inequalities in women's health in the United States: The role of the weathering conceptual framework. *Journal of the American Medical Women's Association, 56*(4), 133–136, 149–50.

Hall, W. J., Chapman, M. V., Lee, K. M., Merino, Y. M., Thomas, T. W., Payne, B. K., Eng, E., Day, S. H., & Coyne-Beasley, T. (2015). Implicit racial/ethnic bias among health care professionals and its influence on health care outcomes: A systematic review. *American Journal of Public Health, 105*(12), e60–e76. https://doi.org/10.2105/AJPH.2015.302903

Health Resources and Services Administration, National Center for Health Workforce Analysis. (2019). *Brief summary results from the 2018 national sample survey of registered nurses*. U.S. Department of Health and Human Services. https://data.hrsa.gov/DataDownload/NSSRN/GeneralPUF18/2018_NSSRN_Summary_Report-508.pdf

Henning-Smith, C., Ramirez, M., Hernandez, A. M., Hardeman, R. R., & Kozhimannil, K. B. (2019). *Differences in preventive care among rural residents by race and ethnicity.* University of Minnesota Rural Health Research Center. https://3pea7g1qp8f3t9ooe3z3npx1-wpengine.netdna-ssl.com/wp-content/uploads/2019/11/UMN-preventive-services-disparities-policy-brief_11.8.19.pdf

Hogarth, R. (2017). *Medicalizing blackness: Making racial difference in the Atlantic world, 1780-1840*. University of North Carolina Press.

JBHE Foundation. (1997). A quarter-century of black progress in medical school education. *The Journal of Blacks in Higher Education, 15*, 18–20. https://doi.org/10.2307/2962669

JBHE Foundation. (2000). A half-century of progress of black students in medical schools. *The Journal of Blacks in Higher Education, 30*, 28–31. https://doi.org/10.2307/2679066

Kania, J., & Kramer, M. (2011). Collective impact. *Stanford Social Innovation Review.* https://ssir.org/articles/entry/collective_impact

Kilbourne, A. M., Switzer, G., Hyman, K., Crowley-Matoka, M., & Fine, M. J. (2006). Advancing health disparities research within the health care system: A conceptual framework. *American Journal of Public Health, 96*(12), 2113–2121. https://doi.org/10.2105/AJPH.2005.077628

King, C. J., & Redwood, Y. (2016). The health care institution, population health and black lives. *Journal of the National Medical Association, 108*(2), 131–136. https://doi.org/10.1016/j.jnma.2016.04.002

Lauderdale, D. S. (2006). Birth outcomes for Arabic-named women in California before and after September 11. *Demography, 43*(1), 185–201. https://doi.org/10.1353/dem.2006.0008

Laurencin, C. T., & McClinton, A. (2020). The COVID-19 pandemic: A call to action to identify and address racial and ethnic disparities. *Journal of Racial and Ethnic Health Disparities, 7*(3), 398–402. https://doi.org/10.1007/s40615-020-00756-0

LaVeist, T. A., Gaskin, D., & Richard, P. (2011). Estimating the economic burden of racial health inequalities in the United States. *International Journal of Health Services, 41*(2), 231–238. https://doi.org/10.2190/HS.41.2.c

LaVeist, T. A., & Nuru-Jeter, A. (2002). Is doctor-patient race concordance associated with greater satisfaction with care? *Journal of Health and Social Behavior, 43*(3), 296–306. https://doi.org/10.2307/3090205

Lawrence, K., & Keleher, T. (2004). Chronic disparity: Strong and pervasive evidence of racial inequalities. *Race and Public Policy Conference.* https://www.racialequitytools.org/resourcefiles/Definitions-of%20Racism.pdf

Lee, I., Monahan, S., Serban, N., Griffin, P. M., & Tomar, S. L. (2018). Estimating the cost savings of preventive dental services delivered to medicaid-enrolled children in six southeastern states. *Health Services Research, 53*(5), 3592–3616. https://doi.org/10.1111/1475-6773.12811

Love, B. L., & Muhammad, G. E. (2017). Critical community conversations: Cultivating the elusive dialogue about racism with parents, community members, and teachers. *The Educational Forum, 81*(4), 446–449. https://doi.org/10.1080/00131725.2017.1350241

Lowery, K. (2017). Bridging the racial divide through cross-racial dialogue: Lessons and reflections from my experience as a facilitator. *Journal of Critical*

Thought and Praxis, 6(2), 114–135. https://lib.dr.iastate.edu/cgi/viewcontent.cgi?article=1140&context=jctp

Maina, I. W., Belton, T. D., Ginzberg, S., Singh, A., & Johnson, T. J. (2018). A decade of studying implicit racial/ethnic bias in healthcare providers using the implicit association test. *Social Science & Medicine, 199*, 219–229. https://doi.org/10.1016/j.socscimed.2017.05.009

Margaret, J., & Came, H. (2019). Organizing—What do white people need to know to be effective antiracism allies within public health? In C. Ford, D. Griffith, M. Bruce, & K. Gilbert (Eds.), *Racism: Science & tools for the public health professional* (1st ed., pp. 315–326). APHA Press.

Moore, A. D., Hamilton, J. B., Knafl, G. J., Godley, P. A., Carpenter, W. R., Bensen, J. T., Mohler, J. L., & Mishel, M. (2013). The influence of mistrust, racism, religious participation, and access to care on patient satisfaction for African American men: The North Carolina-Louisiana Prostate Cancer Project. *Journal of the National Medical Association, 105*(1), 59–68. https://doi.org/10.1016/s0027-9684(15)30086-9

Nardi, D., Waite, R., Nowak, M., Hatcher, B., Hines-Martin, V., & Stacciarini, J. R. (2020). Achieving health equity through eradicating structural racism in the United States: A call to action for nursing leadership. *Journal of Nursing Scholarship, 52*(6), 696–704. https://doi.org/10.1111/jnu.12602

Noel, N., Pinder, D., Stewart, S., & Wright, J. (2019). *The economic impact of closing the racial wealth gap*. McKinsey & Company. https://www.mckinsey.com/~/media/McKinsey/Industries/Public%20and%20Social%20Sector/Our%20Insights/The%20economic%20impact%20of%20closing%20the%20racial%20wealth%20gap/The-economic-impact-of-closing-the-racial-wealth-gap-final.pdf

Noonan, A. S., Velasco-Mondragon, H. E., & Wagner, F. A. (2016). Improving the health of African Americans in the USA: An overdue opportunity for social justice. *Public Health Reviews, 37*, 12. https://doi.org/10.1186/s40985-016-0025-4

Novak, N. L., Geronimus, A. T., & Martinez-Cardoso, A. M. (2017). Change in birth outcomes among infants born to Latina mothers after a major immigration raid. *International Journal of Epidemiology, 46*(3), 839–849. https://doi.org/10.1093/ije/dyw346

O'Brien, R., Neman, T., Seltzer, N., Evans, L., & Venkataramani, A. (2020). Structural racism, economic opportunity and racial health disparities: Evidence from U.S. counties. *SSM – Population. Health, 11*, 100564. https://doi.org/10.1016/j.ssmph.2020.1005644

Office of Disease Prevention and Health Promotion. (2020). *Healthy People 2030: Social Determinants of Health*. U.S. Department of Health and Human Services. https://health.gov/healthypeople/objectives-and-data/social-determinants-health

Ogden, C. (2017). Seeing collective impact efforts with a racial justice lens. *Interaction Institute for Social Change*. https://www.collectiveimpactforum.org/blogs/2426/seeing-collective-impact-efforts-racial-justice-lens

ORS Impact. (2018). *When collective impact has an impact: A cross-site study of 25 collective impact initiatives*. https://www.orsimpact.com/DirectoryAttachments/10262018_111513_477_CI_Study_Report_10-26-2018.pdf

Owens, K., & Walker, A. (2020). Those designing healthcare algorithms must become actively anti-racist. *Nature Medicine, 26*, 1327–1328. https://doi.org/10.1038/s41591-020-1020-3

Paradies, Y., Truong, M., & Priest, N. (2014). A systematic review of the extent and measurement of healthcare provider racism. *Journal of General Internal Medicine, 29*(2), 364–387. https://doi.org/10.1007/s11606-013-2583-1

Pastor, M., Terriquez, V., & Lin, M. (2018). How community organizing promotes health equity, and how health equity affects organizing. *Health Affairs, 37*(3), 358–363. https://doi.org/10.1377/hlthaff.2017.1285

Poma, P. A. (2017). Race/ethnicity concordance between patients and physicians. *Journal of the National Medical Association, 109*(1), 6–8. https://doi.org/10.1016/j.jnma.2016.12.002

Public Health National Center for Innovations. (2020). *10 Essential Public Health Services: EPHS Toolkit, 2020*. Public Health Accreditation Board. http://ephs.phnci.org/toolkit

Reno, R., & Hyder, A. (2018). The evidence base for social determinants of health as risk factors for infant mortality: A systematic scoping review. *Journal of Health Care for the Poor and Underserved, 29*(4), 1188–1208. https://doi.org/10.1353/hpu.2018.0091

Rodríguez, J., Nagda, B. A., Sorensen, N., & Gurin, P. (2018). Engaging race and racism for socially just intergroup relations: The impact of intergroup dialogue on college campuses in the United States. *Multicultural Education Review, 10*(3), 224–245. https://doi.org/10.1080/2005615X.2018.1497874

Rudwick, E. M. (1951). A brief history of Mercy-Douglass Hospital in Philadelphia. *The Journal of Negro Education, 20*(1), 50–66. https://doi.org/10.2307/2965863

Salvitt, T. (1978). *Medicine and slavery: The diseases and health care of blacks in antebellum Virginia*. University of Illinois Press.

Sharma, A. (2010). Diseased race, racialized disease: The story of the negro project of American Social Hygiene Association against the backdrop of the Tuskegee syphilis experiment. *Journal of African American Studies, 14*(2), 247–262. http://www.jstor.org/stable/41819249

Sighoko, D., Murphy, A. M., Irizarry, B., Rauscher, G., Ferrans, C., & Ansell, D. (2017). Changes in the racial disparity in breast cancer mortality in the ten US cities with the largest African American populations from 1999 to 2013: The reduction in breast cancer mortality disparity in Chicago. *Cancer Causes & Control, 28*(6), 563–568. https://doi.org/10.1007/s10552-017-0878-y

Solomon, D., Maxwell, C., & Castro, A. (2019). *Systematic inequality and economic opportunity.* Center for American Progress. https://www.americanprogress.org/issues/race/reports/2019/08/07/472910/systematic-inequality-economic-opportunity/

Stachowiak, S. & Gase, L. (2018). Does collective impact really make an impact? *Stanford Social Innovation Review.* https://ssir.org/articles/entry/does_collective_impact_really_make_an_impact

Street, R. L., O'Malley, K. J., Cooper, L. A., & Haidet, P. (2008). Understanding concordance in patient-physician relationships: Personal and ethnic dimensions of shared identity. *Annals of Family Medicine, 6*(3), 198–205. https://doi.org/10.1370/afm.821

van Dorn, A. V., Cooney, R. E., & Sabin, M. L. (2020). COVID-19 exacerbating inequalities in the US. *Lancet, 395*(10232), 1243–1244. https://doi.org/10.1016/S0140-6736(20)30893-X

Wallace, M., Crear-Perry, J., Richardson, L., Tarver, M., & Theall, K. (2017). Separate and unequal: Structural racism and infant mortality in the US. *Health & Place, 45*, 140–144. https://doi.org/10.1016/j.healthplace.2017.03.012

Watkins, M., Ciofalo, N., & James, S. (2018). Engaging the struggle for decolonial approaches to teaching community psychology. *American Journal of Community Psychology, 62*(3–4), 319–329. https://doi.org/10.1002/ajcp.12295

Webb Hooper, M., Nápoles, A. M., & Pérez-Stable, E. J. (2020). COVID-19 and racial/ethnic disparities. *JAMA, 323*(24), 2466–2467. https://doi.org/10.1001/jama.2020.8598

Williams, D. R., & Cooper, L. A. (2019). Reducing racial inequities in health: Using what we already know to take action. *Journal of Environmental Research and Public Health, 16*(4), 606. https://www.mdpi.com/1660-4601/16/4/606

Wolff, T., Minkler, M., Wolfe, S., Berkowitz, B., Bowen, L., Butterfoss, F., Christens, B.D., Francisco, V. T., Himmelman, A. T., & Lee, K. S. (2016). Collaborating for equity and justice: Moving beyond collective impact. *Nonprofit Quarterly.* https://nonprofitquarterly.org/collaborating-equity-justice-moving-beyond-collective-impact/

World Health Organization. (2020). *Social determinants of health.* https://www.who.int/gender-equity-rights/understanding/sdh-definition/en/

Yancy, C. W. (2020). COVID-19 and African Americans. *JAMA, 323*(19), 1891–1892. https://doi.org/10.1001/jama.2020.6548

Yearby, R. (2018). Racial disparities in health status and access to healthcare: The continuation of inequality in the United States due to structural racism. *The American Journal of Economics and Sociology, 77*(3-4), 1113–1152. https://doi.org/10.1111/ajes.12230

Youngclaus, J., & Roskovensky, L. (2018). An updated look at the economic diversity of U.S. medical students. *Analysis in Brief, 18*, 1–3. https://www.aamc.org/system/files/reports/1/october2018anupdatedlookattheeconomicdiversityofu.s.medicalstud.pdf

20

A Telehealth Antiracist Learning Experience for Nursing and Social Work Students in the Midst of COVID-19

Melissa E. Buckley and Camille R. Jensen

In March 2020, novel coronavirus (COVID-19), a global pandemic, impacted all aspects of life. CDC recommendations to prevent the spread of COVID-19 include social distancing, mask use, and handwashing (CDC, 2020). Risk for severe illness related to COVID-19 increases with age, placing adults age 65 years and older at the highest risk of hospitalization and death (CDC, 2020). According to Plagg et al. (2020), prolonged social isolation leads to loneliness in older adults, negatively impacting quality of life. Protecting older adults' physical health increased the risk of loneliness due to social isolation during COVID-19. Older adults were not only isolated from their communities but were often

M. E. Buckley (✉)
Coppin State University, Baltimore, MD, USA
e-mail: mbuckley@coppin.edu

C. R. Jensen
Michigan State University, East Lansing, MI, USA
e-mail: jense103@msu.edu

© The Author(s), under exclusive license to Springer Nature Switzerland AG 2022

K. Johnson et al. (eds.), *Developing Anti-Racist Practices in the Helping Professions: Inclusive Theory, Pedagogy, and Application*,
https://doi.org/10.1007/978-3-030-95451-2_20

isolated from their families. Telehealth increased dramatically during the pandemic and has proven to be an effective intervention to reach isolated individuals (Zhou et al., 2020). An effective method for supporting older adults, and preventing feelings of loneliness in the community, includes regular remote check-ins (Gorenko et al., 2021). Phone or video calls to provide mental health support are effective telehealth interventions where older adults have access and are able to navigate the technology (Gorenko et al., 2021).

To combat loneliness in adults 65 and older, a community organization in Baltimore City called the Baltimore Neighbors Network (BNN) was formed in March 2020. BNN trained volunteers to make phone calls to older adult "neighbors." This group of neighbors was considered to be vulnerable due to their limited support and access to resources; COVID-19 increased their risk of vulnerability. The goal was to use telehealth as an intervention to provide social support. BNN was a coalition of multidisciplinary Baltimore leaders. At its inception, it included representation from a pro bono counseling agency, university faculty, clergy, members from Healing City Baltimore (HCB), and other local entities. Just a few weeks prior to the shutdown of public places in the state of Maryland, HCB passed a citywide legislation called the Elijah Cummings Healing City Act (Gresh et al., 2021). This act required all city agencies to become trauma-informed by undergoing trauma-informed training and by reevaluating agency policies to ensure they demonstrated awareness and application of trauma-informed care.

It was immediately evident that COVID-19 would have a traumatic impact on all, particularly those deemed to be vulnerable. State Delegate Nick Mosby was quoted in the Baltimore Sun on March 30, 2020 stating, "We've always known that, historically, there's been health disparities in communities of color. It's important to get ahead of it." State Delegate Mosby was the first legislator in the State of Maryland to call upon Governor Hogan to begin tracking COVID-19 cases by geographic location, age, race, and gender.

From a helping professions perspective, vulnerable populations include, but are not limited to, older adults, racial and ethnic minority groups, children and adolescents, and individuals living with comorbidities (Darlington-Pollock et al., 2021; Arasteh, 2021). According to the 2019 U.S. Census report for Baltimore City, 62.7% of the population is Black, 31.8% is White and 5.7% is Hispanic or Latino. Older adults, ages 65 and older, make up 14.5% of the population (U.S. Census, 2019). It was with this understanding that the coalition formed in hopes of reducing the severity of the threat of social isolation that would be caused by COVID- 19.

Partnership with Baltimore Universities: Telehealth Response to COVID

The swift emergence of this public health emergency resulted in a complete shift in everyday lived experiences. An unintended, but overwhelmingly positive, outcome of this virtual community outreach initiative was the development of virtual clinical experiences for both nursing and social work students at a time when in-person experiences were limited due to the pandemic. As with most public spaces, academia was impacted by COVID-19 when colleges and universities were forced to cease campus meetings. This meant that, with little preparation, classes and practicum assignments that were customarily in person were moved to an online platform. This posed challenges for practice-based disciplines such as nursing and social work which have very strict practicum guidelines. For example, the Council on Social Work Education (CSWE), the accrediting body for accredited baccalaureate and graduate social work programs, permitted programs to evaluate students who satisfactorily completed 85% of their required field placement as having met the field placement requirements (CSWE, 2020). Some states reduced the required number of nursing practicum hours and permitted students who had completed at least 75% of their practicum hours to graduate. The American Association of Colleges of Nursing (AACN), following the guidance of the CDC, instituted guidelines for nursing students. Nonclinical classes were suspended while clinical classes and placements were seen as essential and were, in some cases, permitted to develop contingency plans based on the unique circumstances of their learning community (AACN, 2020). Nursing and social work, as front line or essential service professions, made a swift transition to online learning due to the pandemic. Though the simulated learning was a temporary fix, it posed a unique challenge because more than ever before, the needs of the vulnerable needed to be addressed, and students wanted to respond to the growing crisis (Gresh et al., 2020). As a result, programs evaluated which of the current placements were appropriate for in-person placements, ensuring access to personal protective equipment (PPE), while exploring available options for telehealth placements. Prior to COVID- 19, this was unprecedented.

Despite the state of emergency caused by COVID-19, it presented a unique learning opportunity in Baltimore City. Between March 2020 and June 2021, over 800 volunteers were trained, 504 of whom were students from three local universities: Coppin State University College of Behavioral and Social Sciences, Department of Social Work, Johns Hopkins University School of Nursing, University of Maryland, Baltimore School of Social Work, and University of Maryland, Baltimore School of Nursing. Nursing and social work students were instructed in developing and utilizing an Antiracist approach to providing emotional support and facilitating appropriate referrals to community resources for over 1900 adults, aged 65 and older, in the City of Baltimore.

A PhD faculty member supervised Bachelor of Social Work (BSW) students from Coppin State University and both MSW and RN to BSN students from the University of Maryland, Baltimore. Students participated in weekly calls providing emotional support and referrals to community resources. They also developed community outreach projects to engage students, volunteers, older adults, and BNN leadership. Nursing students analyzed referral data gathered during calls to improve and expand community resources available to volunteers. Students met weekly in interdisciplinary supervision groups where they discussed their service learning projects, had guest speakers who addressed a variety of topics including the role of Antiracism in their work, and they had reflective discussions where they processed the understanding of the impact of race and racism. Each supervision was followed by a mindfulness exercise to give students the opportunity to focus on their own journey, self-care and to reduce any feelings of stress caused by the discussion.

A PhD nursing student and faculty from Johns Hopkins University supervised undergraduate nursing students. Students made weekly calls and engaged in service-learning projects to increase volunteer retention through improving the volunteer experience. They created informational flyers for increasing community awareness, and frequently asked questions (FAQ) documents for flu vaccines and voting.

A Doctor of Nursing Practice student and adjunct faculty from the University of Maryland, Baltimore School of Nursing supervised MSN Clinical Nurse Leader students. As a supplement to working in a community vaccine clinic, students made weekly calls and conducted a community health needs assessment based on the target population. The students' observations and experiences during outreach calls led to service-learning projects to improve the volunteer data collection experience, creation of a community awareness poster, and tip sheets for the two most often utilized community resources: Maryland Access Point (MAP) and Baltimore's 211.

Antiracist Service-Learning Projects

According to the National Association of Social Workers (2021), voting is a social work issue and it is important for social workers to provide resources to assist in informing potential voters. Voter suppression is on the rise. Recent local and federal elections have revealed intimidation tactics reminiscent of the practices used in the 1960s (Hardy, 2020). Leading up to, and during the 2020 election, social work and nursing students identified the increased need for voter information: how to register, where to vote, and available transportation. Students created a frequently asked questions (FAQ) resource for student and non-student volunteers to share voter information with the neighbors they were calling. The Voting FAQ included the date of election day, polling site locations, where to find early voting centers, how to vote by mail or the ballot box, and steps to safely vote in person during COVID-19. To create a sense of community and support, students hosted a virtual election day event where they were able to virtually meet other volunteers, community members, and the neighbors they had been calling each week.

Nursing and social work students worked together to host volunteer appreciation events, including a virtual Halloween costume party and holiday season event that included games and "get to know you" activities. Volunteer morale was a primary focus of BNN. Volunteers serve a crucial role to the organization and every effort must be made to ensure they feel like valued members of the organizational structure (Fouzia et al., 2020; Febriani & Selamet, 2020). BNN volunteers were required to undergo intensive training, and based on a survey conducted of the volunteers, the students determined that volunteer retention should be prioritized. This would not only help BNN to be able to make contact with more older adults, it would also ensure that volunteers would feel motivated to do the work, during a time where they were also impacted by the same social conditions that impacted the neighbors they were calling. Hosting volunteer appreciation events may not explicitly be an Antiracist activity, however, it did afford volunteers the opportunity to connect and to share their experiences. The students also worked together to host a virtual fundraising event called "Very Important Baltimoreans." Participants received the ingredients to create a crab cake meal and met virtually to watch a cooking demonstration and participate in their own homes while preparing their individual meals.

Undergraduate nursing students developed important service-learning projects. First, they developed a flyer explaining how to contact BNN if individuals were interested in "a confidential, safe, and supportive way to stay connected." Recognizing barriers to accessing community services, such as lack of internet, technology, and transportation, students collaborated with the Baltimore City Health Department to identify senior housing across Baltimore. They hand distributed 10,000 flyers to 92 senior housing buildings across 24 Baltimore zip codes. With 62.7% of the population identifying as Black and 14.5% identifying as older adults, it was imperative to find additional ways to reach as many older adults as possible.

During flu season, students worked with local pharmacies to verify flu vaccine locations. They developed a Flu Vaccine FAQ and shared it, along with the city's Flu Vaccine Map, with volunteers. The additional flu resources provided volunteers with accurate information to answer questions older adults had about flu vaccines.

MSN students from The University of Maryland, Baltimore completed a 90-hour public health practicum that included community vaccine clinic hours, making weekly calls to older adults, a brief community health needs assessment focused on adults 65 and older, and service-learning projects. The MSN students attended the mandatory Inclusive Listening training. During the weekly clinical experience, students started the day with a pre-conference where new volunteer information was shared and call statistics were reviewed, allowing students to see the impact of the calls volunteers and students were making each week. Each student spent up to three hours making calls to 10–15 older adults. A post-conference session was held where students could share their experiences, ask questions, and debrief after any difficult situations. During the afternoon sessions, students had time to work together on their community health needs assessment project. Guest speakers were brought in from the community who were experts in mental health, elder abuse, and community resources. Students were divided into groups and completed socially distanced windshield surveys. Each group was sent to multiple zip codes in Baltimore. Once the windshield surveys were completed, students were asked to share their observations and engaged in thoughtful conversations about the lack of access to safe housing, nutritious foods, green spaces, and health care. When students observed differences between neighborhoods where they saw more Black people than White people, and there was less green space, lack of grocery stores, fewer children playing outside, and roads and sidewalks were in states of disrepair, they were asked to point out the differences and think about the causes. This led to conversations about structural racism and introduced the students to topics such as the history of redlining in cities. The experiences and interactions students had with neighbors they were calling led to service-learning projects including a quick reference guide for volunteers to improve the call documentation experience, a poster to bring community awareness to BNN, and tip sheets for MAP and Baltimore's 211 that better explained how the volunteer could best share the resources and allowed volunteers to set better expectations with the older adults utilizing them.

Critical Race Theory

Critical Race Theory (CRT) is a grounded theory with origins in the works of Sojourner Truth, W.E.B. DuBois, and Frederick Douglas. Derrick Bell contributed to this body of literature in the 1970s followed by Kimberle Crenshaw, Richard Delgado, and other notable scholars in the 1980s and beyond. CRT became mainstream and controversial in the height of the COVID-19 pandemic due to the former United States President's ban on the use of CRT training in the federal government. In a September 4, 2020 memorandum, Russell Vought, former Director of the United States Office of Management and Budget, under the direction of the former President, claimed that federal dollars had been used to train federal employees to be divisive and anti- American (Vought, 2020). The memorandum referred to CRT as propaganda. It is evident that neither the then president nor his cabinet had an understanding of CRT. Instead of seeking to learn more about racism, which is a principle of Antiracist pedagogy, they reacted to the truths of CRT and attempted to protect their own interests. CRT specifically addresses this behavior in one of its major tenets, "Differential Racialization." This tenet suggests that the needs and attributes of racial groups in the United States have been established based on the needs of the majority racial group. Each of these groups have different histories and struggles and the minority groups are subjected to discriminatory laws and practices that have been enforced by the majority group (Abrams & Moio, 2009). The attempts to ban CRT are based on the needs of people who have benefitted from white privilege and who desire to maintain their privilege, thus they attempt to erase any threat to their privilege through baseless attacks on a theory intended to generate dialogue, awareness and action regarding the eradication of racism.

CRT is a critical examination of the intersection of race, racial justice and the law (George, 2021). It interrogates civil rights by expounding on the varied impacts of the economy, self-interests and historical influences (Delgado, 2017). Unlike traditional civil rights, which embraces incrementalism and step-by-step progress, Critical Race Theory questions the very foundations of the liberal order, including equality theory, legal reasoning, enlightenment rationalism, and neutral principles of constitutional law. CRT is the only body of literature in the academic setting that directly confronts race and racism. Many institutions do not integrate race and racism in their curriculum with intentionality so removing CRT in its entirety poses an academic and social justice threat to all students.

Racial disparities, particularly regarding health access, have always been evident in the United States healthcare system. COVID-19 related mortality emphasized these disparities. For this reason, healthcare and helping professions need more clarity on racial healthcare phenomena. Public Health Critical Race Praxis (PHCRP), the public health application of CRT, was developed for the purpose of studying Antiracism health equity and should be used by helping professionals to better understand the conditions faced by racially disenfranchised groups (Ford, 2020).

Antiracism and Helping Professions

Antiracism builds on CRT through the deliberate actions of counteracting racism. It attempts to dismantle racist structures that continue to oppress disenfranchised and vulnerable groups and replaces those oppressive structures with acceptance, inclusivity, and equity (Kendi, 2019; McCluney et al., 2021). Helping professions need to take a more firm stance against health inequities and in addressing social determinants of health. "Racism is the root cause of underlying widespread disparities in social, economic, and health outcomes, including the ability to stay alive" (South et al., 2020). Health care and helping professions cannot afford to remain silent on issues of racism; the lives of individuals and communities depend on the voices and advocacy of Antiracist helping professionals. South et al. (2020) suggest that adopting a culture of Antiracism among helping professionals would include the integration of Antiracism in training and education, the inclusion of Antiracism in research, financially incentivizing efforts, and revising existing policies. By adopting Antiracist pedagogy, new professionals will enter the workforce with an understanding of the need for Antiracist approaches to practice and the support and services offered to individuals and communities will ultimately be more equitable, resulting in a reduction of the health inequities that currently negatively impact communities of color.

Social work and nursing, as helping professions, have an inherent social justice approach woven into their professional codes of ethics, yet both have a history of silence regarding classroom instruction on the impact of race and racism. Provision 9 of the American Nurses Association Code of Ethics says the profession will "integrate principles of social justice into nursing and health policy" (American Nurses Association, 2015). The National Association of Social Workers Code of Ethics states in its preamble that social justice is one of the core principles of social work practice (National Association of Social Workers [NASW], 2008, preamble). Though the professions say they are committed to social justice, this is not always evident in the curriculum.

Colonized pedagogy is prevalent in higher education and helping professions are ill- equipped to teach their scholars from an Antiracist framework (Blanchet Garneau et al., 2021; Corley & Young, 2018). Research has shown that both social work and nursing have faced pedagogical challenges regarding the inclusion of race and racism in their curriculums (Blanchet Garneau et al., 2018; Van Schalkwyk et al., 2019; Hamilton-Mason & Schneider, 2018). To that end, in September 2020, The Council on Social Work Education (CSWE) formed a task force to conduct an examination of social work pedagogy, and where necessary, offer recommendations to improve and increase diversity and inclusion (Hymans et al., 2020). In order for the recommendations to be effective, they must include Antiracist language and recommendations. Also, they must have clear guidelines that not only help educators to understand but empower them to become Antiracist. Stauffer 2020 research suggests that educators can practice Antiracism by disrupting inequity and addressing the norms that support racist ideologies. The National Academies of Sciences, Engineering, and Medicine (NASEM) et al. (2021), acknowledged that nursing programs cover health equity and social determinants of health, but fail to prepare nurses to practice in non-traditional settings or to work with people from diverse backgrounds. National nursing organizations acknowledge the need for health equity but fall short of identifying when health inequities are caused by structural racism.

Organizations can become Antiracist by adopting a long-term approach to learning about racism. This would include but is not limited to, having ongoing training. Organizations must also accept the discomfort that accompanies racist mistakes. It is not helpful to deny the mistake occurred, to offer excuses for the mistake, or to seek validation from the marginalized group. Admitting the mistake and doing the work of becoming educated prevents recurrence in the future. Lastly, organizations must conduct a systematic analysis of how white supremacy has been sustained within the organizational structure and has oppressed marginalized groups (Kendi, 2019; McCluney et al., 2021). Antiracism in helping professions must be so deeply entrenched into the foundation of practice that professionals will employ Antiracist principles regardless of the racial demographic of the individuals and communities served, but they will also be keenly aware of and responsive to barriers to services encountered by vulnerable populations.

Antiracist Telehealth

Though there was a great deal of uncertainty, it was evident that there would be a surge in telehealth services. This reality birthed the opportunity to partner with local universities to have students join the volunteer team. At that time, there was one faculty member on the BNN organizing team; a black woman who taught at Coppin State University, one of Baltimore city's Historically Black Colleges and Universities (HBCU). She invited local social work programs to assign their students to BNN to complete their 2020–2021 field placements and the Coppin State University Department of Social Work and The University of Maryland, Baltimore School of Social Work accepted the invitation. Over the summer, another faculty member joined the BNN team from the Johns Hopkins School of Nursing and brought a group of students along with her. During the winter of 2020, a third faculty member from The University of Maryland, Baltimore School of Nursing supervised a group of MSN students. By spring of 2021, BNN trained over 500 students as volunteers, many of whom were supervised by these faculty members. Of note is the fact that the social work faculty member supervised both undergraduate nursing and undergraduate and graduate social work students in an interdisciplinary approach. The training the students underwent was informed by an Antiracist perspective. They completed mandatory Inclusive Listening training which teaches strategies for offering support and intervention based on the use of empathetic listening skills. Inclusive Listening skills encourage the listener to identify with the speaker in a neutral way to remove biases and encourage collaboration (CADRE, 2020). In the case of BNN, utilizing Inclusive Listening where callers have no knowledge of the demographics of the neighbors, requires them to promote social justice which is a pillar of Antiracist pedagogy (Blakeney, 2005; Stauffer, 2020).

This chapter detailed a community initiative that was developed in response to the threat of social isolation caused by COVID-19. Nursing and social work students were in a unique situation in March 2020 when many of their field placements came to an early end as a result of the pandemic. One of the initial organizing team members of BNN is a faculty member at a Baltimore City university and was aware of the need for placements for students in her program and saw this as a unique opportunity. A faculty member from another Baltimore City university was seeking out opportunities for her students and was able to onboard her students in the summer of 2020. They became the first cohort of student volunteers. Their roles closely aligned with the roles of traditional BNN volunteers but they were under the supervision of their faculty members who provided guidance. In August of 2020, the BNN organizing team welcomed a cohort of nursing and social work students who worked collaboratively in a cross-disciplinary fashion. Each of their learning activities required them to critically evaluate the impact of Antiracism on the work they were doing and, where necessary, recommendations were made for how to ensure the Antiracist perspective was utilized.

The interdisciplinary collaboration went beyond the boundaries of professional discipline. Some of the students were matriculating at one of Baltimore's Historically Black Colleges and Universities (HBCU) while the others were matriculating at Predominantly White Institutions (PWI). The students were able to contribute their lived experiences as students at their respective institutions to the collaborative learning experience, thus enhancing the Antiracist perspective. Their different perspectives were evident on each of the projects they collaborated on. For example, while researching for the voting event, students from the HBCU did not have access to the same journal articles as the students from the PWI. The HBCU faculty member was able to use this as a teachable moment by explaining the importance of the 14 year historic Maryland HBCU lawsuit. This lawsuit was ultimately about the inequitable funding amongst public universities in Maryland. The fact that the HBCU students did not have the same access to research materials as their cohort members from the PWI was an unfortunate reminder of the inequities, yet it ignited their commitment to social justice and Antiracism.

COVID-19 shifted the way helping professionals perform their duties and the transition to telehealth created opportunities to expand on Antiracist organizational approaches. This community outreach telehealth initiative emphasized a few important points regarding Antiracism. First, organizations have an obligation and must be committed to a long-term approach to learning about racism. It is not enough to have occasional training. This must be a regularly scheduled part of the agency's ongoing commitment to learning. Second, organizations must accept the discomfort they experience when mistakes are made. They must refrain from putting the burden of responsibility to absolve them of those uncomfortable feelings on the marginalized groups. Third, organizations must be committed to the systemic analysis of the presence of white supremacy within the organization and eradicate such oppressive structures (Kendi, 2019; McCluney et al., 2021).

Nursing and social work have always been on the front lines of understanding social determinants of health. They meet people where they are; where they live, work, and the experiences that impact the quality of life. The combined experience, knowledge, and wisdom of these professions position them to lead the charge in Antiracism efforts to achieve health equity.

Reflection Questions

1. How does adding an Antiracism curriculum help with the goal of achieving health equity?

2. What are the benefits of interdisciplinary learning between nursing and social work? Other helping professions?
3. What are the benefits of collaboration between HBCU and PWI institutions?
4. In a telehealth setting, what are some key considerations for an Antiracist approach?
5. Is it possible to employ an Antiracist framework without knowing the racial demographic you are working with?

Quiz Questions

1. What role did telehealth play throughout the COVID-19 pandemic?
2. From a telehealth perspective, what are some barriers to accessing telehealth for vulnerable populations?
3. Telehealth is not accessible to all. By transitioning to telehealth, how did that promote inequities?
4. What evidence exists that nursing and social work are rooted in social justice principles?
5. How can helping professions, as well as organizations, become Antiracist?

References

Abrams, L. S., & Moio, J. A. (2009). Critical race theory and the cultural competence dilemma in social work education. *Journal of Social Work Education, 45*(2), 245. https://doi.org/10.5175/JSWE.2009.200700109

American Association of Colleges of Nursing [AACN]. (2020, March 20). *Considerations for COVID-19 preparedness and response in U.S. schools of nursing.* https://www.aacnnursing.org/News-Information/COVID-19/AACN-Recommendations

American Nurses Association [ANA]. (2015). *Code of ethics with interpretive statements.* Author. Retrieved from http://www.nursingworld.org/MainMenuCategories/EthicsStandards/CodeofEthicsforNurses/Code-ofEthics-For-Nurses.html

Arasteh, K. (2021). Hypertension, diabetes, and poverty among Latinx immigrants in New York City: Implications for COVID-19. *International Journal of Migration, Health and Social Care, 17*(2), 208–241. https://doi.org/10.1108/IJMHSC-09-2020-0088

Blakeney, A. M. (2005). Antiracist pedagogy: Definition, theory, and professional development. *Journal of Curriculum and Pedagogy, 2*(1), 119–132. https://doi.org/10.1080/15505170.2005.10411532

Blanchet Garneau, A., Bélisle, M., Lavoie, P., & Laurent Sédillot, C. (2021). Integrating equity and social justice for indigenous peoples in undergraduate health professions education in Canada: A framework from a critical review of literature. *International Journal for Equity in Health, 20*(1), 1–9. https://doi.org/10.1186/s12939-021-01475-6

Blanchet Garneau, A., Browne, A. J., & Varcoe, C. (2018). Drawing on antiracist approaches toward a critical antidiscriminatory pedagogy for nursing. *Nursing Inquiry, 25*(1). https://doi.org/10.1111/nin.12211

Centers for Disease Control and Prevention [CDC]. Coronavirus disease 2019 (COVID-19) in the U.S. (2020, March 28). https://covid.cdc.gov/covid-data-tracker/

Center for Appropriate Dispute Resolution in Special Education [CADRE]. (2020, July 16). *Inclusive listening: Building understanding, supporting collaboration.* Progress Center | Promoting Progress for Students with Disabilities. Retrieved July 19, 2021, from https://promotingprogress.org/resources/inclusive-listening-building-understanding-supporting-collaboration

Corley, N. A., & Young, S. M. (2018). Is social work still racist? A content analysis of recent literature. *Social Work, 63*(4), 317–326. https://doi.org/10.1093/sw/swy042

Council on Social Work Education. (2020). CSWE and Commission on Accreditation Statement. Retrieved from https://www.cswe.org/accreditation/info/accreditationcovid-19-response/

Darlington-Pollock, F., Dolega, L., & Dunning, R. (2021). Ageism, overlapping vulnerabilities and equity in the COVID-19 pandemic. *TPR. Town Planning Review, 92*(2), 203–207. https://doi.org/10.3828/tpr.2020.40

Delgado, R. (2017). *Critical race theory: An introduction* (3rd ed.). New York University Press.

Febriani, D. M., & Selamet, J. (2020). College students' intention to volunteer for non-profit organizations: Does brand image make a difference? *Journal of Nonprofit & Public Sector Marketing, 32*(2), 166–188. https://doi.org/10.1080/10495142.2019.1656136

Ford, C. L. (2020). Commentary: Addressing inequities in the era of COVID-19: The pandemic and the urgent need for critical race theory. *Family & Community Health, 43*(3), 184–186. https://doi.org/10.1097/fch.0000000000000266

Fouzia Ashfaq, Mattiullah Butt, & Sehrish Ilyas. (2020). Volunteering: what drives and retains it? An analysis of motivational needs together with organizational policies and practices. *Qualitative Research Journal, 21*(2), 189–205. https://doi-org.proxycs.researchport.umd.edu/10.1108/QRJ-04-2020-0024

George, J. (2021, January 12). *A lesson on critical race theory.* American Bar Association. https://www.americanbar.org/groups/crsj/publications/human_rights_magazine_home/civil-rights-reimagining-policing/a-lesson-on-critical-race-theory/

Gorenko, J. A., Moran, C., Flynn, M., Dobson, K., & Konnert, C. (2021). Social isolation and psychological distress among older adults related to COVID-19: A narrative review of remotely-delivered interventions and recommendations. *Journal of Applied Gerontology, 40*(1), 3–13. https://doi-org.proxy-hs.researchport.umd.edu/10.1177/0733464820958550

Gresh, A., LaFave, S., Thamilselvan, V., Batchelder, A., Mermer, J., Jacques, K., Greensfelder, A., Buckley, M., Cohen, Z., Coy, A., & Warren, N. (2020). Service learning in public health nursing education: How COVID-19 accelerated community-academic partnership. *Public Health Nursing.* 38(2), 248–257 ; ISSN 0737-12091525-1446. https://doi.org/10.1111/phn.12796

Gresh, A., LaFave, S., & Thamilselvan, V. (2021). Service learning in public health nursing education: How COVID-19 accelerated community-academic partnership. *Public Health Nursing, 38*, 248–257. https://doi.org/10.1111/phn.12796

Hamilton-Mason, J., & Schneider, S. (2018). Antiracism expanding social work education: A qualitative analysis of the undoing racism workshop experience. *Journal of Social Work Education, 54*(2), 337–348. https://doi.org/10.1080/10437797.2017.1404518

Hardy, L. (2020). Voter suppression post-Shelby: Impacts and issues of voter purge and voter ID laws. *Mercer Law Review, 71*(3), 857–878. https://digitalcommons.law.mercer.edu/cgi/viewcontent.cgi?article=1315&context=jour_mlr

Hymans, D. J., Spence Coffey, D., & McLean, A. (2020, September 25). *We "have a way to go" to achieve racial equity in social work.* Council on Social Work Education (CSWE). https://www.cswe.org/News/General-News-Archives/We-Have-a-Way-To-Go-To-Achieve-Racial-Equity-in

Kendi, I. X. (2019). *How to be an antiracist.* Random House Books.

McCluney, C. L., King, D. D., Bryant, C. M., & Ali, A. A. (2021). From "Calling in Black" to "Calling for Antiracism Resources": The need for systemic resources to address systemic racism. *Equality, Diversity & Inclusion, 40*(1), 49–59. https://doi.org/10.1108/EDI-07-2020-0180

National Academies of Sciences, Engineering, and Medicine [NASEM], National Academy of Medicine, & Committee on the Future of Nursing 2020-2030. (2021). *The future of nursing 2020–2030: Charting a path to achieve health equity*. National Academies Press.

National Association of Social Workers [NASW]. (2008). *Preamble to the code of ethics*. Retrieved July 19,2020 from http://www.socialworkers.org/pubs/Code/code.asp

National Association of Social Workers [NASW]. (2021). *Elections*. NASW – National Association of Social Workers. https://www.socialworkers.org/Advocacy/Political-Action-for-Candidate-Election-PACE/Elections

Plagg, B., Engl, A., Piccoliori, G., & Eisendle, K. (2020). Prolonged social isolation of the elderly during covid-19: Between benefit and damage. Archives of Gerontology and Geriatrics, 89, 104086. https://doi.org/10.1016/j.archger.2020.104086

South, E. C., Butler, P. D., & Merchant, R. M. (2020). Toward an equitable society: Building a culture of antiracism in health care. *The Journal of Clinical Investigation, 130*(10), 5039–5041. https://doi.org/10.1172/JCI141675

Stauffer, R. (2020). Creating an antiracist pedagogy of the oppressed. *Slavic & East European Journal, 64*(4), 595–598.

United States Census Bureau. (2019). *U.S. census bureau quickfacts: Baltimore City, Maryland.* Retrieved July 19, 2021, from https://www.census.gov/quickfacts/fact/table/baltimorecitymarylandcounty/AGE295219

Van Schalkwyk, S. C., Hafler, J., Brewer, T. F., Maley, M. A., Margolis, C., McNamee, L., Meyer, I., Peluso, M. J., Schmutz, A. M., Spak, J. M., & Davies, D. (2019). Transformative learning as pedagogy for the health professions: A scoping review. *Medical Education, 53*(6), 547–558. https://doi.org/10.1111/medu.13804

Vought, R. (2020, September 4). *Memorandum for the heads of executive departments and agencies: Training in the federal government.* Executive Office of the President. https://www.whitehouse.gov/wp-content/uploads/2020/09/M-20-34.pdf?fbclid=IwAR1r7Ej2V0gZ8pNhIEjLtHDDNlfeYvBkzEgUfbrU3cXfot7RP2XKPw nCDe4

Zhou, X., Snoswell, C. L., Harding, L. E., Bambling, M., Edirippulige, S., Bai, X., & Smith, A. C. (2020). The role of telehealth in reducing the mental health burden from COVID-19. *Telemedicine and e-Health, 26*(4), 377–379. https://doi.org/10.1089/tmj.2020.0068

21

Working with Multiracial Individuals: Antiracist Pedagogy, Practices, and Considerations

C. Peeper McDonald and Catherine Y. Chang

Introduction

Given the tumultuous history of race relations within the United States, it is increasingly important for educators and counselors to recognize the growing Multiracial population and to consider the complexities and implications for what it means to be Multiracial and what it means to be an antiracist educator/counselor working with Multiracial individuals. In this chapter, we provide relevant literature related to the Multiracial population, including a discussion of the various Multiracial identity development models and the challenges experienced by this population. We

C. P. McDonald (✉)
Mercer University, Macon, GA, USA
e-mail: Mcdonald_cp@mercer.edu

C. Y. Chang
Georgia State University, Atlanta, GA, USA
e-mail: cychang@gsu.edu

© The Author(s), under exclusive license to Springer Nature Switzerland AG 2022

K. Johnson et al. (eds.), *Developing Anti-Racist Practices in the Helping Professions: Inclusive Theory, Pedagogy, and Application*,
https://doi.org/10.1007/978-3-030-95451-2_21

provide strategies and interventions for educators to engage in culturally responsive antiracist pedagogical practices and strategies for counselors working with Multiracial people.

Background

Multiracial broadly describes a person who identifies as two or more races, whereas *monoracial* describes a person who identifies as only one race (Franco & O'Brien, 2018; Tran et al., 2016). *Biracial* is another common term for someone who does not identify as monoracial, and typically addresses the identification of two races given the *Bi* prefix, which signals two. Other terms that have historically been used to describe the Multiracial population include *Mixed-race*, *Multiple Heritage* (described later on in the chapter), and *Interracial* (though it has become more common for Interracial to refer to couples who do not share the same race where they could either be monoracial, Multiracial, or a combination). In this chapter, *Multiracial* will be used as a means of inclusivity with regard to anyone who does not identify as monoracial. The reader must keep in mind the importance of not labeling others by one's perception of race, but to invite constructive dialogue about how one racially identifies. This will be discussed more later in the chapter regarding *Broaching* and other informed strategies.

Now that *Multiracial* has been operationalized, it is important to understand the complex history of race within the U.S. and how this has contributed to the complexity of what it *means* to be Multiracial (Lou & Lalonde, 2015). Like other racially minoritized groups in the U.S., the Multiracial population is subject to a socio-political history of discrimination based on the social construction of race that privileges those who are White and disempowers those who are not. Some significant milestones related to Multiracial issues are the Loving v. Virginia Supreme Court decision in 1967 that made Interracial marriage legal, the hypodescent or "one-drop rule", and the ability to select more than one race on the U.S. Census in 2000. Specifically, the hypodescent one-drop rule emerged during slavery times and asserted that a person with even one ancestor who was Black (i.e., "one drop") would be considered Black.

This was a direct expression of colonization that served to assign a racial identity to the Multiracial person of the parent or grandparent of the lower social status (Roberts et al., 2020; Young et al., 2020). Fortunately, the U.S. Census Bureau's "check one or more" revision in the 2000 Census affectively marked the legal end to any remaining hypodescent statutes because it allowed Multiracial individuals to identify as non-monoracial. Given this history and the socio-political underpinnings of the construct of race in the U.S., it is not hard to imagine how being Multiracial is complicated. Consistently, researchers posit that Multiracial identity is more than color or phenotype and includes a combination of holidays one celebrates, the language one speaks, and the names one uses (McDonald et al., 2020). Furthermore, the limited research on the role of racial color-blindness in Multiracial people indicates that this construct shows up differently for Multiracial people compared to their monoracial counterparts (see McDonald et al., 2019), further indicating the unique and complex experiences of this group.

Multiracial Identity Models

There are numerous models that attempt to describe Multiracial development and identity experience. The following are some of the most salient.

Poston (1990) was the first scholar to propose a developmental model for understanding non-monoracial individuals. The Biracial Identity Development Model addresses the unique developmental process of being a Biracial individual. The developmental stages are (1) Personal Identity, (2) Choice of Group Categorization, (3) Enmeshment/Denial, (4) Appreciation, and (5) Integration (Poston, 1990). This model recognizes unique experiences and factors related to being Biracial that are irrelevant for monoracial individuals. For example, Poston's model accounts for the possible feelings of guilt when identifying with one racial group over another in Stage 2, Choice of Group Categorization. Although Poston (1990) addressed a need in the literature, there are limitations to the model. This model, consistent with the existing research regarding racial identity for Multiracial people, assumes that one's outward appearance matches the social constructions of race in what it means to *be* or *look* Biracial. Many individuals who self-identify as Biracial or Multiracial may be perceived by others as a singular race. For example, the first author identifies as Native American (Cherokee Tribe) and White and is often perceived by others solely as White. The impact(s) of what it is like to be racially mislabeled by others is not within the scope of Poston's model. Furthermore, given the previous discussion of the many terms used to describe non-monoracial people, Poston's use of the term *Biracial* could be limited in application for anyone who is non-monoracial but does not describe themselves as Biracial.

Root's Ecological Framework (Root, 2001) addresses one of the limitations of Poston's model by focusing on Multiracial identity development. Root's Ecological Framework for understanding Multiracial identity development accounts for the fluidity and nuances of Multiracial identity by exploring the intersectionality of concepts such as community attitudes and racial socialization, ethnicities, and symbolic race within identities, and family functioning. Root also developed the Resolutions of Biracial Identity Tensions Model, which includes four stages, (1) acceptance of the identity society, (2) identification with both racial groups, (3) identification with a single racial group, and (4) identification as a new racial group. Additional helpful resources of Root's include the "Bill of Rights for People of Mixed Heritage" and "50 Experiences of Racially Mixed People" (see Multiracial Resources in Appendix A). These works are significant because they shed important light on the unique challenges that Multiracial people face in the United States using concrete examples. Nonetheless, Root's work has been criticized for focusing too much on adolescent identity, limiting the developmental scope of Multiracial understanding and for the use of mixed language that could lead to confusion (i.e., *Mixed Heritage, Biracial, Mixed People, and Multiracial*) (Evans & Ramsay, 2015).

Poston's and Root's models are foundational for understanding the developmental processes for non-monoracial individuals; however, they are outdated. Scholars also have criticized these models for pathologizing Biracial experiences (i.e., guilty and resentful feelings that are turned inward) and the lack of robust empirical support (Evans & Ramsay, 2015).

Kerwin and Ponterotto's Model of Biracial Identity Development (1995) includes six stages of age-based developmental milestones. Unlike the previous models, this model acknowledges that the individuals' established public racial identity may differ from their private racial identity. The six stages are: (1) *preschool stage*—Biracial children begin to recognize physical differences and similarities, (2) *entry to school stage*—with growing social interaction, Biracial children may be pushed to select a monoracial label, (3) *preadolescence stage*—growing awareness and sensitivity towards race, (4) *adolescence*—growing pressures to identify with the parent of color, (5) *college/young adulthood*—continued immersion with one racial group with growing awareness of race, and (6) *adulthood stage*—continued exploration, awareness, and flexibility related to racial identity.

Expanding our knowledge of Multiracial individuals, in 2009, Cheng and Lee proposed a construct called Multiracial Identity Integration (MII). MII focuses on the negotiation that takes place for Multiracial individuals within their various racial identities, discussed in terms of negative and positive racial experiences. Specifically, the MII construct sheds light on the racial identity negotiation that occurs in Multiracial individuals by describing identity perceptions as conflictual or agreeable to one another (Cheng & Lee, 2009). According to this model, complete integration of one's Multiracial identity leads to better wellness outcomes for the individual.

Henriksen and Paladino developed the Multiple Heritage Identity Development Model (MHID; 2009) that includes a more inclusive and broader attention to identities, including race, ethnicity, gender, sexual orientation, and national origin. This model acknowledges the importance of the intersectionality of identities and that race is not the only identity that is salient for people. The MHID model provides a foundation for understanding the intersectionality of identities, and in doing so, it could minimize the social constructs and systemic oppression that underscore under-represented and minoritized identities. Because this model asserts that every person has multiple heritages, it does not contribute specifically to the understanding of racial identity for Multiracial individuals and in fact may minimize the importance of racial identity. Despite these limitations, the focus of the MHID model on the intersectionality of identities for all people is a starting point with which to understand the complexity of identity and its impacts.

Despite these models and the growing attention to Multiracial individuals, a large portion of Multiracial identity research is based on the existing conceptualizations of monoracial identity, contributing to what is known as the *invisibility* of this population. Multiracial researchers caution the application of these monoracial-based models to Multiracial identity because the monoracial-based models do not have the capacity to recognize the complexity of Multiracial identity and are too linear when it comes to the experience of identity development for Multiracial people. Furthermore, literature focused on the complexity of Multiracial identity shows the influence of environmental factors on identity development and that phenotype is simply one factor in the grand scheme of what it means to be Multiracial (McDonald et al., 2020; Root, 2001). Until recently, assumptions about race were formed from a monoracial system underscored by biology that viewed racial groups as independent and homogenous, rather than complex and interconnected (Franco & O'Brien, 2018). Using this outdated and oversimplified framework to continue to move and interact within the education system or helping professions ultimately invalidates the complexity of Multiracial identity development.

Challenges: Microaggressions

Microaggressions are common and often brief interactions that communicate negative, invalidating, and hostile messages about one's identity(ies). They can be verbal, behavioral, or environmental and exist in any human interaction involving individuals from differing cultural groups. The *microaggressor* often lacks awareness about the impact of the microaggression (Franco & O'Brien, 2018; Sue et al., 2007; Sue, 2010; Tran et al., 2016). The term microaggression was first coined by Dr. Chester Pierce, an African American psychiatrist and Harvard University professor, in 1970 to describe the insults that he routinely witnessed non- Black Americans inflict on African Americans (Pierce, 1970). In 2007, Sue and colleagues introduced the construct to the larger mental health community, and since that time, the term microaggressions has been expanded to include the everyday degradation of any socially marginalized/minoritized group. Negative mental and physical health outcomes (i.e., feelings of invisibility, alienation, and harm to overall well-being) have been highly correlated with microaggressions experienced by Multiracial people (Franco & O'Brien, 2018; Harris, 2017). More specifically, Multiracial people frequently report the common microaggressive experience of others racially categorizing them based solely on phenotype, which has led to personal racial identity insecurity and frustration (Franco & O'Brien, 2018; Harris, 2017; McDonald et al., 2020). Another commonly reported microaggression by Multiracial people includes questions like, "Where are you from?" which sends the message that the Multiracial person appears "foreign" and is an outsider, impacting the belongingness of the microaggressed. An additional common microaggression reported by Multiracial people includes the statement "You don't look Multiracial" which is a judgment based on the microaggressor's view of race that disempowers the Multiracial person by taking away their ability to identify themselves (Tran et al., 2016). Franco and O'Brien (2018) reported that the prevailing ramifications of microaggressions include patterns of detriment to self-esteem, perceptions of self, and motivation. As a result, microaggressions serve to oppress Multiracial individuals in that their expression of identity is consistently subverted by microaggressors' perceptions of what it means and "looks like" to be Multiracial. The need for more investigation of the Multiracial experience as well as training and interventions for the Multiracial population is clear (Franco & O'Brien, 2018; McDonald, 2020; McDonald et al., 2020).

Antiracist Cultural Responsiveness

Antiracist culturally responsive pedagogical and counseling practices are needed for the Multiracial population, an often overlooked and understudied group. Like other minoritized groups, this group is impacted by the systemic bias and stereotyping of educational systems (Frye & Vogt, 2010). As a result, it is imperative that educators and mental health professionals attend to gaps in cultural responsiveness and respond with antiracism so as to not perpetuate the harmful impact (i.e., detriments to self-esteem, perceptions of self, and motivation) and invisibility of the

Multiracial population (Franco & O'Brien, 2018; Harris, 2017). The following sections outline ways that educators and professionals can take steps to practice culturally responsive antiracism.

It Starts with a Personal Antiracist Identity

Though Helms (2008) proposed two schemas (internalization of racism or evolution of a non-racist identity) in her process model of White racial identity, Kendi (2019) takes the schema of a non-racist identity further by claiming that there are only two stances in the world, antiracist and racist. Kendi (2019) defines antiracism as "any idea that suggests that racial groups are equals in all their apparent differences—that there is nothing right or wrong with any racial group. Antiracist ideas argue that racist policies are the cause of racial inequities" (p. 20). Therefore, to be an antiracist is to take actionable steps to dismantle the system that oppresses people of color, and anyone at any time can be practicing racism or antiracism given that every action we take either brings us a step closer to one of the two (Kendi, 2019). The journey towards becoming an antiracist is one that starts with a self-assessment of the ways we are either contributing to or hindering the dismantling of oppressive forces. This self-assessment is continuous and necessary if one wishes to cultivate a long-lasting antiracist identity.

Antiracist Culturally Responsive Pedagogy

Given that racism and other forms of oppression are not only entrenched in our society, but within the bounds of higher education, it is essential that educators move past traditional diversity initiatives designed to only teach tolerance towards actively participating in pedagogy designed at dismantling these systems (Mayhew & Fernández, 2007). Ladson-Billings (1995) defined *Culturally Responsive Pedagogy* as any strategy that supports learners in developing critical thinking skills, affirms learners' cultural identity, and challenges systemic inequalities such as learner achievement gaps, especially within the learning environment.

Furthermore, the culturally responsive educator views the learning environment as a social microcosm of the larger system, through the lens of socio-cultural issues of power and privilege. *Antiracist Pedagogy* then, not only explores and explains the impact of racism but works to counteract it through social justice (Blakeney, 2005). It is specifically defined as "a paradigm located within Critical Theory utilized to explain and counteract the persistence and impact of racism using praxis as its focus to promote social justice for the creation of a democratic society in every respect" (Blakeney, 2005, p. 119). Blakeney (2005) further identifies qualities of Antiracist Pedagogy to include: exploring the historical patterns and constructs that contribute to inequality, an understanding of the impact of privilege and opportunity in order to perpetuate inequality, and challenging both individuals and systemic structures that perpetuate oppression in all its forms including those based on race, ethnicity, class, and power. Ultimately, the aim of antiracist pedagogical endeavors is to create over time an antiracist society. Kishimoto (2018) described Antiracist Pedagogical practices:

> It begins with the faculty's awareness and self-reflection of their social position and leads to the application of this analysis not just in their teaching, but also in their discipline, research, and departmental, university, and community work. In other words, anti-racist pedagogy is an organizing effort for institutional and social change that is much broader than teaching in the classroom (p. 540).

Antiracist Pedagogy also has ties to Freire's Transformational Learning Theory specifically through the framework of *conscientization*. Conscientization describes a level of critical consciousness whereby one views themselves in relation to the world community (Freire, 2000). Upon the realization of one's part in the world community, one can no longer sit idly by with disengagement but instead acts to transform their world community for the better. This transformation takes part through reflection and praxis underscoring the tenets of antiracist pedagogy that seek for people to become critically aware and reflective of the historical and cultural systems of oppression (and the part that they play in these systems) while challenging them to take action to confront oppression.

The antiracist culturally responsive educator intentionally explores the racial context inherent in all curricula within the learning setting. Essentially, the antiracist culturally responsive educator situates the learning content within their political, historical, and economic contexts using an intersectionality lens (exploring the influences of gender identity, sexual identity, and class on racial identity, for example) (Blakeney, 2005; Kishimoto, 2018). The antiracist culturally responsive educator then creates learning opportunities that expose learners to new ways of thinking that challenge how one views themselves and society by engaging learners in reflexivity, community service projects, dialogues and discourse with diverse peers and stakeholders, and role-playing that underscores multiple perspective-taking (Mayhew & Fernández, 2007). In the next section, we provide suggestions for how to implement antiracist cultural responsiveness within educational and professional settings and how to conceptualize them in light of the aforementioned Multiracial considerations.

Language and Interactions

Chen and Yang (2017) offered suggestions on culturally responsive teaching strategies that encourage educators to understand the cultures, values, and beliefs of learners. These same strategies can be applied and adapted within the client-counselor relationship. For this type of cultural understanding to occur, the educator/counselor must be aware of the teacher-student/client-counselor power differential and invite learners/clients to talk about these salient topics within the classroom/counseling setting, listening with a nonjudgmental ear and considering how learners'/clients' cultures, values, and beliefs can contribute to the learning community (or the counseling process). Activities that encourage these conversations include student/client self-introductions, journaling, art projects, activities designed to promote reflection and examine material from alternative perspectives while analyzing societal problems (Chen & Yang, 2017; Mayhew & Fernández, 2007). The following prompts foster self-awareness and can be used in small groups or the larger classroom (adapted from Pope et al., 2020):

1. What are the obvious socially constructed categories in your small group (i.e., race, gender, class, etc.)? Are constructions "real"? What makes them "real" or feel real?
2. Define oppression and privilege. How are oppression and privilege manifested and perpetuated in the U.S.? Oppression is very flexible, which is at least one reason it has endured. Keeping that in mind, how can educators/counselors expose and challenge the durability and flexibility of oppression? How can educators/counselors expose and challenge the facets of privilege?
3. From an educational perspective, what are some realistic teaching visions of social justice, cultural responsiveness, and antiracism? What about from a teacher/counselor educator perspective?
4. How can educators/counselors counterbalance how social norms are appropriated, internalized, and normalized?

These activities have consistently been shown to underscore student learning in diversity and social justice issues (Mayhew & Fernández, 2007). Kishimoto (2018) offers five ways to underscore antiracist approaches and interactions specifically with learners:

> (1) Challenge assumptions and foster students' critical analytical skills; (2) develop students' awareness of their social positions; (3) decenter authority in the classroom and have students take responsibility for their learning process; and (4) empower students and apply theory to practice; and (5) create a sense of community in the classroom through collaborative learning. (p. 546)

Furthermore, adult learning theory underscores the need for educators to create an active learning environment (versus lecture-based passive) and supportive learning community, especially as it is related to teaching and modeling multicultural and social justice competencies (Brown et al., 2014). Considering alternative "ways of knowing" such as indigenous and spiritual ways of learning/knowing and incorporating these into pedagogical frameworks support culturally responsive antiracist practices through inclusivity and by de-centering traditional colonized Western paradigms.

Implications for language abound when working with the Multiracial population, whether in a counseling room or classroom. Culturally responsive language that intentionally seeks to underscore antiracism needs to be used at all levels. One example of this is the need for professionals to consider using words such as "proper" or "correct" when speaking of the written or spoken word in academia. Understanding the intentionality behind these words acknowledges the difference between language used in various environments (e.g., home and academia) but limits the implication that language potentially used at home or within one's family is "wrong." This is extremely important when working with Multiracial individuals for educators and counselors who seek an antiracist identity. In this way, educators and counselors need to pay attention to their colonizing language and seek to deconstruct it.

Broaching is a therapeutic intervention that creates an atmosphere of openness and conveys that the counselor (or educator) is committed to multiculturalism. By proactively addressing issues of diversity, it invites salient identities of the client and counselor to be discussed openly (and re-visited as needed) (Day-Vines et al., 2007, 2021). Foundational to the concept of broaching is that individuals have multiple identities, and these identities are a part of any interaction. Because the identities that we hold can be visible (i.e., phenotype) and invisible (i.e., sexual identity, spiritual identity), it is essential that the counselor/educator initiate the dialogue about identities. Though broaching was first introduced in the counseling field, it has widespread implications and significance for work with anyone, especially Multiracial individuals whose racial identity may not be easily observed or known. Examples of broaching statements used in the training of counselors are, "As counselors our cultural identities will influence our relationship and I wonder if we can spend some time discussing our various identities. What cultural identities do you most identify with? Which cultural identities are important to you?" Educators can certainly engage in the same broaching process by facilitating small groups to encourage critical thinking and reflecting on students' salient identities. Examples of small group prompts that could then be brought back to the larger group for processing include (adapted from McDonald, 2020):

- Share with the group the identities that are most important to you?
- What strengths have you developed as a result of your background?
- In what ways do you see intersectionality occurring regarding your various identities?
- How might these identities impact the learning that will occur in this course?
- There's been a lot going on within the news lately about race and race relations. How might that be affecting you in light of your racial identity? What about your interactions with others?
- How might your identities influence antiracist culturally responsive behaviors inside this course and outside?

The ultimate goal of the broacher is to infuse open dialogue about identities throughout the entire interaction with the person. By continually attending to the person's experience of their identities within an oppressive system(s), the broacher expresses their commitment to acknowledging and working toward the dissolvement of all forms of oppression, underscoring antiracist cultural responsiveness (Day-Vines et al., 2007, 2021).

Knowledge Base

In addition to developing one's own antiracist culturally responsive identity and utilizing antiracist culturally responsive practices with Multiracial individuals, it is also equally important to increase one's knowledge base of competencies and models helpful to this population. The Competencies for Counseling the Multiracial Population developed by the Multiracial/Ethnic Counseling Concerns Interest Network of the American Counseling Association Taskforce were adopted by the American Counseling Association (ACA) Governing Council in 2015 (Kenney et al., 2015). Though these competencies were specially designed to help counselors working with Multiracial individuals, they have implications for anyone wanting to ground their work or teaching with this population in intentionality. The special taskforce designed these competencies within areas of human growth and development, social and cultural diversity, helping relationships, group work, career development, assessment, research and program evaluation, and professional orientation and ethical practice (the eight core areas mandated to be addressed by the Council for Accreditation of Counseling and Related Educational Programs known for short as CACREP). Practical recommendations for how these competencies can be used include:

- Using the competencies as a resource for counselors and educators working with the Multiracial population as the document gives specific recommendations for how Culturally Competent Counselors should interact with the Multiracial population (these recommendations are easily transferable to educators and research);
- Using the competencies as a framework for understanding common factors that influence any work being done with the Multiracial population (including the definition of common terms and acronyms counselors and educators should be aware of); and
- Using the competencies as a foundational piece to effectively advocate for and with the Multiracial population (for example, the competencies outline important considerations regarding transracial adoption that would be helpful for counselors and other helping professionals to mindful when supporting clients going through this process).

Additionally, it is important to consider the role intersectionality plays when practicing antiracist cultural responsiveness with Multiracial individuals. Intersectionality essentially explores the multiple dimensions that make up one's identity (such as gender, race, sexual identity, socioeconomic background, etc.), primarily to support historically marginalized/minoritized people (Ash et al., 2020; Crenshaw, 1989). "Intersectionality challenges the notion of arbitrary binaries placed on race and gender by exploring the complexity of race and gender identities and how such complexities shape people" (Ash et al., 2020, p. 6). Intersectionality, then, moves away from surface-level racial discourse and instead supports antiracist cultural responsiveness because it highlights the complex racial variation in all people, especially needed in the Multiracial population (Ash et al., 2020). A resource that serves as a framework for conceptualizing intersectionality is the Multicultural and Social Justice Counseling Competencies (MSJCC; Ratts et al., 2016).

The MSJCC, endorsed by the ACA Governing Council in 2015, underscores the importance of integrating multicultural and social justice competencies in clinical practice, training, research, and advocacy. Given that the standards rest on integrating multicultural and social justice competencies into all areas of the counseling profession (Chang & Rabess, 2020), this framework is particularly useful when working with Multiracial individuals, given the complexity of what it means to *be* Multiracial. The original multicultural counseling competencies (MCC) focused on the "majority" counselor working with the "minority" client within the domains of awareness, knowledge, and skills. Building on the original MCC, the MSJCC integrates and acknowledges the importance of addressing multicultural and social justice factors. Moving beyond a mono-cultural approach, MSJCC provides a framework for addressing the complicity of multiple identities that both the counselor and client bring to the counseling relationship. The MSJCC conceptual framework includes four quadrants (i.e., privileged counselor-privileged client; privileged counselor-marginalized client; marginalized counselor-privileged client; marginalized counselor-marginalized client), four developmental domains (i.e., counselor self-awareness, client worldview, the counseling relationship (new), and counseling and advocacy interventions (revised to add advocacy), and four areas of competencies (i.e., attitudes and beliefs, knowledge, skills, and action (new)). The MSJCC require that counselors address issues of power, privilege, and oppression in the counseling session, that counselors view client issues within a cultural context, and that counselors implement interventions at the individual and systematic levels. Given that the MSJCC are meant to enhance clinical practice, training, research, and advocacy, it is easily relatable and transferable to pedagogical practices within education (for example, the four quadrants being conceptualized as privileged educator-privileged student; privileged educator-marginalized student; marginalized educator-privileged student; marginalized educator-marginalized student).

Conclusion: A Call to Action for All Helping Professionals

This chapter described the current literature specifically regarding the growth, common terms, various racial identity models (i.e., Cheng & Lee, 2009; Henriksen & Paladino, 2009; Poston, 1990; Root, 2001), and microaggressions of the Multiracial population. Antiracist cultural responsiveness was explored as a best practice for working with Multiracial individuals. Specific praxis includes attending to one's own antiracist identity, paying attention to the language and interactions that inform pedagogical and counseling spaces, and working from an informed knowledge base.

Finally, it is important to remember that all people, especially in the helping professions, are responsible for doing this work. Antiracist cultural responsiveness is social justice and advocacy in action because this type of responsiveness actively works to dismantle systematic oppression by fighting against naivete, apathy, and complacency (Jeffreys & Zoucha, 2017; McDonald, 2020). As a result, through specific suggestions of how to work with Multiracial individuals through an antiracist culturally responsive lens, this chapter is a call to action for all stakeholders working towards an equitable and just society (see Appendix B for additional resources on antiracist and social justice practices). The information and suggestions around praxis can be adapted to fit within any respective professional field. Readers are encouraged to take time to reflect on the following discussion questions and adapt/apply them to their respective field. Additionally, quiz questions are included after the discussion questions section to test the readers' retention of important concepts from the reading.

Multiracial Resources

- *Multiracial Identity and Racial Politics in the United States* (Masuoka, 2017)
- The *Bill of Rights for People of Mixed Heritage* (Root, 1993, www.apa.org/pubs/videos/4310742-rights.pdf)

- *The Multiracial Oath of Social Responsibility* (Root, 2004, https://www.apa.org/pubs/videos/4310742-oath.pdf)
- *50 Experiences of Racially Mixed People* (Root, 2003, https://www.apa.org/pubs/videos/4310742-50.pdf)
- *Critical Mixed Race Studies* (www.criticalmixedracestudies.com)
- *Loving Day* (www.lovingday.org)
- *Mixed Race Studies* (www.mixedracestudies.org)
- *Ackerman Institute for the Family* (www.ackerman.org/research/the-multiracial-family-project/)
- *Competencies for Counseling the Multiracial Population* (https://www.counseling.org/docs/default-source/competencies/competencies-for-counseling-the-multiracial-population-2-2-15-final.pdf?sfvrsn=14)

Antiracist and Social Justice Resources

Books/Handbooks:

- *Readings for Diversity and Social Justice* edited by Adams et al. (2018)
- *The Racial Healing Handbook* by Anneliese Singh
- *Social Justice and Advocacy in Counseling: Experiential Activities for Teaching* edited by Pope et al. (2020)
- When They Call You a Terrorist by Patrisse Khan-Cullors and Asha Bandele
- *Black Feminist Thought: Knowledge, Consciousness, and the Politics of Empowerment* by Patricia Hill Collins
- *White Fragility: Why It's So Hard for White People to Talk about Racism* by Robin DiAngelo
- *Tears we cannot stop* by Michael Eric Dyson
- *Biased: Uncovering the Hidden Prejudice That Shapes What We See, Think, and Do* by Jennifer L. Eberhardt
- *Raising White Kids: Bringing Up Children in a Racially Unjust* America by Jennifer Harvey
- *How to Be an Antiracist* (and related handbook) by Ibram X. Kendi
- *Stamped from the Beginning: The Definitive History of Racist Ideas in America* by Ibram X. Kendi
- *So You Want to Talk About Race* by Ijeoma Oluo

Podcasts:

- Melanin and Mental Health: https://www.melaninandmental-health.com/
- Mental Health Matters Podcast: https://instagram.com/mentalmatterspodcast?igshid=kp04hfooy5cj
- The Anti-Racist Educator Podcast: https://www.theantiracisteducator.com/podcast
- Teaching While White Podcast: https://www.teachingwhilewhite.org/podcast

Websites:

- The Davidson Microaggressions Project resource website (https://davidsonmicroaggressionsproject.org/, 2020)
- Antiracism Resources in Higher Education: (https://libguides.merrimack.edu/antiracism/HE, 2021)
- Anti-Racism and Anti-Oppression: Teaching Resources: (https://library.cod.edu/antiracism/resources, 2021)
- Anti-Racism Research & Resource Guide: (https://libraryguides.binghamton.edu/antiracism/decolonizingcurricula, 2021)

Guiding Questions

1. What stood out to you most about the chapter you just read? How does learning about the Multiracial population impact how you view your current professional role? What action steps do you need to take in your role as educator/counselor as a result of what you read?

   What are the wider implications of this knowledge for other minoritized/marginalized groups in your professional sphere?
2. Sue et al. (2007) expanded the definition of *microaggressions* to include the everyday degradation of any socially marginalized/minoritized group. Given that most of us hold both privileged and marginalized identities, what personal experiences might you have with microag-

gressions? How do these experiences build your own empathy for Multiracial individuals' experiences of microaggressions? Discuss ways in which you yourself may have perpetuated a microaggression(s) and how you can take steps to mitigate these in the future.

3. The journey towards becoming antiracist is one that starts with a self-assessment of the ways we are either contributing to or hindering the dismantling of oppressive forces. This self-assessment is continuous and necessary if one wishes to cultivate a long-lasting antiracist identity. Do a self-assessment and discuss with group members ways that you have contributed to dismantling oppressive systems in your role as an educator or helping professional. In what ways have you fallen short of this goal and what action steps can you take to rectify this?
4. The *Language and Interactions* section of the chapter reminds us that implications for language abound when working with the Multiracial population. Culturally responsive language that intentionally seeks to underscore antiracism needs to be used at all levels. Think about the everyday language you use as a counselor or educator. In what ways does this language underscore antiracism and in what ways could it be improved to more clearly align with culturally responsive antiracism? What action steps need to be taken?
5. Review the Competencies for Counseling the Multiracial Population (Kenney et al., 2015) and the Multicultural and Social Justice Counseling Competencies (MSJCC; Ratts et al., 2016). After reviewing, think about how you could integrate this information in your role as a counselor or educator with the Multiracial people with which you work. How could you utilize these resources to influence your interactions with your clients or students for the purpose of culturally responsive antiracist practice?

Quiz Questions

Answer whether the below 5 statements (items 1–5) are *True* or *False*. If *False*, explain why.

1. *Mixed-race, Multiple Heritage, and Interracial* are all terms that have been used synonymously with the term *Multiracial,* therefore a culturally responsive antiracist educator/helper uses the terminology self-identified by the student or client.
2. Significant milestones related to Multiracial issues are the Loving v. Virginia Supreme Court decision in 1967, the hypodescent or "one-drop rule", and the ability to select more than one race on the U.S. Census in 2000.
3. Research has shown that Multiracial identity is by and large about skin-color/presenting phenotype.
4. Since Multiracial identity is a part of the greater human experience, there are no specific competencies or standards that need to be considered as a counselor or educator working with this population.
5. Specific praxis of culturally responsive antiracism includes attending to one's own antiracist identity, paying attention to the language and interactions that inform pedagogical and counseling spaces, and working from an informed knowledge base.

Fill in the blank below for the following 5 questions (items 6–10) with the correct vocabulary word from the chapter.

6. ________ are common and often brief interactions that communicate negative, invalidating, and hostile messages about one's identity(ies). They can be verbal, behavioral, or environmental and can exist in any human interaction that involves individuals from differing cultural groups.
7. ________ is any idea that suggests that racial groups are equals in all their apparent differences—that there is nothing right or wrong with any racial group. This ideology argues that racist policies are the cause of racial inequities.
8. ________ not only explores and explains the impact of racism, but works to counteract it through social justice and is specifically defined as a paradigm located within Critical Theory utilized to explain and counteract the persistence and impact of racism using praxis as its focus to promote social justice for the creation of a democratic society in every respect.

9. ________ is a therapeutic intervention that creates an atmosphere of openness and conveys the message that the counselor (or educator) is committed to multiculturalism. By proactively addressing issues of diversity, it invites salient identities of the client and counselor (student-educator) to be discussed openly (and re-visited as needed).
10. ________ essentially explores the multiple dimensions that make up one's identity (such as gender, race, sexual identity, socioeconomic background, etc.), especially to support historically marginalized/minoritized people and challenges the notion of arbitrary binaries placed on race and gender by exploring the complexity of race and gender identities and how such complexities shape people (Ash et al., 2020).

References

Adams, M., Blumenfeld, W. J., Catalano, D. C. J., DeJong, K. S., Hackman, H. W., Hopkins, L. E., Love, B. J., Peters, M. L., Shlasko, D., & Zúñiga, X. (Eds.). (2018). *Readings in diversity and social justice*. Routledge.

Ash, A. N., Hill, R., Risdon, S., & Jun, A. (2020). Anti-racism in higher education: A model for change. *Race and Pedagogy Journal: Teaching and Learning for Justice, 4*(3), 1–35.

Blakeney, A. (2005). Antiracist pedagogy: Definition, theory, and professional development. *Journal of Curriculum and Pedagogy, 2*(1), 119–132. https://doi.org/10.1080/15505170.2005.10411532

Brown, C. B., Collins, S., & Arthur, N. (2014). Fostering multicultural and social justice competence through counsellor education pedagogy. *Canadian Journal of Counselling and Psychotherapy, 48*(3), 300–320.

Chang, C. Y., & Rabess, A. (2020). Response to signature pedagogies: A framework for pedagogical foundations in counselor education: Through a multicultural and social justice competencies lens. *Teaching and Supervision in Counseling, 2*(2), 20–27. https://doi.org/10.7290/tsc020203

Chen, D., & Yang, X. (2017). Improving active classroom participation of ESL students: Applying culturally responsive teaching strategies. *Theory of Practice in Language Studies, 7*(1), 79–86. https://doi.org/10.17507/tpls.0701.10

Cheng, C., & Lee, F. (2009). Multiracial identity integration: Perceptions of conflict and distance among multiracial individuals. *Journal of Social Issues, 65*(1), 51–68. https://doi.org/10.1111/j.1540-4560.2008.01587.x

Crenshaw, K. (1989). *Demarginalizing the intersection of race and sex: A Black feminist critique of antidiscrimination doctrine, feminist theory, and antiracist politics*. University of Chicago Legal Forum.

Day-Vines, N. L., Cluxton-Keller, F., Agorsor, C., & Gubara, S. (2021). Strategies for broaching the subjects of race, ethnicity, and culture. *Journal of Counseling and Development, 99*(3), 348–357. https://doi.org/10.1002/jcad.12380

Day-Vines, N. L., Wood, S. M., Grothaus, T., Craigen, L., Holman, A., Dotson-Blake, K., & Douglass, M. J. (2007). Broaching the subjects of race, ethnicity, and culture during the counseling process. *Journal of Counseling & Development, 85*, 401–409. https://doi.org/10.1002/j.1556-6678.2007.tb00608.x

Evans, A. M., & Ramsay, K. (2015). Multiracial and biracial individuals: A content analysis of counseling journals, 1991–2013. *Journal of Multicultural Counseling & Development, 43*(4), 262–274. https://doi.org/10.1002/jmcd.12020

Franco, M. G., & O'Brien, K. M. (2018). Racial identity invalidation with multiracial individuals: An instrument development study. *Cultural Diversity and Ethnic Minority Psychology, 24*(1), 112–125. https://doi.org/10.1037/cdp0000170

Freire, P. (2000). *Pedagogy of the oppressed*. Continuum.

Frye, B. J., & Vogt, H. A. (2010). The causes of underrepresentation of African American children in gifted programs and the need to address this problem through more culturally responsive teaching practices in teacher education programs. *Black History Bulletin, 73*(1), 11–17.

Harris, J. C. (2017). Multiracial college students' experiences with multiracial microaggressions. *Race, Ethnicity and Education, 20*(4), 429–445. https://doi.org/10.1080/13613324.2016.1248836

Helms, J. E. (2008). *A race is a nice thing to have: A guide to being a White person or understanding the white persons in your life* (2nd ed.). Microtraining Associates.

Henriksen, R. C., & Paladino, D. A. (2009). *Counseling multiple heritage individuals, couples, and families*. American Counseling Association.

Jeffreys, M. R., & Zoucha, R. (2017). Revisiting "The invisible culture of the multiracial, multiethnic individual: A transcultural imperative". *Journal of Cultural Diversity, 24*(1), 3–5.

Kendi, I. X. (2019). *How to be an antiracist*. Random House Publishing Group.

Kenney, K. R., Kenney, M. E., Alvarado, S. B., Baden, A. L., Brew, L., Chen-Hayes, S., Crippen, C. L., Harris, H. L., Henriksen Jr., R. C., Malott, K. M., Paladino, D. A., Pope, M. L., Salazar, C. F., & Singh, A. A. (2015). *Competencies for counseling the multiracial population*. https://www.counseling.org/docs/default-source/competencies/competencies-for-counseling-the-multiracial-population-2-2-15-final.pdf?sfvrsn=10

Kerwin, C., & Ponterotto, J. G. (1995). Biracial identity development: Theory and research. In J. G. Ponterotto, J. M. Casas, L. A. Suzuki, & C. M. Alexander (Eds.), *Handbook of multicultural counseling* (pp. 199–217). Sage Publications, Inc.

Kishimoto, K. (2018). Anti-racist pedagogy: From faculty's self-reflection to organizing within and beyond the classroom. *Race, Ethnicity and Education, 21*(4), 540–554. https://doi.org/10.1080/13613324.2016.1248824

Ladson-Billings, G. (1995). Toward a theory of culturally relevant pedagogy. *American Educational Research Journal, 32*(3), 465–491. https://doi.org/10.3102/00028312032003465

Lou, E., & Lalonde, R. N. (2015). Signs of transcendence? A changing landscape of multiraciality in the 21st century. *International Journal of Intercultural Relations*, 45, 85–95. https://doi.org/10.1016/j.ijintrel.2015.01.004

Mayhew, M., & Fernández, S. (2007). Pedagogical practices that contribute to social justice outcomes. *Review of Higher Education, 31*(1), 55–80. https://doi.org/10.1353/rhe.2007.0055

McDonald, C. P. (2020). When worlds collide: Culturally responsive practices for multiracial students and families. In T. Crosby-Cooper (Ed.), *Implementing culturally responsive practices in education* (pp. 211–229). IGI Global Publishing.

McDonald, C. P., Chang, C., Dispenza, F., & O'Hara, C. (2019). The relationships among multiracial identity, color-blind racial ideology, and discrimination in multiracial individuals: Implications for professional counseling and counselor education. *Journal of Counseling & Development, 97*, 75–85. https://doi.org/10.1002/jcad.12237

McDonald, C. P., Chang, C., O'Hara, C., Guvensel, K., & Parker, L. (2020). Racial mislabeling in multiracial individuals: Implications for professional counseling and education. *Teaching and Supervision in Counseling, 2*(1), 13–23. https://doi.org/10.7290/tsc020102

Pierce, C. (1970). Offensive mechanisms. In F. B. Barbour (Ed.), *The Black seventies* (pp. 265–282). Porter Sargent.

Pope, M., Gonzalez, M., & Cameron, E. R. (2020). In N., & Pangelinan, J. S. (Ed.), *Social justice and advocacy in counseling: Experiential activities for teaching*. Routledge.

Poston, W. (1990). The biracial identity development model: A needed addition. *Journal of Counseling & Development, 69*(2), 152–155. https://doi.org/10.1002/j.15566676.1990.tb01477.x

Ratts, M. J., Singh, A. A., Nassar-McMillan, S., Butler, K., & McCullough, J. R. (2016). Multicultural and social justice counseling competencies: Guidance for the counseling profession. *Journal of Multicultural Counseling and Development, 44*, 28–48.

Roberts, S. O., Ho, A. K., Gülgöz, S., Berka, J., & Gelman, S. A. (2020). The roles of group status and group membership in the practice of hypodescent. *Child Development, 91*(3), e721–e732. https://doi.org/10.1111/cdev.13279

Root, M. P. (2001). Reconstructing race, rethinking ethnicity. In A. Bellack & M. Hersen (Eds.), *Comprehensive clinical psychology: Sociocultural and individual differences* (Vol. 10, pp. 141–160). Elsevier.

Sue, D. W. (2010). Microaggressions, marginality, and oppression: An introduction. In D. W. Sue (Ed.), *Microaggressions and marginality: Manifestation, dynamics, and impact* (pp. 3–22). Wiley.

Sue, D. W., Capodilupo, C. M., Torino, G. C., Bucceri, J. M., Holder, A. M. B., Nadal, K. L., & Esquilin, M. (2007). Racial microaggressions in everyday life: Implications for clinical practice. *American Psychologist, 62*(4), 271–286. https://doi.org/10.1037/0003066X.62.4.271

Tran, A. G. T. T., Miyake, E. R., Martinez-Morales, V., & Csizmadia, A. (2016). "What are you?" Multiracial individuals' responses to racial identification inquiries. *Cultural Diversity and Ethnic Minority Psychology, 22*(1), 26–37. https://doi.org/10.1037/cdp0000031

Young, D. M., Sanchez, D. T., Pauker, K., & Gaither, S. E. (2020). A meta-analytic review of hypodescent patterns in categorizing multiracial and racially ambiguous targets. *Personality and Social Psychology Bulletin*. https://doi.org/10.1177/0146167220941321

22

Epilogue

Kaprea F. Johnson, Narketta M. Sparkman-Key,
Alan Meca, and Shuntay Z. Tarver

Racism is as complex as trying to understand the depths of our universe and yet there have been people invested since the beginning of time working to unravel the mysteries that exist in outer space. Momentum related to understanding outer space has never slowed even in periods of little discovery, there are still millions of dollars and hours dedicated to simply understanding what's up there. We make no quorums about the

K. F. Johnson (✉)
Department of Educational Studies, Counselor Education Program,
The Ohio State University, Columbus, OH, USA
e-mail: Johnson.9545@osu.edu

N. M. Sparkman-Key • S. Tarver
Department of Counseling and Human Services, Old Dominion University,
Norfolk, VA, USA
e-mail: nsparkma@odu.edu; smccoy@odu.edu

A. Meca
Department of Psychology, The University of Texas at San Antonio,
San Antonio, TX, USA
e-mail: alan.meca@utsa.edu

© The Author(s), under exclusive license to Springer Nature Switzerland AG 2022

K. Johnson et al. (eds.), *Developing Anti-Racist Practices in the Helping Professions: Inclusive Theory, Pedagogy, and Application*,
https://doi.org/10.1007/978-3-030-95451-2_22

complexity of outer space; we acknowledge that it's complicated and yet we persist. Many in our society have become comfortable with the excuse that racism is too complex to understand, solve, and eradicate; and unlike outer space, racism directly impacts every facet of our society every day. Racism is the root cause of inequity, health disparities, economic disenfranchisement, education inequality, violence, and other shameful ills of society. It creates long lasting physiological and psychological effects on societies and people impacted, making the eradication of racism one of the most important tasks of our pre-pluralistic society.

As a reminder, a pluralistic society is one that has diversity, embraces different groups (i.e., tolerant), power is shared amongst multiple groups (i.e., communication), and there is a commitment to autonomy and building social bonds. In the United States, we have had leaders, advocates, scholars, and engaged citizens fighting to eradicate racism and to create a pluralistic society, for centuries. These radical, fearless people who were fighting for a better world, were often subjected to violence, isolation, imprisonment, economic deprivation, and other tactics to disrupt their forward momentum; and yet the fight persisted. The sacrifices were not in vain, as their hard work and dedication is the foundation that has moved society closer to acknowledging and addressing racism. We must persist and continue to build upon the work of our past and current anti-racist leaders. The current reckoning within our society presents us with an opportunity to eradicate racism. We have the skills, knowledge, and awareness of the true impact of racism which can lead us toward a pluralistic society in which all people are celebrated, respected, and able to thrive.

In a world that's constantly evolving and wrestling with racial injustices, we have to be guided by non-deceptive strategies to eradicate racism. These strategies are action oriented, forward thinking, momentum building, fearless, audacious, equity centered, and justice focused. As written, by Audre Lorde, "we can't use the masters' tools to dismantle the master's house"; ideals such as respectability politics and appealing to the heart of racist are deceptive strategies from the 'masters house' to keep the movement stagnate. Today's youth have coined the term "stay woke", to highlight the need for critical thinking and critical awareness of the issues and events around us. In order to move closer to an anti-racist society, we must recognize when tools from the master's toolbox are being utilized to distract us (i.e., turning a blind eye etc.). These tools are typically an excuse for us to increase our own comfort at the expense of the collective fight to eradicate racism. Be mindful of sentiments that seem in line with the fight but could also have adverse consequences, like fighting for tolerance. Tolerance is akin to being "not racist" and as Dr. Ibram Kendi has noted "just being not racist isn't enough". Instead of tolerance, let's strive for embracing, celebrating, and loving others, so that we can all thrive in this society.

We invite you to be your 'ancestors wildest dreams', for those of you who have ancestors who were fighting to eradicate racism in all its forms. Your ancestor from centuries ago probably could have never imagined that you would be reading a book on anti-racism, which you can directly utilize to influence the eradication of racism within your sphere of influence and power. And for those who have ancestors who were fighting to maintain racism, we invite you to be your 'ancestor's wildest nightmares'! Your ancestors from centuries ago probably could have never imagined that you would be amid a fight to dismantle a structure that they fought so hard to maintain. For all of us, we must be compelled to fight for the eradication of racism in all its forms and within all structures of our society. Decentering ourselves and centering the collective good. Reflected in the collection of chapters that make up this book, we all have an entrance into the fight to eradicate racism. Contributing authors provided new tools and strategies in the areas of pedagogy and practice that can be utilized in this collective fight. The foundation of the book is that collectively we can build our antiracist identities and put our knowledge and awareness toward action in our spheres of work, power, and influence to eradicate racism and racist structures that permeate our society. It is our hope that you take this text and reflect on your next steps toward becoming antiracist. Expand on this work by implementing these strategies in other helping environments and engage in interprofessional collaborative relationships that challenge systems and lead the way for new antiracist practices. Apply these theories in the environments you encounter and assess the impact. Together we can end racism, but it takes innovation and dedication.

As helping professionals, we fight for the wellbeing of others, and like those that have come before us, we must continue to fight racism, the root causes of a variety of pervasive disparities. So, the question becomes what will you do? What will you do in your community locally, regionally, nationally, and globally to eradicate racism in all forms? Ask yourself, who are you willing to fight for? What cause are you willing to put yourself on the line for and why? Every member of society has a role in dismantling this system, but those who are entrusted with 'helping others' should have a unique and invested interest in ensuring that racism is dismantled within every structure of this society. You are a helping professional because you want to see people thrive and you want change - perhaps you didn't realize that you are the person to make that change happen, but you are! Envision what you want society to be and know that it can happen.

Answer Key

Chapter 3

1. B
2. B
3. D
4. C
5. B
6. C
7. D

Chapter 4

1. Grounded in the mission, to prepare all English Learners in the state of California to learn, thrive and lead, SEAL is a research-based systems change model grounded in teachers' professional development and focused on preschool through 6th grade. The model coalesces around four pillars: academic language, the creation of rich and affirming environments, alignment of the preschool and elementary

© The Author(s), under exclusive license to Springer Nature Switzerland AG 2022

K. Johnson et al. (eds.), *Developing Anti-Racist Practices in the Helping Professions: Inclusive Theory, Pedagogy, and Application*,
https://doi.org/10.1007/978-3-030-95451-2

systems and articulation across grades, and partnerships between families and schools.

2. Inequitable access to appropriately trained teachers, inequitable access to appropriate assessment, inadequate instructional time, inequitable access to instructional materials and curriculum, and extensive segregation into schools that place them at high risk for education failure. Additionally, not only are many DLLs/ELs not given the opportunity to fully develop academic language in English, but in English-only school environments, many of them also lose their home language.
3. Lau v. Nichols (1974): The United States Supreme Court ruled that students, primarily Chinese-speakers, were being denied access to equal educational opportunity because they lacked the English skills to understand and participate in educational programs. In the decades since, EL education has been required nationally by all K-12 systems, including those in California.
4. Pathway to Biliteracy displays and activities, home language interviews, student language biographies and poems, language portfolios, multilingual resources, community language studies, multilingual team names and chants, home-school connections, and multilingual celebrations. Students across grade levels are encouraged to set their sights on earning the California Seal of Biliteracy. Teachers are provided with training on key issues of language transfer between English and students' home languages. For older students, teachers are equipped with strategies to talk with students about the connections between language and power, analyzing why and how language is deployed in their school, their community, and in the larger world. Bilingual convenings with discussions of the relationship between language and power. Family school partnerships.
5. Structured read-alouds, chants, songs, and libraries that include rich literature in the home language and English, dramatic play and hands-on activities encourage children to learn through play, Persona Dolls, partnerships with families. By educating them about the historical context and policies that have contributed to schooling that fails ELs/DLLs. Helps with articulation and alignment. Provides leadership

convenings, instructional rounds (reflection on SEAL implementation in the classroom with the support of SEAL staff), check-ins, bilingual program design meetings, attendance at teacher training modules, pre- and post-module communication, technical assistance and family-school partnership modules. Provides research on best practices for DLLs/ ELs, guidance on strategic leveraging of state policy, bilingual program support, Bilingual Teacher Professional Development Program.

Chapter 5

Content/Quiz Answers

1. Actively fighting racism by lobbying for reforms in the political, economic, and social spheres. Our overlapping identities may hold distinct unique power dynamics in society, privileges, prejudices, stereotypes; all of which will impact our relative position of privilege and power based on the scenario and the identities of people around us.
2. An individual's desire to contribute to and actively engage in a community's battle for justice and equality makes them allies, partners, and comrades of that community, even if they are not initially a part of it. Self-reflection is required. Not only should prospective allies recognize and use their advantage, but if all groups recognize their own forms of oppression, they may be able to fight jointly against everyone's oppression.
3. Human beings are complicated, interrelated, and multifaceted creatures that can only be completely comprehended in the context of our groups and civilizations. The **I-ARC Framework**, in turn, takes measures to unravel, comprehend, and alter the intricacies of how we shape society and how society shapes us.
4. It is critical that as a co-conspirator, you apply each Principle as it relates to the **I-ARC Framework** to your life. Within Principle 1, one can remember not to generalize experiences. It is systemic and personal. Within Principle 2, the holistic practice of co-conspiratorship

requires engaging and acknowledging members of all oppressed communities regardless of race, sexual origin, and/or gender identity. Principle 3 is a reminder that the continuous work of enacting changes and dismantling repressive systems will not happen overnight. However, the commitment requires grit as a foundation in challenging inequities across the globe. Lastly, Principle 4 prompts that you may never receive recognition for the work you do. Instead, know that the systemic change in which you have committed to ensuring is the reward itself.

5. To begin, understand the difference between speaking for someone and communicating with someone; where possible, commit to conversation rather than discussion. Teachers must try to understand and use multicultural teaching techniques, create an explicitly antiracist curriculum, and be devoted to discussing identity development in the classroom. Multiracial solidarity is directed toward areas of intersection, not a false universalism or fake unity, and does not imply that everyone thinks similarly.

Chapter 6

1. a seemingly race-conscious frame that acknowledges and ostensibly condemns a system of White privilege and racial inequity, but does so in ways that legitimize and reinforce racist attitudes, policies, and practices.
2. False
3. perfectionism, sense of urgency, defensiveness, quantity over quality, worship of the written word, only one right way, paternalism, either/or thinking, power hoarding, fear of open conflict, individualism, I'm the only one, progress is bigger—more, objectivity, and right to comfort
4. exceptionalism and respectability politics
5. To promote Progressive relationships and prevent Regressive, Crossed, and oppressive Parallel dynamics.

Chapter 8

Quiz Answer Key

1.

Mainstream model framework	Antiracist framework
The use of marginalized language features by white teachers as a means of rapport-building and humor	*The inclusion of multicultural works in the classroom (books, interviews, artists, etc.) and the subsequent discussion and celebration of language differences*
Mentor texts exclusively written by speakers of Mainstream English	*Discussing language as a tool for enslavement during relevant history lesson*
Celebrate native language norms in relaxed settings (e.g. classroom discussion), advocate for temporary language abandonment for achievement of mastery	*Elimination of forced code- switching in the classroom*

2. In the space below, identify the four linguistic facts of life as developed and explicated by Lippi-Green (2012):

   a. All spoken language changes over time. Language change is natural and unavoidable.
   b. All dialects (both stigmatized and mainstream/standard) are "equal in linguistic terms." This means that all dialects are fully functioning and fully developed languages.
   c. Written language and spoken language are different.
   d. Spoken language shows variation at every level. Spoken language is inherently variable.

3. In the space below, identify the four "linguistic gospel truths" outlined in this chapter:

   a. Linguistic mother tongues provide formative identity work.
   b. It is essential to foster positive language attitudes in the classroom.
   c. Standardized English is the language of privilege because **what** is not allowed is reflective of **who** is not allowed.

d. Diversity is more than having a variety of student identities in your classroom, it must also include the acceptance of diverse language varieties.

4. In considering the Anti-Racist Model of Language Education (Table 8.3), which of the following practices would be an example of the way a teacher could *confront the language of mainstream cultural hegemony?*

    a. Celebrating the language of BBVE speakers by allowing them to explore their language norms through written classroom assignments
    b. Working collaboratively with students to establish classroom norms with respect to language inclusivity
    c. Stress that language abandonment need only be practiced during summative assessment
    d. **Explicitly naming common language myths and dispelling them using student-friendly language**

5. In considering the Mainstream Model of Language Education, which of the following practices would be an example of an *overt* practice utilized by educators to maintain hegemonic practices of language in the classroom?

    a. **The teacher positions oneself as an arbiter of language use—to be used as a tool to bridge the gap between inferior dialects and prestigious white mainstream varieties of English.**
    b. Rewards speakers who speak how they write
    c. Celebrates the adoption of ME conventions
    d. Uses linguistic appropriation to bond/relate to students of color

Chapter 9

1. False
2. Western, European, Industrial, Rich and Democratic
3. True
4. Color-evasiveness
5. False

Chapter 10

1. A non-racist program is one that takes a passive stance against racism. This means, they will do things such as promoting the Black Lives Matter message or hosting a Black History Month event. An Antiracist program is one that implements theoretical frameworks such as CRT throughout the pedagogy.
2. a) helping professionals must have an understanding of social inequities so they can avoid the continued marginalization of those who are directly impacted by social inequities.

   b) helping professionals who lack the understanding of systematic oppression and social inequities will fail to understand the challenges faced by the client and the community.
3. The narrow focus on pathology without the integration of holistic, asset based, and historical analysis have not prepared students of color to understand their lived experiences, nor the systemic challenges faced by clients and communities.
4. Answer must discuss more than one of the tenets
5. Eurocentrism seeks to impose a European perspective into the consciousness of other people across the world (Asante, 2012). The Eurocentric ideology makes its way into every aspect of other people's lives, assimilating them into and erasing the diverse history of those who are considered other. This process started with the European conquest of the Americas and has unfortunately continued to this day. Eurocentric education affects all people but in very different ways. It influences their worldviews, their culture, their self-esteem, and their physical, mental and spiritual well-being by reproducing the racist status quo and reinforcing racist beliefs that people of color have less rights to agency and self-determination.
6. Eurocentrism seeks to impose a European perspective into the consciousness of other people across the world (Asante, 2012). The Eurocentric ideology makes its way into every aspect of other people's lives, assimilating them into and erasing the diverse history of those who are considered other. This process started with the

European conquest of the Americas and has unfortunately continued to this day. Eurocentric education affects all people but in very different ways. It influences their worldviews, their culture, their self-esteem, and their physical, mental and spiritual well-being by reproducing the racist status quo and reinforcing racist beliefs that people of color have less rights to agency and self-determination.

7. Race-based judgments, evaluations, and practices are rooted at every level of the society and are embedded in the everyday life of individuals. The prescriptions and stereotypes about race and inter-racial or intra-racial relations are absorbed by the individual through culturalization and socialization processes. These prescriptions and stereotypes are put into practice in their daily activities and feed the loop indefinitely by the repeated thoughts, words, and actions (Abrams, Moio, 2009).
8. HBCUs created spaces for former slaves to obtain skills and networks to transition towards some type of independence after years of enslavement, trauma and exploitation.
9. Inherent racism teaches us that, when laying the foundations of the helping relationship with Black clients, social workers have to pay extra-attention to the risk of allowing their own stereotypes to permeate their professional decisions
10. Social justice, Dignity and worth of the person, and Importance of human relationships

Chapter 11

1. C
2. B
3. A
4. D
5. C

Chapter 12

1. D
2. A
3. A
4. C
5. D

Chapter 13

1. B, C
2. D
3. A
4. A, B, D
5. D

Chapter 14

1. B
2. D
3. A
4. C
5. B
6. B
7. A
8. C
9. D
10. A
11. B
12. C
13. D
14. A
15. B

Chapter 15

1. B
2. A
3. A
4. B
5. A

Chapter 16

1. B
2. C
3. A
4. B
5. TRUE

Chapter 17

1. False
2. C
3. D
4. A
5. True
6. C
7. A
8. D

Chapter 18

1. **False.** The Race-Class Lens argues that when White people (and some people of color) support politicians who are empowered into office by peddling racial fear, these politicians enact policies that harm communities of color, but also harm White people. However, although the harm to White people and people of color are related, it is *disproportionate* and

unequal. The Race-Class Lens helps us understand how the "wages of Whiteness" gain value among Whites (and some people of color) as a salve for the effects of economic inequality, and how a message of multiracial working class solidarity can help us render the wages of Whiteness *less valuable* compared to the solidarity dividend we stand to gain.

2. **True**. While research findings on DEI training are mixed, there is evidence that when training is framed as forwarding institutional and personal goals and values, is grounded in a shared institutional identity, and allows opportunity for positive contact across difference, such training can be effective. Intergroup Dialogue (IGD) is a unique DEI intervention that "stands out" from other forms of training in that it includes training in communication and conflict resolution skills prior to engaging in dialogue on issues of power and privilege. Hence, it includes many of the traits that make DEI maximally effective.
3. **False**. While economic inequality and racial inequality are related, it is not that one "causes" the other. Rather, economic inequality is made possible by the creation of a racial hierarchy that serves to rationalize and maintain the power of wealthy elites. The Race-Class Lens shows how racial hierarchy is the foundation of capitalist exploitation. Therefore, any economic justice project that does not address racial injustice at its core will be ineffective in actualizing meaningful change--all a right-wing project has to do is weaponize race to devastate the multiracial working class coalition necessary to enact such change. A Race-Class Message, by contrast, helps "inoculate" White people and some people of color against the allure of racial fear messages and points out the benefits of coming together across race to build a government that works for all of us.

Chapter 19

1. B
2. D
3. C
4. A
5. D
6. B
7. D

Chapter 20

1. Telehealth allowed nursing and social work professions to reach people who may not have had access to mental health or other health care services. Additionally, telehealth effectively provided social support during a period of social isolation. Telehealth can be as advanced as video conferencing with patients and families or as simple as telephone calls.
2. a. Access to a device (phone, smartphone, tablet, PC)
   b. Access to the internet.
   c. Possessing the skills and abilities to navigate technology
3. There are communities that do not have internet access.
4. The professional code of ethics for both disciplines speaks to the commitment to social justice.
5. a. By having ongoing training.
b. By accepting the discomfort that accompanies racist mistakes.
c. By conducting a systemic analysis of how white supremacy has been sustained within the organizational structure and has oppressed marginalized groups.

Chapter 21

Quiz Answers

1. True
2. True
3. *False*. Research has shown that Multiracial identity is more than color or phenotype and includes a combination of holidays one celebrates, the language one speaks, and the names one uses (McDonald et al., 2020).
4. *False*. Due to the complexity of what it *means* to be Multiracial, there are numerous resources available to counselors and educators that can support work with Multiracial individuals. Examples include:

The Competencies for Counseling the Multiracial Population developed by the Multiracial/Ethnic Counseling Concerns Interest Network of the American Counseling Association Taskforce (adopted by the American Counseling Association (ACA) Governing Council in 2015; Kenney et al., 2015) and the Multicultural and Social Justice Counseling Competences (MSJCC; Ratts et al., 2016) that serves as a framework for conceptualizing intersectionality.

5. True
6. Microaggressions
7. Antiracism
8. Antiracist Pedagogy
9. Broaching
10. Intersectionality

Index[1]

[1] Note: Page numbers followed by 'n' refer to notes.

© The Author(s), under exclusive license to Springer Nature Switzerland AG 2022

K. Johnson et al. (eds.), *Developing Anti-Racist Practices in the Helping Professions: Inclusive Theory, Pedagogy, and Application*,
https://doi.org/10.1007/978-3-030-95451-2

W

X

The manufacturer's authorised representative in the EU is Springer Nature Customer Service Centre GmbH, Europaplatz 3, 69115 Heidelberg, Germany. If you have any concerns regarding our products, please contact ProductSafety@springernature.com

Printed and bound by CPI Group (UK) Ltd, Croydon, CR0 4YY
28/09/2026
02224060-0013